CARDIAC VALVE
DISEASE
IN CHILDREN

CARDIAC VALVE DISEASE IN CHILDREN

Editor

JEFFREY M. DUNN, MD
Professor
Department of Surgery
Temple University School of Medicine
Director
Pediatric Heart Institute
Saint Christopher's Hospital for Children
Philadelphia

Elsevier
New York • Amsterdam • London

Elsevier Science Publishing Co., Inc.
52 Vanderbilt Avenue, New York, New York 10017

Distributors outside the United States and Canada:
Elsevier Science Publishers B.V.
P.O. Box 211, 1000 AE Amsterdam, the Netherlands

Library of Congress Cataloging in Publication Data

Cardiac valve disease in children.
Includes index.
1. Heart valve diseases in children.   I. Dunn,
Jeffrey M.   [DNLM: 1. Heart Valve Diseases — in infancy &
childhood. WS 290   C2666]
RJ426.V3C37 1987   618.92′125   87-13508

ISBN 0-444-01243-5

Current printing (last digit):
10 9 8 7 6 5 4 3 2 1

Manufactured in the United States of America

Dedicated to Linda, David, and Kathryn

Contents

Preface

Cardiac valve disease in infants and children is a major challenge for the pediatric cardiologist and surgeon. The subject of valve disease in the pediatric population is not well represented in current literature. It is in an attempt to fill this void that we began this project. The contributors to this book are leaders in this area and their excellent contributions have made our task a simple one. Because of our emphasis on diagnosis and treatment of congenital cardiac valve disease, we expect that this book will be important for pediatric cardiologists and thoracic surgeons.

I wish to thank the many contributors to this book whose excellent manuscripts reflect the current state of knowledge in their respective subjects. I especially would like to thank Mrs. Marguerite Gonzalez who helped collect, review, and assemble the various manuscripts.

Contributors

Robert H. Anderson, MD, FRC Path
Joseph Levy Professor of Paediatric Cardiac Morphology, Department of Paediatrics, Cardiothoracic Institute, Brompton Hospital, London

Rohinton K. Balsara, MBBS, FACS, FCCP
Associate Professor of Surgery, Temple University, and Department of Pediatric Cardiac Surgery, Saint Christopher's Hospital for Children, Philadelphia

Lee N. Benson, MD, FRCP (C), FACC
Associate Professor of Pediatrics (Cardiology), and Director, The Variety Club, Cardiac Catheterizations Laboratories, Department of Pediatrics, Division of Cardiology, The Hospital for Sick Children, Toronto

A. Michael Borkon, MD
Assistant Professor of Surgery, Department of Cardiac Surgery, Johns Hopkins University School of Medicine, Baltimore

Edward L. Bove, MD
Associate Professor of Surgery, Pediatrics, and Communicable Diseases, University of Michigan Medical Center, Ann Arbor, Michigan

John W. Brown, MD
Associate Professor of Surgery, Section of Cardiothoracic Surgery, Indiana University School of Medicine, Indianapolis

James W. Buchanan, DVM, M Med Sci
Professor of Cardiology, Department of Clinical Studies, School of Veterinary Medicine, University of Pennsylvania, Philadelphia

Catherine Bull, MD, MRCP
Senior Lecturer in Paediatric Cardiology, Institute of Child Health, London

Randall L. Caldwell, MD
Associate Professor of Pediatrics, Section of Pediatric Cardiology, Indiana University School of Medicine, Indianapolis

Alain Carpentier, MD, PhD
Professor of Cardiac Surgery; Chief, Département de Chirurgie Cardiovasculaire, Hôpital Boussais, Paris

Sylvain Chauvaud, MD
Cardiac Surgeon, Département de Chirurgie Cardiovasculaire, Hôpital Broussais, Paris

Jerald L. Cooper
Indiana University School of Medicine, Indianapolis

Gordon K. Danielson, MD
Professor of Surgery, Mayo Medical School, and Consultant, Thoracic and Cardiovascular Surgery, Mayo Clinic and Mayo Foundation, Rochester, Minnesota

William R. Deschner, MD
Resident in Surgery, Section of Cardiothoracic Surgery, Indiana University School of Medicine, James Whitcomb Riley Hospital for Children, Indianapolis

Richard M. Donner, MD
Associate Professor of Pediatrics, Department of Pediatrics, Temple University School of Medicine, Saint Christopher's Hospital for Children, Philadelphia

Kim F. Duncan, MD, MS, FRCSC
Assistant Professor, Department of Surgery, University of Manitoba, Winnipeg, Manitoba, Canada

Jeffrey M. Dunn, MD
Professor, Department of Surgery, Temple University School of Medicine, and Director, Pediatric Heart Institute, Saint Christopher's Hospital for Children, Philadelphia

Paul A. Ebert, MD
Department of Surgery, University of California, Moffet, San Francisco

Robert M. Freedom, MD, FRCP (C), FACC
Head, Division of Cardiology, and Professor of Paediatrics and Pathology, Hospital for Sick Children, University of Toronto, Toronto

Timothy J. Gardner, MD
Professor of Surgery, Department of Surgery, Johns Hopkins University School of Medicine, Baltimore

Donald A. Girod, MD
Professor of Pediatrics, Section of Pediatric Cardiology, Indiana University School of Medicine, Indianapolis

Siew Yen Ho, PhD
Senior Lecturer, Department of Paediatrics, Cardiothoracic Institute, London

P. Horvath, MD
Senior House Officer, Thoracic Unit, The Hospital for Sick Children, London

Roger A. Hurwitz, MD
Professor of Pediatrics, Section of Pediatric Cardiology, Indiana University School of Medicine, Indianapolis

Rae-Ellen W. Kavey, MD
Divisions of Cardiopulmonary Surgery and Pediatric Cardiology, State University of New York Upstate Medical Center, Syracuse, New York

Harold King, MD
Chief, Department of Surgery, Section of Cardiothoracic Surgery, Indiana University School of Medicine, James Whitcomb Riley Hospital for Children, Indianapolis

Josef Koncz, MD
Professor of Surgery, Emeritus, Clinic for Thoracic and Cardiovascular Surgery, University of Goettingen, Goettingen, Germany

Marc R. de Leval, MD
Consultant Cardiothoracic Surgeon, Cardiothoracic Unit, The Hospital for Sick Children, London

F.J. Macartney, MA, MB, BCh, FRCP, FACC
Vandervell/British Heart Foundation Professor of Paediatric Cardiology, Institute of Child Health, and Honorary Consultant in Pediatric Cardiology, The Hospital for Sick Children, London

Louis M. Marmon, MD
Chief Surgical Resident, Department of Surgery, Temple University School of Medicine, Philadelphia

Boyd Marts
Indiana University School of Medicine, James Whitcomb Riley Hospital for Children, Indianapolis

Walter H. Merrill, MD
Assistant Professor, Department of Cardiac and Thoracic Surgery, Vanderbilt University School of Medicine, Nashville, Tennessee

Simcha Milo, MD
Director, Department of Cardiac Surgery, Rambam Medical Center, Haifa, Israel

William I. Norwood, MD, PhD
Professor of Surgery, University of Pennsylvania, and Chief of Cardiovascular Surgery, Children's Hospital of Philadelphia, Philadelphia

Albert D. Pacifico, MD
J.W. Kirklin Professor of Surgery, and Director, Division of Cardiothoracic Surgery, Department of Surgery, University of Alabama at Birmingham, Birmingham, Alabama

Houshang Rastan, MD
Professor of Surgery, Medical Heart Center, Cardiac Surgery, Teheran, Iran

Peter J. Robinson, MB, FRACP
Consultant Cardiologist, Royal Alexandra Hospital for Children, Camperdown, and Saint George Hospital, Kogarat, New South Wales, Australia

Robert J. Robison, MD
Assistant Professor of Surgery, Section of Cardiothoracic Surgery, Indiana University School of Medicine, Indianapolis

Gerhard Rupprath, MD
Director of the Pediatric Clinic, Stadtisches Krankenhaus, Kaiserslautern, Germany

Hartzell V. Schaff, MD
Associate Professor of Surgery, Mayo Medical School, and Consultant, Thoracic and Cardiovascular Surgery, Mayo Clinic and Mayo Foundation, Rochester, Minnesota

Jeffrey F. Smallhorn, MD, FRACP, FRCP (C)
Associate Professor of Pediatrics, and Director, Echocardiography Laboratory, Division of Cardiology, University of Toronto, The Hospital for Sick Children, Toronto

Jaroslav Stark, MD, FRCS
Consultant Cardiothoracic Surgeon, Cardiothoracic Unit, The Hospital for Sick Children, London

I. Sullivan, B Med Sci, MB, FRACP
Senior Registrar, Thoracic Unit, The Hospital for Sick Children, London

James F.N. Taylor, MD, FRCP, FACC
Consultant Paediatric Cardiologist, The Hospital for Sick Children, London

E. Rainer de Vivie, MD
Professor of Surgery, Chief of Pediatric Surgery, Clinic for Thoracic and Cardiovascular Surgery, University of Goettingen, Goettingen, Germany

Johannes Vogt, MD
Department of Pediatric Cardiology, University of Goettingen, Goettingen, Germany

James R. Zuberbuhler, MD, FACC
Director, Department of Pediatric Cardiology, Department of Pediatrics, Children's Hospital of Pittsburgh, Pittsburgh

Section I

THE AORTIC VALVE

CHAPTER 1

The Morphology of the Aortic Valve with Regard to Congenital Malformations

Siew Yen Ho, PhD, and
Robert H. Anderson, MD, FRC Path

SUMMARY

The normal aortic valve is more complex than its simple trifoliate arrangement suggests. The concept of an aortic annulus is simplistic because the aortic leaflets are attached to the aortic wall along their semilunar margins. The ventriculoarterial junction is therefore shaped like a three-pronged crown — the zeniths being the commissural attachments and the nadirs the leaflet troughs. The areas between the arcs of leaflet attachment are the triplicated interleaflet fibrous triangles. The commissural ridge is a circumferential region of the aortic wall joining the three commissural attachments. The aortic valve is in fibrous continuity with the aortic leaflet of the mitral valve.

Obstructive lesions are the most common diseases of the aortic root in childhood. The etiology of the diffuse and discrete forms of subvalvar stenosis and their categorization are contentious. It is preferable to describe these lesions morphologically as the fibrous shelf, the tunnel lesion, aneurysmal tissue tags, anomalous insertion of the atrioventricular valve apparatus, and deviation of the outlet septum. Valvar stenosis is more commonly due to the shape of the leaflets rather than numerical aberrations. The dome-shaped, unicommissural unileaflet, and the dysplastic trifoliate variants are inherently stenotic, whereas the bifoliate valve becomes stenotic with age. Classically described as a narrowing of the ascending aorta just above the aortic valve, some cases of supravalvar stenosis may be more accurately classified as valvar due to an accentuation of the commissural ridge.

3

INTRODUCTION

In hearts with concordant ventriculoarterial connections, diseases affecting the outflow from the left ventricle are mainly obstructive. The obstructions are generally considered at subvalvar, valvar, and supravalvar levels. Before embarking on descriptions of these types of aortic outflow stenosis, however, it is essential to give an account of the anatomy of the normal valve, which is, to our eyes, much more complex than some recent reviews would suggest. Moreover, in keeping with Harlan et al,[1] it seems to us that many of the so-called supravalvar lesions are no more than stenosis at the level of the valve commissures.

NORMAL ANATOMY

The left ventricular outflow tract has part muscular and part fibrous borders (Fig. 1.1). Its fibrous border is made up of the extensive area of aortic–mitral fibrous continuity, which forms the aortic vestibule. Posteriorly this area has an extensive diverticulum that separates the mitral valve from the muscular ventricular septum; we have previously described this part of the septum as

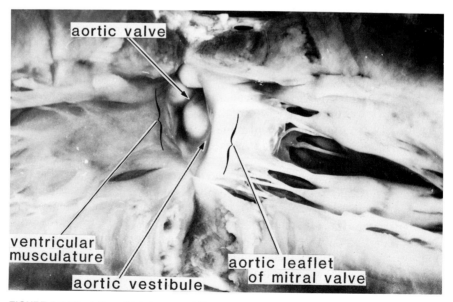

FIGURE 1.1 The left ventricle is opened like a clam to show the borders of the aortic outflow tract. Note the extensive area of aortic–mitral fibrous continuity.

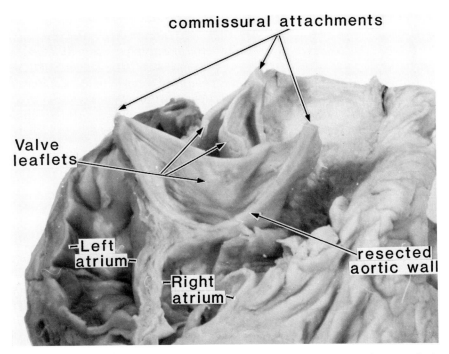

FIGURE 1.2 Resection of the aortic wall to the attachment of the valve leaflets reveals the three-pronged appearance of the aortic crown.

the "inlet septum." On its right aspect it is certainly bordered by the inlet of the right ventricle. The presence of the posterior diverticulum, however, means that its left side forms the wall of the subaortic outflow tract. Most of the muscular septum in this region of the normal heart, therefore, is really an inlet–outlet septum. The left ventricular outflow tract itself terminates at the level of the aortic valve leaflets, which guard the aortic orifice.

The architecture of the aortic valve is more complicated than the simple trifoliate arrangement of the leaflets. The entire valve complex is composed of the leaflets and their commissural attachments, which are subtended between the struts of a three-pronged crown (Fig. 1.2). The leaflets are arranged within this crown in semilunar fashion. The aortic wall above the leaflets forms part of the valve complex to the level of the commissural ring. This supraleaflet region is itself expanded in triple fashion to form the sinuses of Valsalva. There is a further triplicated zone beneath the leaflets that forms the reciprocating area of outflow tract wall from the zenith of the commissures to the nadir of the leaflet attachments. Because of the crescentic attachments of the valve leaflets to the aortic wall, the plane of the aortic valve extends from zenith to nadir depending on whether the commissural attachment or the deepest trough of the leaflet is taken as the reference point.

When this complex architecture is considered as an entity, it emerges that the aortic valve in no way possesses an "annulus" comparable to that of the mitral valve. Despite the recognition of morphology as described above, the valve is suggested in almost all texts to have a "ring" or "annulus" (Fig. 1.3a). Even McAlpine, who pioneered the description as given above,[2] continues to use the term "annulus" for want of a better term; it is extremely unlikely that the term will ever pass from the surgical vocabulary. It is vital, therefore, to understand the precise architecture of the structures that govern the presence of the so-called annulus. As described above, the three semilunar leaflets are attached to struts of fibrous aggregations that extend upwards from the ventricular myocardium to the extracardiac region. When the aortic wall is removed to the level of the leaflets, this arrangement becomes readily apparent (Fig. 1.2). It is the aortic wall removed to reveal this crownlike arrangement that makes up the sinuses. The three aortic sinuses are more prominent than those of the pulmonary trunk. Their dilations extend along the aortic wall to just above the free margins of the valve leaflets (Fig. 1.3b, 1.3c). Above this dilated portion, the aortic wall shows a well-defined, circumferential commissural ridge that is particularly evident when one looks down from the arterial aspect (Fig. 1.3). The commissural ridge can be traced as a circle joining the apices of the three fibrous struts (the apices marking the positions of the three aortic valve commissural attachments). It is this ring that realistically is the most obvious annulus, even though not usually described in that fashion. The orifices of the coronary arteries usually arise on or beneath the commissural ridge, although they may sometimes arise above.

In the closed position, the aortic leaflets have an overlap of their free edges. This is because the total leaflet area is considerably greater than the aortic cross-sectional area.[3] In clinical practice the leaflets are named right coronary, left coronary, and noncoronary, in relation to the origins of the coronary arteries (Fig. 1.3c). In anatomic terms, however, the leaflets may be named anterior, left posterior, and right posterior, respectively. The right posterior sinus, then, corresponds to the noncoronary leaflet and the anterior sinus to the right coronary leaflet. Within normal hearts, there is considerable variability in the relative sizes of each leaflet.[4] All three leaflets meet at their nodules. These are fibrous aggregations at the midpoint of the free edge of each leaflet and become increasingly more prominent with age. The remaining leaflet tissue (the lunule) is thin, translucent, and may occasionally be fenestrated. The close apposition of the nodules and the free edges of the adjacent leaflets seen in plane view gives the characteristic appearance of a Mercedes-Benz logo. When the valve is in open position, the free margin of each leaflet straightens and the aortic orifice becomes triangular in outline.

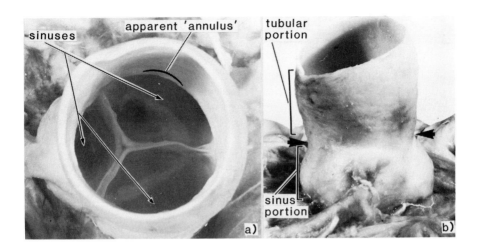

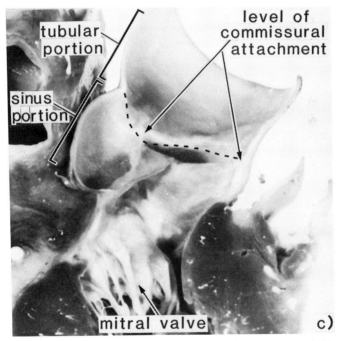

FIGURE 1.3 (a) When the aortic root is viewed from above the commissural ridge gives the appearance of an aortic annulus. **(b)** A side view shows a narrowed region *(arrows)* between the dilated sinus portion and the tubular portion of the aorta. **(c)** A longitudinal section shows the narrowed region *(broken line)* corresponding to the commissural attachments of the leaflets. (Photographs courtesy of Dr. A. Angelini.)

When viewed from the ventricular aspect, the closed aortic valve is seen to be supported by the subvalvar crown, which itself has part muscular and part fibrous origins. The crown itself forms a ringlike structure that, at the level of the commissures, has considerable depth. It is this apparent ring that is the "surgical" aortic ring, and its size has little functional significance.[3] When examined closely, it can be seen that, in addition to the obvious region of aortic–mitral valve fibrous continuity, there are further fibrous areas upon which the aortic leaflets insert; these are the interleaflet triangles.[5] McAlpine,[2] in his detailed examination of the "aorto-ventricular membrane," called these triangular areas the "fibrous trigones." In describing the structures as fibrous trigones, however, they can easily be confused with the better known left and right fibrous trigones. The latter structures are the collagenous thickenings at either extreme of the fibrous continuity between the aortic and mitral valves. The left fibrous trigone is attached to the ventricular musculature that forms the left margin of the inner heart curvature. The right fibrous trigone is fused to the membranous septum and together they make up the so-called central fibrous body of the heart.

It is the semilunar line of attachment of the three leaflets that results in the three additional fibrous triangles, which have their apex at the commissural insertions (Fig. 1.4). (For the reasons given above, we prefer to describe

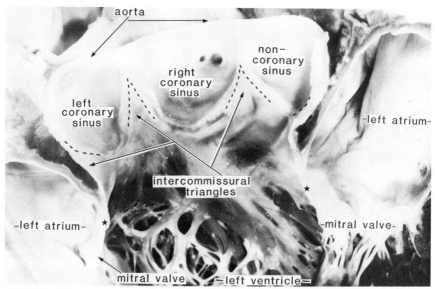

FIGURE 1.4 The aortic root displayed after cleaving the aortic leaflet of the mitral valve *(asterisks)* and removing the semilunar leaflets. The intercommissural fibrous triangles are situated between the broken lines.

these structures as interleaflet triangles rather than fibrous trigones.) The triangle between the right and noncoronary leaflets is situated above the interventricular part of the membranous septum. As the commissure is located well onto the aortic wall, the upper part of this triangle is in potential communication with the outside of the heart. The triangle between the noncoronary and left coronary leaflets is along the region of aortic–mitral fibrous continuity. Its upper part abuts on the transverse sinus of the pericardium. Less extensive than the others is the fibrous triangle between the left and right coronary leaflets.

All of this area is in potential communication with extracardiac space, because both aortic and pulmonary leaflets are supported in part on a sleeve of outflow tract musculature. There is an extensive tissue plane between the facing surfaces of the aortic and pulmonary trunks. Taken as a whole, it can be seen that the left ventricular outflow tract is partly muscular and partly fibrous. Neither an aortic annulus nor ring exists as a discrete structure in one plane. Each leaflet has a semilunar attachment to the ventriculoarterial junction. Each of the three fibrous triangles of interleaflet tissue in the subaortic outflow tract is above the level of ventricular musculature. McAlpine[2] has rightly pointed to these areas as potential sites for aneurysm formation.

THE AORTIC VALVE COMPLEX IN DISEASE

Obstruction of flow from the left ventricle to the aorta is the most frequent form of aortic root disease in childhood. Taking the aortic valve as a reference point, the obstruction can be considered at subvalvar, valvar and supravalvar levels.

Subvalvar Stenosis

In a study of 99 patients under the age of 1 year with congenital heart disease, Freedom et al[6] observed a wide variety of anatomic substrates for subaortic stenosis. The most common derangements were due to intracardiac malformations such as a malalignment of the outlet septum; in only three patients did the Toronto team observe a relatively discrete form of subaortic stenosis. In hearts with normally positioned aortic outflow tracts, the subvalvar stenosis has been described as comprising discrete and diffuse types. Opinions differ, however, with regard to the types of lesions constituting either form. The latter usually refers to lesions in hearts with hypertrophic cardiomyopathy. Although Edwards[7] distinguished hearts with localized muscular hypertrophy of the ventricular septum in the subaortic area from the diffuse form related to generalized hypertrophy of the myocardium, he pointed out that the two may be variants of the same pathologic process. He also included hearts with glycogen storage disease with the diffuse form.

The more common variety of subvalvar aortic stenosis is frequently described as "congenital discrete subvalvar stenosis." This form can appear either as a shelf or as a more extensive tunnel. It can be associated with lesions of the mitral valve or found in combination with complex heart malformations. When considering hearts with normally placed aortic outflow tracts, it appears that there is some overlap between those with discrete fibrous shelves and those with diffuse myocardial involvement. Secondary endocardial thickening may overlie the protruding myocardium in the subaortic region. Roberts[8] made careful distinction between the endocardial thickening found with discrete subaortic stenosis from that found with muscular septal hypertrophy. Endocardial plaques in the latter, he observed, never extended more apically than the level corresponding to the free margin of the aortic leaflet of the mitral valve. Owing to the close proximity of the mitral valve to the subaortic outflow tract, it is to be anticipated that certain conditions affecting the mitral valve may cause subaortic stenosis and vice-versa.[7]

In view of the dynamic nature of congenital heart disease, Somerville[9] contends that the shelf variant of subaortic stenosis is a progressive disorder acquired in postnatal life. This contention is supported by the hemodynamic and angiographic studies of Freedom et al.[10,11] Furthermore, Somerville[12] correctly challenges the standard descriptions of the obstructive lesion as a membrane or diaphragm. According to her investigations, the membrane has never been demonstrated either at surgery or at necropsy. Instead, a ridge of irregular fibroelastic tissue is usually found. This tissue is attached to thickened endocardium that overlies a bulging ventricular septal myocardium. We agree with her observations and therefore describe the lesion as a shelf. The term "discrete" is also contentious because these lesions are usually associated with secondary involvement of the myocardium and the aortic valve.[12] Relative to the controversy of what constitutes a "discrete" or "diffuse" lesion and whether it is congenital in origin is the proposal by Rosenquist et al[13] that an increased separation between aortic and mitral valves during early heart development might contribute to the etiology of discrete subaortic stenosis. Perhaps these differences can best be summarized by Edwards'[7] succinct statement that "subaortic stenosis is a complicated subject." Nonetheless, the lesions that cause outflow obstruction in the immediate subvalvar region can be considered in terms of several morphologic types. These include the fibrous shelf, the tunnel lesion, aneurysmal tissue tags, anomalous insertion of atrioventricular valve apparatus and deviations of the outlet septum.

The Fibrous Shelf

Although often described as a thin membrane or circumferential diaphragm situated immediately underneath the aortic valve leaflets, most illustrations show a crescentic shelf of fibrous tissue extending from just below the non-coronary aortic leaflet to fuse with the aortic leaflet of the mitral valve. This shelf may be superimposed upon thickened endocardium extending some distance apically beneath the aortic valve (Fig. 1.5). It may also be seen in the left ventricle in hearts with discordant ventriculoarterial connections (in which case it is in subpulmonary position) or found in the already narrowed outflow tract of an atrioventricular septal defect.

The Tunnel Lesion

Instead of being in the form of a protruding shelf, the tunnel form of obstruction involves a length of the outflow tract (Fig. 1.6). It is usually due to hypertrophy of the septal myocardium upon which a thick layer of fibrous tissue may be superimposed. It is suggested that this lesion may be related to idiopathic myocardial hypertrophy, which may be familial.[14] Although typi-

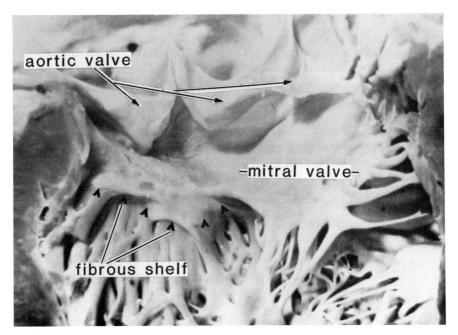

FIGURE 1.5 A fibrous shelf *(arrowheads)* in continuity with the aortic leaflet of the mitral valve causes outflow obstruction. (Photograph courtesy of Prof. A. Becker.)

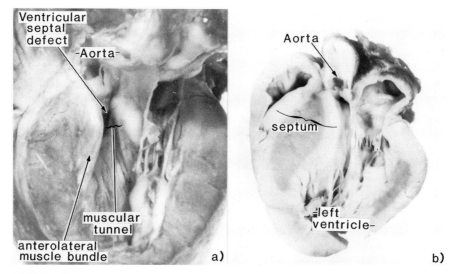

FIGURE 1.6 Tunnel lesions in two hearts. **(a)** The lesion is caused by an anomalous anterolateral muscle bundle in a heart associated with interruption of the aortic arch. **(b)** Another heart, from a patient with glycogen storage disease, is sectioned to show the septal bulge encroaching upon the aortic outflow tract.

cally associated with an abnormally small aortic annulus,[15] this need not be a cardinal feature.[14]

Aneurysmal Tissue Tags

Tags of fibrous tissue arising either from the membranous septum or arising as a duplicated atrioventricular valve leaflet can aggravate an intrinsically narrow aortic outflow tract, for instance in hearts with atrioventricular septal defect and concordant ventriculo-arterial connections[16] (Fig. 1.7). In hearts with a discordant ventriculoarterial connection, these tissue tags are also significant hemodynamically because the pressure differential favors protrusion into the left ventricular and subpulmonary outflow tract.

Anomalous Insertion of the Atrioventricular Valve Apparatus

This anomaly is most frequently seen in hearts with atrioventricular septal defect. Papillary muscles or chords supporting the left component of the atrioventricular valve can encroach upon the outflow tract.

Deviation of the Outlet Septum

In hearts with concordant ventriculoarterial connections, leftward deviation of the outlet septum in association with a ventricular septal defect is a common cause of left ventricular outflow obstruction (Fig. 1.8). In such cases, there is a significant association with coarctation or interruption of the aortic arch.[17,18] In hearts with complete transposition, the deviated outlet septum is the commonest cause of left ventricular (and therefore subpulmonary) outflow obstruction.

Valvar Stenosis

The most common form of left ventricular outflow obstruction is at the level of the aortic valve.[8] Aberrations in the number of aortic valve leaflets seldom

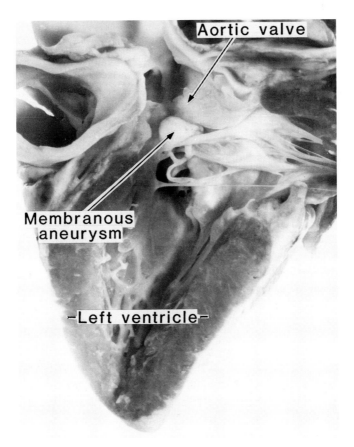

FIGURE 1.7 A left ventricular view of a heart with atrioventricular septal defect shows an aneurysm of the membranous septum protruding into the aortic outflow tract. (Photograph courtesy of Dr. S. Banik.)

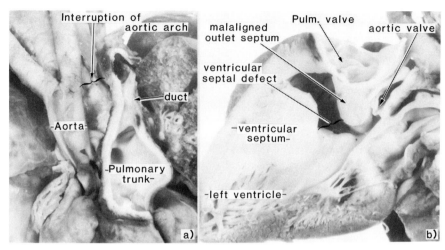

FIGURE 1.8 A heart with interruption of the aortic arch **(a)** has an associated ventricular septal defect with deviation of the outlet septum **(b)**. (Photograph courtesy of Dr. A. Smith.)

present with problems in children. Of more significance is the shape of the valve. Most congenitally malformed valves are not stenotic at birth but stenosis is acquired with age.[4,8] The acquired fibrosis and subsequent calcification can affect either a congenitally malformed or a normally formed valve, both of which previously functioned normally. Commissural fusion may also be congenital or acquired postnatally. It may be exceedingly difficult to distinguish the two forms.[19] Nonetheless, we shall consider the valve in terms of the dome-shaped lesion, the unicommissural unileaflet valve, the bifoliate arrangement, the dysplastic trifoliate valve, and the normal trifoliate valve with its intrinsic variations.

The Dome-Shaped Valve

Aptly named, this lesion is characterized by a dome-shaped membrane with a central perforation of restricted size making the valve intrinsically stenotic (Fig. 1.9). Three (or, rarely, two or four) shallow raphes may be recognizable at the base of the dome. Indeed, this valve has also been described as "acommissural" to distinguish it from the unicommissural valve.[20] This type of morphology occurs more frequently in pulmonary rather than aortic position.

The Unicommissural Unileaflet Valve

The single leaflet is attached circumferentially and at its commissure to the aortic wall, thus leaving a characteristic eccentrically located orifice (Fig.

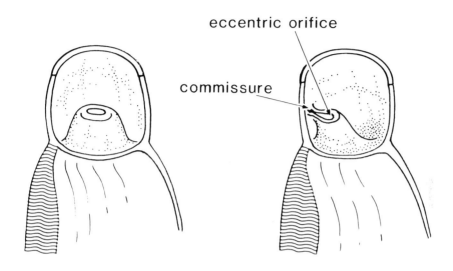

eccentric orifice

commissure

Dome-shaped valve   Unicommissural valve

FIGURE 1.9 Diagram showing the central orifice of an acommissural dome-shaped valve in contrast to the eccentric orifice of an unicommissural valve.

1.10). It is arguable as to whether the valve is truly unicommissural. Most frequently, two raphes may be distinguished radiating from the stenotic ostium, suggesting undeveloped commissures of a trileaflet valve.[21] The leaflet tissue is usually thickened. Being intrinsically stenotic, this morphology is one of the most common causes of isolated aortic valve stenosis in children.

The Bifoliate Valve

There are two basic types depending on the orientation of the leaflets.[8] When the leaflets are arranged in left–right position, a coronary artery arises from each sinus and a raphe is present in the right leaflet. When orientated in anteroposterior position, then both coronary arteries arise from the anterior sinus and the raphe is located in the anterior leaflet. These two types are equally common in patients with congenitally bifoliate aortic valve.[21] The valve malformed in this fashion can be subdivided into two other types: those with almost equal sized leaflets and those with one leaflet larger than the other (Fig. 1.11). Apart from a predilection for valvar stenosis, the latter form may also manifest with prolapse of the larger leaflet. In a series of 85 cases, Roberts[21] found that 72% had stenotic valves with or without aortic regurgitation, 13% had pure regurgitation, and 15% had normal function.

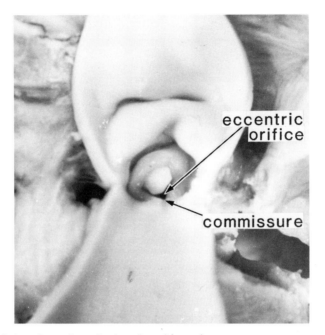

FIGURE 1.10 An unicommissural valve, viewed from above.

The true incidence of the bifoliate aortic valve is unknown because they are not intrinsically stenotic unless dysplastic. Dysplastic leaflets are thickened, rolled, and redundant. Obstruction is then due to the abnormal exuberant leaflet tissue rather than commissural fusion.[22] The bifoliate valve becomes stenotic only as it thickens and becomes calcified. Such a valve is estimated to occur in 50%–80% of hearts with coarctation.[23,24]

The Dysplastic Trifoliate Valve

The dysplastic valve has a gelatinous appearance with thickening of all three leaflets (Fig. 1.12) which have a mucoid tissue core. Although the changes tend to obscure the valve commissures, the obstruction to flow is caused by the swollen leaflets rather than commissural fusion. This type of valve stenosis is seldom amenable to surgical correction.

The Trifoliate Valve

As mentioned earlier, the three leaflets of the normal aortic valve are rarely of equal size.[4] Several reports[25,26] have indicated that the stenotic trifoliate valve shows changes at the cellular level which represent an accentuated

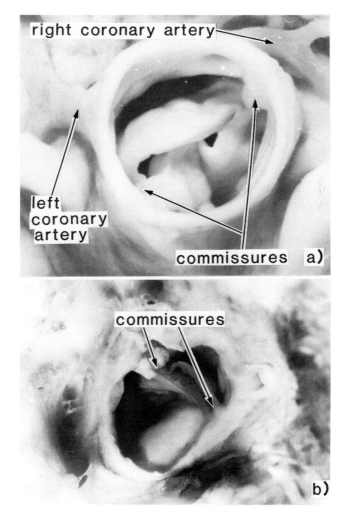

FIGURE 1.11 A bifoliate valve with two nearly equal-sized leaflets **(a)** and another with dispar-ity in leaflet size **(b)**.

aging process. With this in mind, Vollebergh and Becker investigated the initial suggestion by Roberts[21] that minor inequalities in leaflet size could underlie isolated aortic stenosis. They expanded this concept, providing evidence that leaflet inequality (along with other factors such as individual tissue variations in reaction to haemodynamic changes) probably played a significant role in the pathogenesis of isolated aortic stenosis.

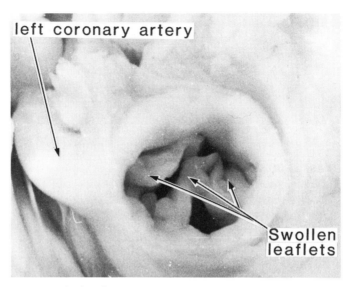

FIGURE 1.12 A dysplastic valve.

Supravalvar Aortic Stenosis

Of the three levels of aortic stenosis, the so-called supravalvar type is least frequently observed.[27] Since Chevers'[28] original description in 1842, supravalvar aortic stenosis has become recognized as a narrowing of the ascending aorta just above the aortic valve and coronary orifices. The malformation can be inherited as an autosomal dominant trait,[29] as part of William's syndrome[30] in association with mental retardation and distinctive physical characteristics or as part of a generalized disorder associated with infantile hypercalcemia.[31]

Supravalvar aortic stenosis is conventionally described as taking one of three forms: an hour-glass deformity, a fibrous membrane with central orifice, and a diffusely hypoplastic ascending aorta[7] (Fig.1.13). The elastic units in the aortic media are thickened, fragmented, and show a disorganized pattern that is said to reflect a localized response to wall stress.[32] As the coronary arteries originate beneath the region of aortic narrowing they are subjected to elevated pressures, and it is this pressure that is thought to account for the tortuosity and premature atherosclerotic lesions of the coronary arteries.

Recently, an entity has been described as a variant of congenital aortic stenosis that is characterized by an asymmetrically small left aortic sinus associated with a supravalvar ridge above the left coronary orifice.[1] This morphology has considerable significance to the surgical repair of supraval-

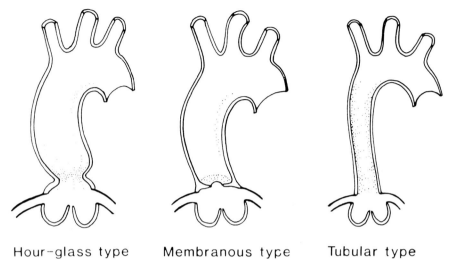

Hour-glass type   Membranous type   Tubular type

FIGURE 1.13 The forms of supravalvar aortic stenosis.

var aortic stenosis. Although Rastelli et al[33] alluded to the fact that abnormalities of the aortic leaflets were present in just less than half their patients with supravalvar stenosis, they did not elaborate further. This observation brings into question whether supravalvar stenosis is in some cases valvar due to a malformation of the leaflets (Fig. 1.14) In their description of the hour-

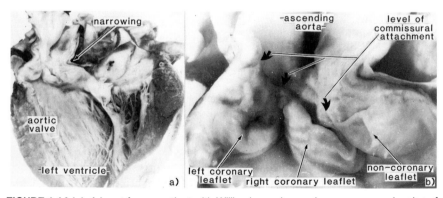

FIGURE 1.14 (a) A heart from a patient with William's syndrome shows a narrowed region of the aorta. **(b)** A close-up view of the aortic valve region shows the narrowed region corresponding to an accentuation of the level of commissural attachment. A tissue shelf protrudes across the opening of the right coronary leaflet. In addition, the left coronary leaflet has no free margin being adherent to the aortic wall. A small orifice in the leaflet permits flow to the left coronary ostium.

glass deformity of the pulmonary trunk with bottle-shaped sinuses, Milo et al[34] pointed out that the pulmonary stenosis is at the level of the commissural attachment of the valve leaflets. The leaflets appear as deep pockets with relatively narrow openings. The appearance described by Harlan et al[1] is remarkably similar to one of Milo's "pockets." In these cases at least, it seems to us that the lesions are best considered at commissural ridge level (and therefore part of the valve) rather than supravalvar.

ACKNOWLEDGMENT
We are grateful to the help given by our colleagues in obtaining some of the illustrative material.

REFERENCES

1. Harlan JL, Clark EB, Doty DB. Congenital aortic stenosis with hypoplasia of the left sinus of Valsalva. J Thorac Cardiovasc Surg 1985;89:288-294.
2. McAlpine WA. Heart and Coronary Arteries. An Anatomical Atlas for Clinical Diagnosis, Radiological Investigation and Surgical Treatment. Springer-Verlag, New York, 1975, pp 154-159.
3. Davies MJ. The aortic valve. Pathology of Cardiac Valves. Butterworth, London, 1980, pp 1-7.
4. Vollebergh FEMG, Becker AE. Minor congenital variations of cusp size in tricuspid aortic valves. Possible link with isolated aortic stenosis. Br Heart J 1977;39:1006-1011.
5. Anderson RH, Devine WA, Zuberbuhler JR. The anatomy of the subaortic region of the normal human left ventricle. Int J Cardiol (in press).
6. Freedom RM, Dische MR, Rowe RD. Pathologic anatomy of subaortic stenosis and atresia in the first year of life. Am J Cardiol 1977;39:1035-1044.
7. Edwards JE. Pathology of left ventricular outflow tract obstruction. Circulation 1965;31:586-599.
8. Roberts WC. Valvular, subvalvular, and supravalvular aortic stenosis: morphologic features. Cardiovasc Clin 1973;5:97-126.
9. Somerville J. Congenital heart disease—changes in form and function. Br Heart J 1979;41:1-22.
10. Freedom RM, Fowler RS, Duncan WJ. Rapid evolution from "normal" left ventricular outflow tract to fatal subaortic stenosis in infancy. Br Heart J 1981;45:605-609.
11. Freedom RM, Pelech A, Brand A, et al. The progressive nature of subaortic stenosis in congenital heart disease. Int J Cardiol 1985;8:137-143.
12. Somerville J. Fixed subaortic stenosis—a frequently misunderstood lesion. Int J Cardiol 1985;8:145-148.
13. Rosenquist GC, Clark EB, McAllister HA, et al. Increased mitral-aortic separation in discrete subaortic stenosis. Circulation 1979;60:70-74.
14. Maron BJ, Redwood DR, Roberts WC, et al. Tunnel subartic stenosis. Left ventricular outflow tract obstruction produced by fibromuscular tubular narrowing. Circulation 1976;54:404-416.
15. Kelly DT, Wulfsberg BA, Rowe RD. Discrete subaortic stenosis. Circulation 1972;46:309.
16. Piccoli GP, Ho SY, Wilkinson JL, et al. Left sided obstructive lesions in atrioventricular septal defects. J Thor Card Surg 1982;83:453-460.

17. Van Praagh R, Bernhard WF, Rosenthal A, et al. Interrupted aortic arch:surgical treatment. Am J Cardiol 1971;27:200–211.
18. Moulaert A, Bruins CC, Oppenheimer-Dekker A. Anomalies of the aortic arch and ventricular septal defects. Circulation 1976;53:1011–1015.
19. Waller BF, Carter JB, Williams HJ Jr, Wang K, Edwards JE. Clinicopathologic correlations. Bicuspid aortic valve, comparison of congenital and acquired types. Circulation 1973;58:1140–1151.
20. Roberts WC, Morrow AG. Congenital aortic stenosis produced by a unicommissural valve. Br Heart J 1965;27:505–511.
21. Roberts WC. The congenitally bicuspid aortic valve. A study of 85 autopsy cases. Am J Cardiol 1970;26:72–83.
22. Chietlin MD, Fenoglio JJ, McAllister HA, et al. Congenital aortic stenosis secondary to dysplasia of congenital bicuspid aortic valves without commissural fusion. Am J Cardiol 1978;42:102–107.
23. Becker AE, Becker MJ, Edwards JE. Anomalies associated with coarctation of the aorta. Particular reference to infancy. Circulation 1970;41:1067–1075.
24. Edwards JE. The congenital bicuspid aortic valve. Circulation 1961;23:485–95.
25. Sell S, Scully RE. Aging changes in the aortic and mitral valves. Histologic and histochemical studies, with observations on the pathogenesis of calcific aortic stenosis and calcification of the mitral annulus. Am J Pathol 1965;46:345–365.
26. Roberts WC, Perloff JK, Constantino T. Severe valvular aortic stenosis in patients over 65 years of age. A clinicopathologic study. Am J Cardiol 1971;27:497–506.
27. Peterson TA, Todd DB, Edwards JE. Supravalvular aortic stenosis. J Thor Cardiovasc Surg 1965;50:734–741.
28. Chevers N. Observations on the diseases of the orifice and valves of the aorta. Guys Hosp Rep 1842;7:387–427.
29. Noonan JA. Syndromes associated with cardiac defects. Pediatric Cardiovascular Disease. 1981;108.
30. Williams JCP, Barratt-Boyes BG, Lowe JB. Supravalvular aortic stenosis. Circulation 1961;24:1311–1318.
31. Garcia RE, Friedman WF, Kaback MM, et al. Idiopathic hypercalcemia and supravalvar aortic stenosis. N Engl J Med 1964;271:117–120.
32. O'Connor WN, Davis JB, Geissler R, et al. Supravalvar aortic stenosis. Clinical and pathologic observations in six patients. Arch Pathol Lab Med 1985;109:179–185.
33. Rastelli GC, McGoon DC, Ongley PA, et al. Surgical treatment of supravalvar aortic stenosis. J Thor Cardiovasc Surg 1966;51:873–882.
34. Milo S, Fiegel A, Shem-Tov A, et al. Isolated pulmonic stenosis: anatomical aspects and surgical implications. Valvular pulmonic stenosis (in press).

CHAPTER 2

Evaluation of
Aortic Valve Disease

Richard M. Donner, MD

Diseases of the aortic valve account for approximately 4% of all congenital heart disease,[1] but they continue to pose a major clinical problem for the cardiologist. Because surgical therapy is limited and carries considerable risk, the evaluation of the severity of disease and proper selection of patients for invasive study or surgery, or both, assume tremendous importance. In current practice, this is accomplished by examining those factors influencing the prognosis in groups of patients with similar disease. Many variables contribute to the outcome, but sufficient knowledge exists to discuss their relationship to the prognosis of aortic stenosis in older infants and children. In addition, some information is available regarding aortic regurgitation in older children and young adults. The subject of significant aortic valve disease in newborns requires different analysis and is discussed elsewhere.

AORTIC STENOSIS IN OLDER INFANTS AND CHILDREN

The development of practical management criteria in the older infant or child with aortic stenosis depends upon the nature and quality of the information gathered by both invasive and noninvasive means. Although there is some overlap, it is customary to regard noninvasive information as either supporting or rejecting the need for invasive study, while invasive criteria are used to evaluate the need for surgery.

Invasive Procedures

Data obtained by invasive means (i.e., cardiac catheterization) is generally considered the "gold standard," better illustrates the physiology of obstruc-

22

tive disease, and provides a standard by which noninvasive data is evaluated. Most invasive criteria used to judge severity of disease may be placed into one of the following four groups: *(a)* anatomy; *(b)* hemodynamics; *(c)* pump performance and muscle function; or *(d)* muscle perfusion

Anatomy

The type and location of left ventricular outflow obstruction greatly influences the immediate and long-term surgical results. A recommendation for surgery, therefore, must be founded on accurate anatomic information. Although surgery for valvar obstruction may be indicated in a given set of circumstances, the relatively poorer results for supravalvar narrowing may force postponement of this recommendation.[2] Diffuse, muscular, or tubular subvalvar stenosis requiring extensive reconstruction of the left ventricular outflow tract or an apico–aortic conduit might fall into this same category.[3,4] In contrast, the progressive nature of aortic stenosis and regurgitation and more favorable outcome associated with discrete, fibrous subaortic stenosis might advance a recommendation for surgery in the presence of less severe criteria.[5] Though anatomic description and Doppler estimation of the site and severity of obstruction may be initiated by echocardiography, catheterization is usually necessary to confirm the site and significance of the lesion. This is particularly relevant when it is suspected that more than one site of obstruction or other associated defects may be present (e.g., peripheral pulmonary artery narrowings associated with supravalvar aortic stenosis or Williams syndrome). Axial cineangiography is probably best suited for obtaining both static and dynamic anatomic information.[6] The latter is most useful when coupled with retrograde pressure recordings made during a pullback maneuver from left ventricular apex to distal ascending aorta. When single-side-hole or micromanometer-tipped catheters are employed for this use, the presence and individual significance of multiple or complex obstructions may be more accurately diagnosed.

Hemodynamics

Historically, measurement of hemodynamic variables — such as left ventricle-to-aortic gradient, left ventricular end-diastolic pressure, cardiac index, and aortic valve area — has provided the core of data upon which management decisions are based. This is not surprising because their determination is relatively simple. Interpretation of these data, however, may vary considerably. Four major studies that followed changes of left ventricular-to-aortic gradient in children with principally valvar obstruction[7-10] are listed in Table 2.1. Three of the four studies show a significant progression of the disease during the study interval, and in two of them, a large number of children entered a "severe" catagory. Although there are some qualifica-

TABLE 2.1 Left Ventricle-to-Aortic Gradient in Serial Studies

Study	Mean Follow-Up Period (yr)	Mean Increase (mm Hg)	% Severe* (mm Hg)
Friedman et al, 1971	6.8–13.1	33	55% (>50)
El-Said et al, 1972	7.0–11.0	27	—
Cohen et al, 1972	8.5–15.1	18	40% (>50)
Hurwitz et al, 1973	9.0–14.0	3	12% (>80)

*The percent of patients entering the "severe" group at the time of follow-up study.

tions, these findings suggest that severity of obstruction, as reflected by left ventricle-to-aortic gradient, is often progressive and should be reassessed in some manner at approximately 6-year intervals. The definition of "severe" obstruction is arbitrary but ranges from 50 mm Hg to 70 mm Hg or greater.

In four studies of left ventricular–end-diastolic pressure[8,11–13] shown in Table 2.2, only one suggested a relationship between its value and the severity of obstruction, assessed by left ventricular-to-aortic gradient. This parameter may have other important determinants, but at present its role in decision making is unclear. Changes in cardiac index and aortic valve area during serial studies[7–9] are illustrated in Table 2.3. No clear cut pattern of change is established. This may result from a variation of the compensatory mechanism among patients or simple inaccuracies inherent in their measurement and computation. The study of Friedman et al[7] may have encouraged the general acceptance of 0.7 cm² as a marker for a "critical" valve area, representing a severe degree of obstruction.

Pump Performance and Muscle Function

Evaluation of cardiac contractile muscle function and pump performance may be carried out during cardiac catheterization[14,15] and some noninvasive

TABLE 2.2 Left Ventricular End-Diastolic Pressure in Serial Studies

Study	LVEDP (mm Hg)	Comments
Braunwald et al, 1963	>13 in 21/100	9/11 with LVEDP >17 mm Hg had a gradient >90 mm Hg
El-Said et al, 1972	10.2–11.7	No change at follow-up despite increased gradient
Hossack et al, 1979	7.5 (mild) 8.7 (mod) 9.2 (severe)	No relation to severity
Donner et al, 1983	9.2	No relation to gradient

Abbreviation: LVEDP = left ventricular end-diastolic pressure.

TABLE 2.3 Cardiac Index and Aortic Valve Area in Serial Studies

Study	Cardiac Index	AVA Index	Critical AVA
Friedman et al, 1971	Normal with no change	Decreased 2/4	<0.7 cm
El-Said et al, 1972	Decreased	Decreased 13/18	—
Cohen et al, 1972	Normal with no change	Decreased in at least 4/15	—

Abbreviation: AVA = aortic valve area.

techniques[16] with increasing sophistication. Contractile function reflects the current state of the myocardium and its ability to perform independent of loading conditions; it is frequently assessed by performing loading experiments and measuring quantities such as Vmax or the slope of the end-systolic pressure-volume points. Pump performance simply measures the ability of the heart to eject blood under fixed conditions; determinations of ejection fraction, mean velocity of circumferential fiber shortening, and stroke-work index are most often used to evaluate it. Contractile muscle function, interacting on a given afterload ("afterload match"), determines the level of pump performance. In moderate or severe congenital aortic stenosis, contractile function is normal while afterload is reduced, resulting in enhanced pump performance that is usually manefestated by an ejection fraction between 70% and 95%.[13] The reduced afterload is due to pronounced muscle hypertrophy and diminished wall stress throughout the cardiac cycle.[13] Thus, enhanced pump performance and an elevated ejection fraction are to be expected in children with well-compensated obstruction. These findings persist at least into the third decade of life, but they differ from "acquired" obstruction in the adult, in which muscle function and pump performance may be normal or reduced. In acquired obstruction it is suggested that diminished pump performance (caused by reduced muscle function or inadequate hypertrophy and elevated wall stress) may return to normal after successful valve replacement.[17] The finding of reduced or even normal pump function in a child with aortic stenosis suggests inadequate compensation that might be reversed with surgical therapy. However, the response to such therapy and the role of muscle function and pump performance analysis in clinical decision making is yet to be determined.

Muscle Perfusion

The invasive evaluation of myocardial blood flow in aortic stenosis is closely linked to the original investigations of this important subject. Although there may be many metabolic factors involved, ischemia of the myocardium is probably related closely to factors that affect cornary blood flow. Figure 2.1 shows that the normal transmural pressure gradients across the left ventricu-

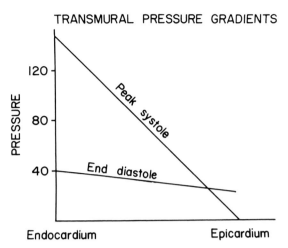

FIGURE 2.1 Transmural pressure gradients at peak systole and end diastole. Subendocardial pressure equal to or greater than systemic pressure during much of systole makes subendocardial perfusion dependent upon diastolic flow.

lar wall in systole and diastole place restrictions on subendocardial blood flow. Perfusion of this region is greatly dependent upon flow occuring during diastole. Factors that alter oxygen delivery in diastole, such as tachycardia, anemia, or decreased perfusion pressure, are initially compensated for by a decrease in coronary vascular resistance in the subendocardium. When coronary vasodilatation is maximal and perfusion time and/or pressure drops further, ischemia results. The laboratory and clinical investigation of these phenomena are well described.[18] An index of subendocardial blood flow may be calculated simply from aortic and left ventricular pressure recordings by taking the ratio of the area between aortic and left ventricular pressure in diastole (diastolic pressure–time index, or DPTI) to the area under the left ventricular pressure curve in systole (systolic pressure–time index or SPTI)[19] (Fig. 2.2). The "myocardial oxygen supply/demand ratio" is obtained by multiplying this fraction by the blood oxygen carrying capacity. A supply/demand ratio of more than 8–10 signifies roughly uniform oxygen delivery across the myocardial wall; below this, oxygen delivery to subendocardial muscle is compromised.[18,20] In children with severe valvar aortic stenosis and a valve area less than $0.7cm^2/m^2$ mycoardial supply/demand ratios tended to be less than 10; but ratios greater than 10 were found in nearly all of these subjects whose heart rate was less than 100 beats/min.[21] This suggests that tachycardia is an important determinant of subendocardial ischemia. Its presence or absence needs to be considered when using this index as a criterion for recommending surgery.

Noninvasive Procedures

Data obtained by noninvasive means may be organized into one of the following three groups: *(a)* clinical symptoms and physical examination; *(b)* resting and exercise electrocardiography; and *(c)* echocardiography.

Clinical Symptoms and Physical Examination

Patient history and physical examination are the traditional methods used to triage patients for further study. However, the small but significant incidence of sudden death in children with aortic stenosis brings about periodic reevaluation of clinical criteria. Although most children are asymptomatic, it is difficult to validate the incidence of true symptoms in older infants and young children. Phenomena such as dyspnea on exertion, angina pectoris, and even syncope are often inaccurately interpreted or confused with normal events. In some investigations, the incidence of symptoms ranges between 20% and 60%, however, though there may be some correlation between the presence of symptoms and the degree of stenosis, the absence of symptoms in a given patient does not exlude the possibility of severe hemodynamic obstruction.[10-12] It is generally agreed that the presence or strong

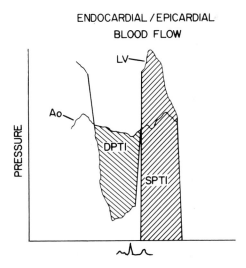

FIGURE 2.2 Quantitation of subendocardial blood flow. Subendocardial flow occurs primarily during diastole and is proportional to the "diastolic pressure–time index," the area under the aortic pressure–time curve. Subepicardial flow occurs mostly in systole and is proportional to the "systolic pressure-time index", the area under the left ventricle pressure–time curve. The ratio of diastolic to systolic time indices estimates the fraction of subendocardial to subepicardial blood flow. Abbreviations: Ao = aorta; DPTI = diastolic pressure–time index; LV = left ventricle; SPTI = systolic pressure–time index.

suspicion of symptoms is an absolute indication for further study.[2,10-12] Findings on physical examination that suggest significant obstruction include palpation of a thrill (gradient >25 mm Hg), a left ventricular lift, a narrow pulse contour, paradoxical splitting of the second sound, disappearance of an ejection click, a fourth heart sound, and a harsh murmur that peaks late in systole.[2,12] Although any one or more of these findings may suggest that invasive study is indicated, the absence of these in no way eliminates the possibility of severe stenosis.[2,10-12]

Resting and Exercise Electrocardiography

The severity of obstruction is generally reflected by the presence and degree of left ventricular hypertrophy on the resting ECG; the correlation between the two is further strengthened by examining the vectorcardiogram. However, the number of false-positive and -negative diagnoses for severe stenosis is too high to rely on this finding alone.[2,10-12,22] Certainly, severe aortic stenosis may exist in the presence of a normal resting ECG. The addition of ST segment depression and T-wave abnormalities to criteria for left ventricular hypertrophy improves the sensitivity of the resting ECG for detecting severe stenosis,[2,12,22] and there is good correlation between the presence of T-wave changes and an oxygen supply/demand ratio less than 10.[22] The ST-segment and T-wave changes after maximal exercise identify severe obstruction in nearly all cases and further improve sensitivity.[23,25]

Echocardiography

The predicatable response of left ventricular wall thickening to increased aortic obstruction permits M-mode echocardiography to estimate the left ventricular peak systolic pressure.[26-28] Alterations of pump performance may be observed by measuring the shortening fraction or estimating the ejection fraction. Pulsed and continuous-wave Doppler techniques can provide good estimation of the peak instantaneous left ventricular-to-aortic gradient in most patients.[29,30] The success of the latter method, however, often depends on the skill and experience of the technician. Both M-mode and Doppler methods are probably best utilized to follow the course of disease with serial examinations in order to establish a trend.

Decisions to recommend invasive study or surgical therapy in a given child with aortic stenosis must be made on an individual basis after consideration of all available data. It is probably not wise to develop a rigid system of criteria that attempts to direct the care of all patients. Instead, the following guidelines are offered to assist evaluation and management of the child with aortic stenosis:

Guidelines for Recommending Invasive Study

1. Periodic routine catheterization is probably not necessary, but should be performed if there is any question regarding severity.
2. Catheterization is indicated if symptoms are present or strongly suspected, or there is evidence on physical examination of moderate or severe obstruction.
3. Catheterization is indicated if there is evidence for resting or exercise ischemia, particularly in the absence of anemia or tachycardia.
4. Catheterization is indicated if there is echocardiographic evidence of increasing obstruction or impaired or inappropriate pump performance.

Guidelines for Recommending Surgical Therapy

1. There is no absolute left ventricular to aortic gradient at which surgery must be performed, regardless of other findings. However, many centers consider a gradient of 50–70 mm Hg sufficient for this recommendation.
2. An aortic valve area less than 0.7 cm/m^2 is generally considered critical and is sufficient to recommend surgery.
3. Abnormal or inappropriate pump performance or muscle function is a strong but, at present, not an absolute indication for surgery.
4. An oxygen supply/demand ratio less than 8–10 is a strong indication for surgery.

AORTIC REGURGITATION IN OLDER CHILDREN AND YOUNG ADULTS

Much of the data concerning evaluation, prognosis, and management of chronic aortic regurgitation is derived from adult populations. Criteria for and outcome of surgery are seldom analyzed in early childhood because relatively few children are believed to require this therapy. In older children and young adults there is less distinction between criteria to recommend invasive study and those needed to recommend surgery; therefore, it is best to consider only general principles regarding findings and prognosis. Three factors are most often related to outcome: *(a)* the presence or absence of symptoms; *(b)* pump performance and/or muscle function; and *(c)* the presence or absence of muscle ischemia. It is generally agreed that asymptomatic patients with normal pump performance and muscle function have a favorable prognosis.[31,32] To a large extent, this may be independent of heart size or degree of regurgitation as estimated by aortic root angiography.[31] In such a patient, the subsequent appearance of either symptoms (dyspnea on exertion, angina pectoris, syncope) or evidence for pump or muscle dysfunction is considered sufficient criteria to recommend surgery[31-33]; the surgical outcome and long term results appear acceptable.[31,33] Surgical results in the presence of both symptoms and pump or muscle dysfunction are generally poor.[31,33]

Because it is relatively independent of preload, left ventricular end–systolic volume has been proposed as a convenient measure of muscle function; it is related to postoperative left ventricular performance, and it is superior to preoperative determination of pump performance (ejection fraction)[34]. Similarly, the echocardiographic left ventricular end–systolic dimension correlates with surgical results in symptomatic patients.[35] Although the latter has been proposed as a criterion for surgery in asympatomatic patients (end-systolic volume greater than 55mm),[36] much caution must be exercised.[32,37] The role of exercise-induced left ventricular pump dysfunction in asymptomatic patients remains to be defined. When assessed by radionuclide techniques, it may precede or predict the occurance of symptoms or dysfunction at rest.[31,38]

Evidence of myocardial ischemia at rest by electrocardiography is uncommon in children with aortic regurgitation. However, it may be elicited with exercise in some patients; the magnitude of ST-segment abnormalities roughly parallels the degree of regurgitation as measured by left ventricular end–diastolic volume.[39] Little has been written concerning ischemia in chronic aortic regurgitation but evidence for this may be considered sufficient to recommend surgical therapy.[32]

As in the case of aortic stenosis, criteria for invasive study and surgery must be evaluated on an individual basis. The following guidelines are offered:

Guidelines for Recommending Invasive Study or Surgical Therapy

1. In the absence of symptoms or left ventricular pump or muscle dysfunction, there is no indication to recommend surgery solely to prevent the occurance of symptoms or dysfunction.
2. The presence of symptoms, left ventricular dysfunction or evidence of muscle ischemia is sufficient to procede with invasive investigation and surgery.
3. The role of exercise induced dysfunction or ischemia is unclear. The presence of these phenomena may suggest more frequent monitoring.

REFERENCES

1. Keith JD, Rowe RD, Vlad P. Heart Disease in Infancy and Childhood. MacMillan, New York, 1978, p 3.
2. Friedman WF, Pappelbaum SJ. Indications for hemodynamic evaluation and surgery in congenital aortic stenosis. Pediatr Clin North Am 1971;18:1207–1223.
3. Konno S, Imai Y, Nakajima M, Tatsuno K. A new method for prosthetic valve replacement in congenital aortic stenosis associated with hypoplasia of the aortic valve ring. J Thorac Cardiovasc Surg 1975;70:909–917.
4. DiDonato RM, Danielson GK, McGoon DC, Driscoll DJ, Julsrud PR, Edwards WD. Left ventricle–aortic conduits in pediatric patients. J Thorac Cardiovasc Surg 1984;88:82–91.
5. Sommerville J, Stone S, Ross O. Fate of patients with fixed subaortic stenosis after surgical removal. Br Heart J 1980;43:629.
6. Bargeron LM, Elliot LP, Soto B, Bream PR, Curry GC. Axial Cineangiography in congenital heart disease. Circulation 1977;56:1075–1093.
7. Friedman WF, Modlinger J, Morgan JR. Serial hemodynamic observations in asymptomatic children with valvar aortic stenosis. Circulation 1971;43:91–97.
8. El-Said G, Galiato FM Jr, Mullins CE, McNamara DG. Natural history of congenital aortic stenosis in childhood. Am J Cardiol 1972;30:6–12.
9. Cohen LS, Friedman WF, Braunwald E. Natural history of mild congenital aortic stenosis elucidated by serial hemodynamic studies. Am J Cardiol 1972;30:1–5.
10. Hurwitz RA. Valvar aortic stenosis in childhood: clinical and hemodynamic history. J Pediatr 1973;82:228–233.
11. Braunwald E, Goldblatt A, Aygen MM, Rockoff SD, Morrow AG. Congenital aortic stenosis. I. Clinical and hemodynamic findings in 100 patients. II. Surgical treatment and results of operation. Circulation 1963;27:426–462.
12. Hossack KF, Neutze JM, Lowe JR, Barratt-Boyes BG. Congenital valvar aortic stenosis. Natural history and assessment for operation. Br Heart J 1980;43:561–573.
13. Donner R, Carabello B, Black I, Spann JF. Left ventricular wall stress in compensated aortic stenosis in children. Am J Cardiol 1983;51:946–951.
14. Grossman W, Braunwald E, Mann T, McLauren LP, Green LH. Contractile state of the left ventricle in man as evaluated from end-systolic pressure–volume relations. Circulation 1977;56:845–852.
15. Mehmel HC, Stockins B, Ruffmann K, von Olshausen K, Schuler G, Kubler W. The linearity of the end-systolic pressure–volume relationship in man and its sensitivity for assessment of left ventricular function. Circulation 1981;63:1216–1222.
16. Colan SD, Borow KM, Neumann A. Left ventricular end–systolic wall stress-velocity of fiber shortening relation: a load-independent index of myocardial contractility. J Am Coll Cardiol 1984;4:715–724.
17. Kennedy JW, Doces J, Stewart DK. Left ventricular function before and following aortic valve replacement. Circulation 1977;56:944–950.
18. Hoffman JIE. Determinants and prediction of transmural myocardial perfusion. Circulation 1978;58:381–391.
19. Buckberg GD, Fixler DE, Archie JP, Hoffman JIE: Experimental subendocardial ischemia in dogs with normal coronary arteries. Circ Res 1972;30:67.
20. Brazier J, Cooper N, Buckberg G. The adequacy of subendocardial oxygen delivery. The interaction of determinants of flow, arterial oxygen content and myocardial oxygen need. Circulation 1974;49:968–977.

21. Lewis AB, Heymann MA, Stanger P, Hoffman JIE, Rudolph AM. Evaluation of subendocardial ischemia in valvar aortic stenosis in children. Circulation 1974;49:978–984.
22. Hugenholtz PG, Lees MM, Nadas AS. The scalar electrocardiogram, vectorcardiogram, and exercise electrocardiogram in the assessment of congenital aortic stenosis. Circulation 1962;26:79–91.
23. Whitmer JT, James FW, Kaplan S, Schwartz DC, Knight MJS. Exercise testing in children before and after surgical treatment of aortic stenosis. Circulation 1981;63:254–263.
24. Halloran KH. The telemetered exercise electrocardiogram in congenital aortic stenosis. Pediatr 1971;47:31–39.
25. Chandramouli B, Ehmke DA, Lauer RM. Exercise-induced electrocardiographic changes in children with congenital aortic stenosis. J Pediatr 1975;87:725–730.
26. Blackwood RA, Bloom KR, Williams CM. Aortic stenosis in children. Experience with echocardiographic prediction of severity. Circulation 1978;57:263–268.
27. Bass JL, Einzig S, Hong CY, Moller JH. Echocardiographic screening to assess the severity of congenital aortic valve stenosis in children. Am J Cardiol 1979;44:82–87.
28. Donner RM, Black I, Spann JF, Carabello BA. Improved prediction of peak left ventricular pressure by echocardiography in children with aortic stenosis. J Am Coll Cardiol 1984;3:349–355.
29. Hatle L, Angelsen BA, Tromsdal A. Non-invasive assessment of aortic stenosis by Doppler ultrasound. Br Heart J 1980;43:284–292.
30. Young JB, Quinones MA, Waggoner AD, Miller RR. Diagnosis and quantification of aortic stenosis with pulsed Doppler echocardiography. Am J Cardiol 1980;45:987–994.
31. Bonow RO, Rosing DR, McIntosh CL, Jones M, Maron BJ, Lan G, Lakatos E, Bacharach SL, Green MV, Epstein SE. The natural history of asymptomatic patients with aortic regurgitation and normal left ventricular function. Circulation 1983;68:509–517.
32. O'Rourke RA, Crawford MH. Timing of valve replacement in patients with chronic aortic regurgitation (editorial). Circulation 1980;61:493–495.
33. Clark DG, McAnulty JH, Rahimtoola SH. Valve replacement in aortic insufficiency with left ventricular dysfunction. Circulation 1980;61:411–420.
34. Borrow KM, Green LH, Mann T, Sloss LJ, Braunwald E, Collins JJ Jr, Cohn L, Grossman W. End-systolic volume as a predictor of postoperative left ventricular performance in volume overload from valvular regurgitation. Am J Med 1980;68:655–663.
35. Henry WL, Bonow RO, Borer JS, Ware JH, Kent KM, Redwood DR, McIntosh CL, Morrow AG, Epstein SE. Observations on the optimum time for operative intervention for aortic regurgitation. I. Evaluation of the results of aortic valve replacement in symptomatic patients. Circulation 1980;61:471–483.
36. Henry WL, Bonow RO, Rosing DR, Epstein SE. Observations on the optimum time for operative intervention for aortic regurgitation. II. Serial echocardiographic evaluation of asymptomatic patients. Circulation 1980;61:484–492.
37. Fioretti P, Roelandt J, Bos RJ, Meltzer RS, van Hoogenhuijze D, Serruys PW, Nauta J, Hugenholtz PG. Echocardiography in chronic aortic insufficiency. Is valve replacement too late when left ventricular end–systolic dimension reaches 55 mm? Circulation 1983;67:216–220.
38. Borer JS, Bacharach SL, Green MV, Kent KM, Henry WL, Rosing DR, Seides SF, Johnston GS, Epstein SE. Exercise-induced left ventricular dysfunction in symptomatic and asymptomatic patients with aortic regurgitation: assessment with radionuclide cineangiography. Am J Cardiol 1978;42:351–357.
39. Goforth D, James FW, Kaplan S, Donner R, Mays W. Maximal exercise in children with aortic regurgitation: an adjunct to noninvasive assessment of disease severity. Am Heart J 1984;108:1306–1311.

CHAPTER 3

Critical Aortic Stenosis in Infancy

Jaraslav Stark, MD, FRCS,
Kim F. Duncan, MD, MS, FRCSC,
I. Sullivan, B Med Sci, MB, FRACP,
Peter J. Robinson, MB, FRACP,
P. Horvath, MD, and Marc R. de Leval, MD

Patients with critical aortic stenosis often present in the neonatal period. Many are critically ill on admission and emergency or urgent surgery offers the only chance of survival. Like in other critically ill neonates, several factors influence survival:

1. Preoperative condition
2. Severity of the lesion
3. Associated cardiac defects

Some of our patients were admitted with severe congestive heart failure, and had been intubated and ventilated since admission to the referring hospital. Others presented with incipient or fully developed renal failure that required preoperative peritoneal dialysis.

To improve the preoperative condition, or at least to avoid further deterioration, we have adopted the following protocol in recent years:

1. If the patient is in severe heart failure with low cardiac output, prostaglandin infusion is started to keep the ductus arteriosus opened or to try to reopen it.[1]
2. *Diuretics* are given if required and catecholamine infusion, usually dopamine, is started.
3. The patient is intubated, ventilated, and usually paralyzed.

33

4. If severe oliguria or anuria is present, early peritoneal dialysis is considered.
5. Diagnosis is established by careful clinical examination, evaluation of chest x-ray, electrocardiogram, cross-sectional echocardiography, and Doppler ultrasound studies.[2] Thickened, usually poorly mobile valve can be visualized, and additional cardiac lesions excluded. Left ventricular function is also assessed. Measurement of a gradient at cardiac catheterization is known to be unreliable because of the low cardiac output and poor left ventricular function. Manipulation of the catheter and angiocardiography may precipitate ventricular fibrilation and the contrast medium with a high solute load may be detrimental to the kidneys, which may already be in incipient renal failure.
6. Operation is performed urgently, allowing a few hours for the measures mentioned above to improve the child's condition. If there is a rapid and steady improvement, delaying the operation for 12–24 hours may be advantageous. When improvement is not observed, emergency operation is recommended.

OPERATION

Our current operative technique of choice is transventricular valvotomy (TVV) through the left anterolateral thoracotomy. In the past we have used hypothermic cardiopulmonary bypass (CPB), and more recently, valvotomy under normothermic inflow occlusion (IO).[3] Our reason for changing from CPB to IO was the simplicity of the operation and, in our particular circumstances where only one operating room is available, it was easier to organize nonbypass rather than bypass surgery. Death on the table occurred in only one 7-day-old baby, who was operated on under IO. Severe endocardial fibroelastosis was found at autopsy. This compares well with four patients dying during operation during cardiopulmonary bypass.

In 1983 we were encouraged by the reports of Binet et al[4] and started to use transventricular valvotomy, which is currently our technique of choice. This technique was originally reported by Trinkle et al in 1975.[5] We use an anterolateral thoracotomy through intercostal space 5–6. The chest is entered at the level of the apex impulse. The pericardium is opened in front of the phrenic nerve and left thymic lobe is mobilized and resected. One-half percent of lignocaine is injected into the pericardial cavity. A purse string suture of 4-0 prolene is placed at the apex, care being taken to avoid the left anterior descending and any other major branches of the coronary arteries. Through a stab incision, Hegar dilators are passed through the valve in increasing sizes, starting with No. 3. The passage of the Hegar is guided by the index finger placed over the root of the aorta. We use increasing sizes until either the gradient is abolished or a Hegar one size smaller than the aortic root measured on echocardiography is passed. The purse string is then tied, pericardium loosely closed and chest closed with a drain.

RESULTS

Between September 1983 and October 1984, we operated on 12 infants, aged 1 day to 49 days (mean, 21.2 days). There were no intraoperative deaths but three patients died later.

One 16-day-old infant died of empyema, necrotising enterocolitis, and septicemia 2 weeks after the operation. Another baby, age 28 days, had undergone valvotomy under IO earlier. A TVV was performed as a reoperation. Left ventricular function did not improve after valvotomy, and a residual gradient of 35 mm Hg persisted. Although it was felt that aortic annulus was too small, another valvotomy, this time while the patient was on cardiopulmonary bypass, was attempted 2 weeks later, but the patient died. Autopsy showed dysplastic mitral valve and endocardial fibroelastosis. The third death occurred in a 12-day-old baby whose gradient actually increased from 15 to 30 mm Hg after valvotomy. After initial improvement, however, his left ventricular function deteriorated. He required intermittent positive pressure ventilation and died 6 weeks after operation.

Comparison of aortic valvotomy done under CPB, IO, and TVV is shown on the Table 3.1. The three series are not strictly comparable, as the three techniques were used chronologically. There was no statistically significant difference between hospital mortality in the three groups. It is perhaps interesting to note that no intraoperative death occurred using TVV and only one in the IO group, compared with four in the CPB group. However, we believe that this is related more to the improvement in pre- and intraoperative care rather than to the actual technique of the operation.

Recently Messina et al[6] reported excellent results with 10 survivors of 11 neonatal valvotomies performed while using cardiopulmonary bypass. The

TABLE 3.1 Critical Aortic Stenosis in Infants, 1971–1984

Operation	Bypass	Inflow Occlusion	Transventricular
Number	20	11	10
Age (days)[a]	64	31	21
Died	7 (35%)	3 (27%)	2 (20%)
Follow-up (months)[a]	106	36	6

[a]Mean.

only death occurred in an infant with narrowed aortic annulus, small left ventricle, and associated coarctation of the aorta and mitral stenosis. Severe associated anomalies including endocardial fibroelastosis and atrioventricular valve malformations were present in all three groups in our series. Similar findings were reported by others.[7] For this reason, we believe that the mortality for this condition will remain elevated.

REFERENCES

1. Leoni F, Huhta JC, Douglas J, Mackay R, de Leval MR, Macartney FJ, Stark J. Effect of prostaglandin on early surgical mortality in obstructive lesions of the systemic circulation. Br Heart J 1984;52:654–659.
2. Stark J, Smallhorn J, Huhta J, de Leval M, Macartney FJ, Rees PG, Taylor JFN. Surgery for congenital heart defects diagnosed with cross-sectional echocardiography. Circulation 1983;68:(suppl 2):II-129–138.
3. Sink JD, Smallhorn JF, Macartney FJ, Taylor JFN, Stark J, de Leval M. Management of critical aortic stenosis in infancy. J Thorac Cardiovasc Surg 1984;87:82–86.
4. Losay J, Planche CL, Binet JP, Hvass U, Belhaj M, Bruniaux J. Valvular aortic stenosis in infancy. Palliative surgery. Thorac Cardiovasc Surg 1982;30:96–97.
5. Tinkle JK, Norton JB, Richardson JD, Grover FL, Noonan JA. Closed aortic valvotomy and simultaneous correction of associated anomalies in infants. J Thorac Cardiovasc Surg 1975;69:758–762.
6. Messina LM, Turley K, Stanger P, Hoffman JIE, Ebert PA. Successful aortic valvotomy for severe congenital valvular aortic stenosis in the newborn infant. J Thorac Cardiovasc Surg 1984;88:92–96.
7. Lakier JB, Lewis AB, Heymann MA, Stanger P, Hoffman JIE, Rudolph AM. Isolated aortic stenosis in the neonate. Natural history and hemodynamic considerations. Circulation 1974;50:801–808.

CHAPTER 4

Aortic Valvotomy for Critical Aortic Stenosis in Neonates

John W. Brown, MD, Robert J. Robison, MD, Boyd Marts, and Harold King, MD

Congenital aortic stenosis represents 1%–15% of congenital cardiac malformations requiring surgical treatment.[1] Patients with critical aortic stenosis in the neonatal period make up less than 10% of this group, and usually present with intractable congestive heart failure and a severe low cardiac output.[2] The goal of surgery for critical aortic stenosis in the neonate is to acutely relieve the left ventricular outflow obstruction and interrupt the rapidly fatal course. More definitive procedures on the aortic valve are reserved for older, larger patients with less valvular dysplasia.

There have been two surgical approaches to aortic valvotomy in neonates, open and closed. Each approach has certain advantages and vocal advocates. The purpose of this report is to review our surgical experience with both open and closed aortic valvotomy in this critically ill neonatal group.

MATERIALS AND METHODS

Aortic valvotomy was performed in 30 neonates with critical aortic stenosis from August 1971 to August 1986. There were 25 males and 5 females, with a mean age of 20 days and mean weight of 3.7 kg. All patients presented with severe congestive heart failure and other clinical manifestations of a low cardiac output. Urgent cardiac catheterization was performed in 28 of 30 patients and demonstrated severe left ventricular (LV) outflow obstruction in each patient. Two patients underwent echocardiography as their only preoperative diagnostic procedure. In 9 of 28 (32%) patients catheterized, the

37

stenotic aortic valve could be crossed permitting measurement of transvalvular gradients; the gradients ranged from 15 to 65 mm Hg. Associated cardiac anomalies were demonstrated in 97% and are listed in Table 4.1. A small left ventricle was present in 17 (47%), while the remaining 16 patients had normal, nearly normal, or dilated left ventricles. Since 1980, neonates suspected of having critical aortic stenosis were started on prostaglandin-E_1 to maintain ductal patency.

Twenty of the 30 infants required emergent operation because of hemodynamic instability (20 patients), acidosis (16 patients), or preoperative cardiac arrest (8 patients). Twenty-five of the 30 patients were approached through a median sternotomy, and five were approached through a left thoracotomy. Fifteen patients (50%) underwent a closed transventricular aortic valvotomy, 10 via a sternotomy, and 5 via left thoracotomy. In closed valvotomy patients, a pledgeted mattress suture of 4-0 polypropylene was placed at the left ventricular apex. A small stab wound was made in the apex and a series of Hegar dilators, starting with the 3-mm and ending with the 7-mm dialator, were guided up through the aortic valve with finger palpation of the aortic root (Fig. 4.1). In five of the 15 closed valvotomy patients, the valvotomy was performed using a transventricular 6–7-mm × 2-cm ballooned Gruntzig catheter, placed through the apex and guided through the aortic valve by finger palpation. Details of Gruntzig catheter technique have been previously described (Fig. 4.2).[1,3] Four of the five Gruntzig valvotomies were performed via a left thoracotomy and in two, an associated severe coarctation was repaired by using a subclavian flap. Seven of the 15 patients undergoing closed aortic valvotomy performed via sternotomy developed ventricular fibrillation during elevation of the cardiac apex and required

TABLE 4.1 Associated Cardiac Anomalies

Abnormality	Number	Percent
PDA	18	60
Small left ventricle	14	47
Endocardial fibroelastosis	8	27
Coarctation	7	23
Hypoplastic arch	6	20
ASD	3	10
Pulmonary stenosis	2	7
VSD	1	3
Mitral stenosis	1	3
Mitral insufficiency	1	3

Abbreviations: PDA = Patent ductus arteriosus; ASD = Atrial septal defect; VSD = Ventricular septal defect.

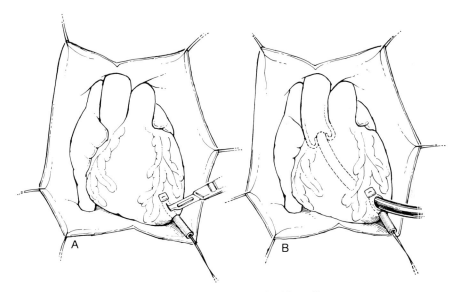

FIGURE 4.1 Technique of closed aortic valvotomy using blunt dilators.

placement on standby cardiopulmonary bypass for resuscitation. The other eight patients remained stable through the closed valvotomy. None of the five patients undergoing closed valvotomies done via a left thoracotomy fibrillated and manipulation of the heart was minimized with this approach.

Fifteen neonates underwent open transaortic valvotomy during standard cardiopulmonary bypass via a median sternotomy. The severely dysplastic aortic valves were opened with a scapel and/or spread with a clamp. The aorta was closed with a single row of fine running polyproylene. Hypothermia and/or cardioplegia were not used routinely, and the ischemic period was usually less than 10 minutes.

Hospital survivors were followed-up at regular intervals, and eight underwent postoperative catheterization at a mean period of 36 months after operation. No subsequent surgical procedures have thus far been required.

RESULTS

Eighteen of the 30 (60%) neonates operated on died during initial hospitalization. Six died in the operating room, five died within 24 hours of operation, two died between 1 and 7 days, and five died between 7 and 21 days after operation. The mean age of the survivors was 27 days, and 18 days in

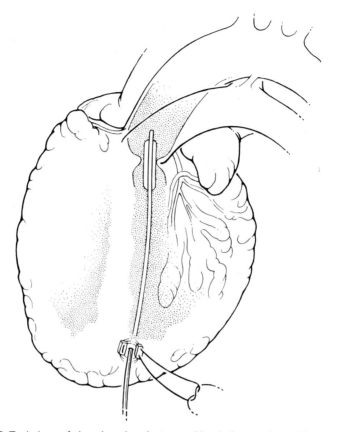

FIGURE 4.2 Technique of closed aortic valvotomy with a balloon catheter dilator.

nonsurvivors. Twelve of 14 (86%) of patients with small left ventricles died while 10 of 16 (63%) patients with normal or dilated LVs survived. Seven of eight patients operated on prior to 1978 by open aortic valvotomy died, which prompted us to adopt a closed approach in most subsequent cases.

The cause of early death was persistent postoperative low cardiac output in 13, sudden and unexplained in 4, and as a result of preoperative renal failure in 1.

The 12 survivors improved dramatically after surgery and were subsequently discharged from the hospital. They have been followed-up from 1 to 68 months. One patient expired at 9 months of presumed pneumonia. The other 11 patients have done well; two required cardiac medications. Cardiac catheterization has been performed in 10 patients. This revealed transvalvular gradients, ranging from 12 to 44 mm Hg, and mild aortic insufficiency was seen in two patients.

Patient survival was assessed with regards to the presence of severe associated cardiac anomalies, left ventricular size, time period of surgery, and technique of surgery (Table 4.2). Mortality during operation was higher in patients with severe associated cardiac defects, in particular those with small left ventricles.

DISCUSSION

The treatment of congenital aortic stenosis in neonates is largely palliative. The goal of early surgery is to relieve the severe heart failure by reducing the left ventricular outflow obstruction. At an older age, further procedures will likely be needed when more definitive surgical repair can be accomplished. Those patients who require surgery within the first few weeks of life are a particularly high risk group.

The results of surgery for aortic stenosis in neonates is compiled in Table 4.3.[1,2,4-13] Surgical mortality is high, ranging up to 75%. There are three factors that lead to this appreciable morbidity. First, the degree of left ventricular outflow tract obstruction is usually severe, setting a clinical stage of severe congestive heart failure and low cardiac output. The surgeon is often

TABLE 4.2 Mortality Rates and Various Clinical Features

Clinical Features	Mortality Rate
Severe associated cardiac anomalies	
Present	80% (16/20)
Not present	20% (2/10)
	$P < 0.01$[a]
Small left ventricle	
Present	86% (12/14)
Not present	38% (6/16)
	$P < 0.02$[a]
Operative period	
Prior to 1978	88% (7/ 8)
After 1978	50% (11/22)
	NS[b]
Operative technique	
Open	67% (10/15)
Closed	53% (8/15)
	NS[b]

[a]As determined by χ-square analysis.
[b]NS = not significant.

TABLE 4.3 Results of Aortic Valvotomy in Neonates

Author	Institution	Year Published	No. of Patients	Age	Technique	Mortality (%)
Lakier et al[4]	U.C. SF	1974	10	<1 mo	open	80
Keane et al[2]	Boston Childrens	1975	28	<6 mo	open IO[a]	29
Chiariello et al[1]	Buffalo	1976	4	<2 mo	open	75
Trinkle et al[5]	San Antonio	1978	4	<3 mo	closed	0
Kugler et al[6]	T.H.I.	1979	21	<2 mo	open	52
Edmunds et al[7]	Philadelphia	1980	14	<1 mo	open	50
Sandor et al[8]	Toronto	1980	25	<6 mo	open	52
Sade et al[9]	S. Carolina	1981	7	<3 mo	open IO	43
Armstead et al[10]	Brompton Eng.	1982	8	<1 mo	open	62
Mocellin et al[11]	Munich FRG	1983	30	<2 mo	open in 22	40
Messina et al[12]	San Francisco	1984	11	<1 mo	open (28°)	9
Sink et al[13]	GOS-London	1984	6	<2 mo	open IO	12
Brown et al	Ind. Univ.	1986	30	<2 mo	open	67
					closed	53

[a]Open IO = Open valvotomy with inflow occlusion.

faced with an acidotic, oliguric patient in severe respiratory distress or requiring a ventilator. Second, left ventricular hypoplasia may be present. Moller et al[14] have described two forms of aortic stenosis in the first year of life. In one form the left ventricle and aorta are of normal size, and the obstruction is usually valvular; in the other form the left ventricle and aorta are hypoplastic and peripheral perfusion is through reversed ductus arteriosus flow. As expected, the surgical results in this latter group are poor, only 14% of our patients with small left ventricles survived. Third, other significant cardiac defects are often present. We noted associated defects in 97% of our patients; in 67% of the patients these were considered severe and the operative mortality rate was higher in the group.

Aortic valvotomy usually relieves the left ventricular outflow obstruction and allows for patient survival and growth. There are two techniques of aortic valvotomy, the open and closed methods. The open aortic valvotomy usually involves cardiopulmonary bypass (or use of inflow occlusion), aortotomy, and direct valvotomy. The majority of aortic valvotomies reported have been performed using the open technique during bypass. Advocates of this method stress the advantage of precise valvotomy under controllable conditions.[6-13] Prior to 1978, we had only 1 out of 8 (13%) patients survive aortic valvotomy using the open method in conjunction with bypass. This prompted us to consider closed aortic valvotomy.

Closed aortic valvotomy was first described in 1953 by Larzelere and Baily[15] for use in adults. Marquis and Fagan[16] later used this technique in six teenagers and young adults. The method was revised again by Trinkle et al,[17] who in 1974 reported its use in four neonates. Blunt dilatation was used in three patients while a valvulotome was used in one. A follow-up report in 1978 revealed that three of the four (75%) patients were still alive.[5] The one patient in whom the valvulotome was used developed significant aortic insufficiency and died while undergoing aortic valve replacement. The three patients in whom blunt dilatation was used were reported to be thriving. Cardiac catheterization was performed in two patients demonstrating transvalvular gradients of 5–25 mm Hg without significant aortic insufficiency. We have had similar good clinical experience with closed aortic valvotomy, with seven of 15 (47%) long-term survivors from this critically ill group of patients. Palliation has been effective following closed valvotomy, with all seven patients thriving, five of whom do not require any cardiac medications. We, too, have favored blunt dilatation using either metal or balloon dilators. Blunt dilatation seems effective in acutely relieving the valvular stenosis without producing significant insufficiency and the results appear to be long lasting. Figure 4.3 shows the postmortum view of the aortic valve after transventricular balloon catheter dilitation of an infant who died 2 weeks after operation of pre-existant renal failure. Splits occurred precisely

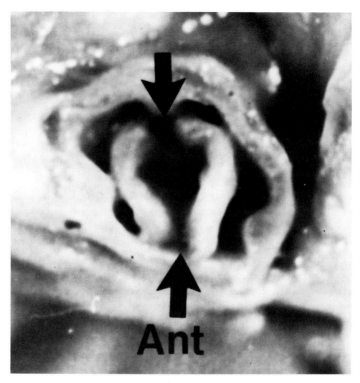

FIGURE 4.3 Necropsy close-up view of a neonates aortic valve following transventricular balloon angioplasty. *Arrows* show separation of cusps at commissures.

at the commissures. In addition coarctation repair can be performed at the same operation if closed valvotomy is done via a left thoracotomy which is our currently favored approach.

In summary we have described our experience with aortic valvotomy for critical aortic stenosis in the first 2 months of life. This is a high-risk group because the patients are frequently critically ill, and there is a significant association of small left ventricles and other severe cardiac defects. In our early experience, we had an extremely high mortality with open valvotomy, which prompted us to attempt closed valvotomy. We have been encouraged by this experience and currently favor closed aortic valvotomy via a left thoracotomy for critical aortic stenosis in neonates for these reasons: *(a)* cardiopulmonary bypass and hypothermic cardiac arrest are not required in these small, severely ill neonates; *(b)* effective and long-lasting relief of stenosis is obtained without producing significant insufficiency; and *(c)* the approach can be performed through a lateral thoracotomy, allowing for concomitant coarctation repair if needed.

REFERENCES

1. Chiariello L, Agosti J, Vlad P, Subramanian S. Congenital aortic stenosis: experience with 43 patients. J Thorac Cardiovasc Surg 1976;72:182.
2. Keane JR, Bernhard WF, Nadas AS. Aortic stenosis in infancy. Circulation 1975;52:1138.
3. Brown JW, Robison RJ, Waller BF. Transventricular balloon catheter aortic valvotomy in neonates. Ann Thorac Surg 1985;39:376.
4. Lakier JB, Lewis AB, Heymann MA, et al. Isolated aortic stenosis in the neonate. Circulation 1974;50:801.
5. Trinkle JK, Grover FL, Arom KV. Closed aortic valvotomy in infants. J Thorac Cardiovasc Surg 1978;76:198.
6. Kugler JD, Campbell E, Vargo TA, et al. Results of aortic valvotomy in infants with isolated aortic valvular stenosis. J Thorac Cardiovasc Surg 1979;78:553.
7. Edmunds LH, Wagner HR, Heymann MA. Aortic valvulotomy in neonates. Circulation 1980;61:421.
8. Sandor GGS, Olley PM, Trusler GA, et al. Long-term follow-up of patients after aortic valvotomy for congenital valvular aortic stenosis in children: a clinical and actuarial follow-up. J Thorac Cardiovasc Surg 1980;80:171.
9. Sade RM, Crawford FA, Hohn AR. Inflow occlusion for semilunar valve stenosis. Ann Thorac Surg 1982;33:570.
10. Armistead SH, Lane I, McFarland R, Paneth M. The surgery of aortic valve disease in neonates, infants, and children. J Cardiovasc Surg 1982;23:140.
11. Mocellin R, Simon SB, Comazzi M, Sebening F, Buhlmeyer K. Reduced left ventricular size and endocardial fibroelastosis as correlates of mortality in newborns and young infants with severe aortic valve stenosis. Pediatr Cardiol 1983;4:265.
12. Messina LM, Turley K, Stanger P, Hoffman JIE, Ebert PA. Successful aortic valvotomy for severe congenital valvular aortic stenosis in the newborn infant. J Thorac Cardiovasc Surg 1984;88:92.
13. Sink JD, Smallhorn JF, Macartney FJ, Taylor JFN, Stark J, de Leval MR. Management of critical aortic stenosis in infancy. J Thorac Cardiovasc Surg 1984;87:82.
14. Moller JH, Nakik A, Eliot RS, Edwards JE. Symptomatic congenital aortic stenosis in the first year of life. J Pediatr 1966;69:729.
15. Larzelere HB, Paily CP. Aortic commissurotomy. J Thorac Cardiovasc Surg 1953;26:31.
16. Marquis RM, Logan A. Congenital aortic stenosis and its surgical treatment. Br Heart J 1955;17:373.
17. Trinkle JK, Norton JB, Richardson JD, et al. Closed aortic valvotomy and simultaneous correction of associated anomalies in infants. J Thorac Cardiovasc Surg 1975;69:758.

CHAPTER 5

Aortoventriculoplasty in Small Aortic Annulus

E. Rainer de Vivie, MD,
Houshang Rastan, MD, Johannes Vogt, MD,
Gerhard Rupprath, MD, and Josef Koncz, MD

SUMMARY

The aortoventriculoplasty (AVP) is an established operative procedure for enlargement of different types of congenital aortic stenosis, including the small aortic annulus. Between 1974 and 1985, 72 patients underwent 75 AVPs. The early mortality was 9.3% (7/75). Of the last 55 patients, only two died (3.6%). There was one late death due to rhythm disturbances, resulting in a late mortality of 1.3%. Three patients underwent subsequent operation: one patient due to aortic aneurysm dissecans, one due to right ventricular outflow tract obstruction, and one due to out-grown prosthesis (Björk-Shiley 21). The mean preoperative gradient of 88 ± 27 mm Hg (50–160 mm Hg) over the left ventricular and flow tract was reduced by AVP to 12 ± 12 mm Hg. Most of the patients (65/72) had sinodial rhythm after AVP; three patients required pacemakers for a permanent aortoventricular block.

INTRODUCTION

Until a few years ago the treatment of a congenitally small aortic annulus posed a difficult problem for the surgeon.[1-8] Performing a commissurotomy of a valvular aortic stenosis with small aortic annulus achieved only a temporary hemodynamic improvement by decreasing the gradient between the left ventricle and aorta.[9-11] This operative procedure can, therefore, only be

46

regarded as palliative. Outflow tract stenoses of the left ventricle, either isolated in the subvalvular area or as so-called multilevel stenosis, are regarded as similarly problematic.[12-14] The long-term results of resection of the subvalvular stenotic segment are unsatisfactory, and the same is true for the myotomy and myectomy of Bigelow and Morrow for the treatment of hypertrophic obstructive cardiomyopathy (HOCM), especially the so-called tunnellike subaortic stenosis.[15-18] The development of new operative procedures for the enlargement of a small aortic annulus and/or various left ventricular outflow tract stenoses has led to a significant improvement in the surgical treatment of these complex congenital cardiac defects. Some of these procedures have reached the level of routine operations nowadays.[2,13,19-23]

This chapter presents a critical analysis of the clinical and long-term hemodynamic results (after recatheterization) of aortoventriculoplasty. The advantages and disadvantages of other surgical methods are discussed and compared with those of AVP.

HISTORY AND METHODS

After experimental trails, in 1974, Rastan and Koncz[20,21] performed an aortoventriculoplasty for the first time on a 12-year-old boy with a tunnel-shaped subaortic stenosis, which had already been operated on. The first publications followed in 1975.[15,24] Independent of this, Konno et al[19] described the same technique in 1975 for prosthetic valve replacement in a case of congenital aortic stenosis with hypoplastic aortic annulus.

Briefly, the surgical procedure is as follows: The aorta is opened lengthwise in the direction of the commissures between the right and left coronary ostia as far as the annulus. Then a transverse opening is made in the right ventricle below the pulmonary valve so that the two incisions join, thereby transecting the aortic annulus in the commissure. The cut is continued into the ventricular septum until the left ventricular outflow tract is sufficiently enlarged (Fig. 5.1). After resection of the aortic valve, the V-shaped cleft in the septum is widened with a triangular shaped prosthetic patch, which achieves enlargement of the aortic annulus at the same time. Implantation of the aortic valve and closure of the ascending aorta with a suitable vascular prosthesis follows. The right ventricular outflow tract is then reconstructed with a second triangular-shaped patch. The vascular prostheses are sealed with fibrin glue to avoid bleeding. The various types of left ventricular outflow tract stenoses are illustrated in Figure 5.2.

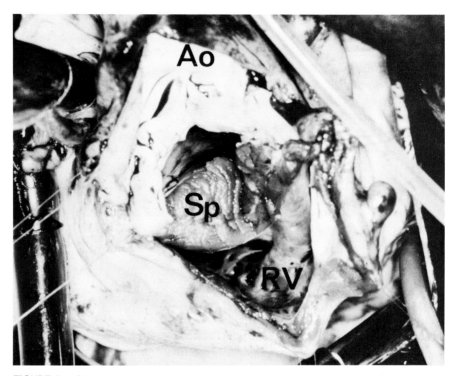

FIGURE 5.1 Operative situs after incision into the ventricular septum. The aortic annulus is enlarged to twice of its size. Abbreviations: Ao = aorta; Sp = septum; RV = right ventricle.

PATIENTS

Between 1974 and 1985 in the Clinic for Thoracic and Cardiovascular Surgery, 75 aortoventriculoplasties were performed in 72 patients; three reoperations were necessary. Most patients were in their midteens (average, 14.2 ± 0.7yrs); the youngest patient was 5 years and the oldest was 32 years old; there were 25 female and 47 male patients. The total number of the various aortic stenoses are important for a clear picture of the patient population: since 1961, 1220 patients were diagnosed in the Department of Pediatric Cardiology, University of Goettingen, of whom 547 have been operated on. In this surgical group 303 had valvular aortic stenoses, 59 had supravalvular aortic stenoses, and 185 had subvalvular aortic stenoses (Table 5.1). We divided our patient population into five groups on the basis of the preoperative angiographic diagnoses (Table 5.2).

Most patients had undergone one or more previous operations, AVP being the first surgery in only 11. The type and number of previous operations are listed in Table 5.3. Most of the patients received valves 25 – 27 mm

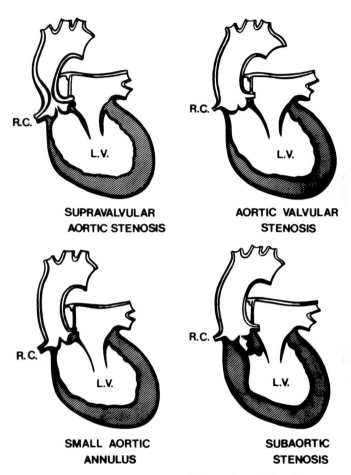

FIGURE 5.2 Different types of aortic stenosis. Abbreviations: RC = right coronary artery; LV = left ventricle.

TABLE 5.1 Congenital Aortic Stenosis

	Number of Patients
Cardiological diagnosis	1220
Total operations	547
Valvular AS[a]	303
Subvalvular AS	185
Supravalvular AS	59
Aortoventriculoplasty	75

[a]Aortic stenosis.

TABLE 5.2 Aortoventriculoplasty

Diagnosis	Patients	Mortality
Valvular aortic stenosis with narrow annulus	16	0
Diffuse SAS	26	4
Tunnellike 16		
(With Shone Complex 7)		
Multilevel stenosis	22	2
Outgrown prothesis	7	1
HOCM-Reop	4	0
TOTAL	75	7

Abbreviations: SAS = subaortic stenosis; HOCM = hypertrophic obstructive cardiomyopathy.

in diameter, the distribution of the prosthetic valve size compared to the age of the patients is shown in Figure 5.3.

MORTALITY

There were seven deaths after 75 operations, giving an early mortality of 9.3%. In the early phase (1974 to 1977), 5/20 patients died (25%); this high proportion was due to problems with operative technique and difficulties in establishing the indication (Table 5.4). Only two out of the last 55 patients

TABLE 5.3 Previous Operation Prior to Aortoventriculoplasty

	No. of Patients
Previous procedure	
Resection of SAS	21
Commissurotomy	20
Myotomy and/or myectomy	8
AVR	7
VSD – closure	4
Supravalvular	
Patchplasty	3
MVR	1
No previous procedure	11
Total	**75**
Aortoventriculoplasty used as	
First procedure	11
Second procedure	48
Third procedure	16
Total	**75**

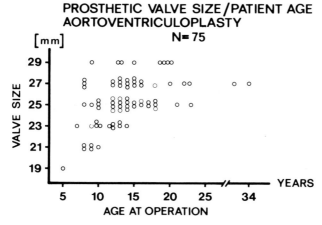

FIGURE 5.3 Size distribution of the prostheses implanted plotted to the age of the patients.

died, which represents a mortality of 3.6%. The causes of death were as follows; three patients died of myocardial failure, two of pulmonary insufficiency with pulmonary hypertonia, one of renal failure, and one myocardial infarction with an associated coronary anomaly. There was also one late death: One patient died due to a technical failure of the pacemaker 8 years after the initial operation; the cause of death was a total aortoventricular block after operation.

FOLLOW-UP EXAMINATIONS

All surviving patients were examined by using 2-dimensional echocardiography during follow-up cardiological examinations. In 39 patients, a complete catheterization in both the right and left sides of the heart was performed between 1 month and 3.5 years (average, 10.5 months) after operation. On average, the gradient in the patients was significantly reduced (from 88 ± 27

TABLE 5.4 Mortality from Aortoventriculoplasty

	No. of Patients/ Total Patients	%
Time period		
1974–1977	5/20	25
1977–1985	2/55	3.6
Early mortality	7/75	9.3
Late mortality	1/75	1.3

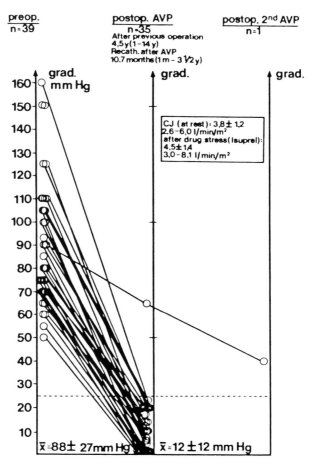

FIGURE 5.4 Preoperative and postoperative gradients between left ventricle and aorta after aortoventriculoplasty. Abbreviation: CI = cardiac index.

mm Hg to 12 ± 12 mm Hg) following AVP. Only one patient had a residual gradient of 65 mm Hg as a result of an outgrown Björk-Shiley prosthesis (21 mm) (Fig. 5.4); the prosthesis, implanted when the patient's age was 8 years, had to be exchanged for a 25-mm Björk-Shiley prosthesis 8 years after the original operation and after further dilatation of the annulus.

After drug stress testing (0.1 μg/kg isoproterenol) the gradients remained low. Left ventricular end diastolic pressure (LVEDP) levels remained in the normal range or could be reduced in 75% of the patients, while in 25% the postoperative LVEDP levels were unchanged or were pathological in comparison to the preoperative values. Among survivors, cardiac

TABLE 5.5 Incremental Risk Factors of Aortoventriculoplasty

	n	Medical Course	Mortality
Thrombembolic event	0		
Obstruction of RVOT (patch shrinking)	1	Reoperation	
Outgrown prosthesis (BS 21)	1	Reoperation	
Aeurysm dissecans	1	Reoperation	
Total AV block	3	Pacemaker	1 (late)
VSD	3	Qp/Qs — 1.2:1, 1.3:1 No reoperation	
Mild paravalvular leak	6	No reoperation	

Abbreviations: RVOT = right ventricular outflow tract; BS 21 = Björk-Shiley 21; AV = aortoventricular; VSD = ventricular septal defect.

index (CI) at rest averaged of 3.8 $\pm$ 1.2 L/min per m^2 (2.6–6.0 L/min per m^2) and rose approximately 18% after drug stress testing.

INCREMENTAL RISK FACTORS

Analysis of the long-term results of the patients, after an observation time of more than 10 years, allows for the following evaluation of AVP (Table 5.5):

1. No patient has had a thromboembolic event or valve dysfunction due to valve thrombosis.

2. The implanted vascular prosthesic material has obviously not undergone essential degenerative changes after 10 years. Only one patient had to be reoperated because of an increased gradient of 40 mm Hg between the right ventricle and the pulmonary artery; however this patient had questionable endocarditis during the first postoperative year. Shrinkage of the right ventricular outflow patch was seen on reoperation.

3. The aortoventriculoplasty had to be exchanged in only one patient, after 8 years, because of a Björk-Shiley prosthesis (21 mm) that had become too small.

4. A dissecting aneurysm of the ascending aorta occurred in one patient 6 months after AVP as the result of a suture dehiscence. Reoperation on this 18-year-old patient was successful.

5. A total aortoventricular block occurred after AVP in three patients, all of whom received transvenous pacemakers. Each of them had been operated on once or twice before, and the intracardiac anatomic conditions were complicated. One of these patients died 8 years after AVP, apparently as the result of a technical failure of the pacemaker. Most of the

patients (63/75) had sinusoidal rhythm after AVP, 13 developed complete right bundle branch block (RBBB), and another 15 developed RBBB and/or left anterior hemiblock.

When critically evaluating the above-mentioned points in order to estimate the risk factors, it must first be stressed that no thromboembolic complications occurred during our use of mechanical valve prostheses, even in children. In the follow-up studies of our AVP series we have encountered no serious bleeding complications, although all patients received anticoagulation therapy. In childhood, problems arise from the regulation of anticoagulation therapy and the higher risk of injuries with bleeding complications; therefore, some authors believe that anticoagulation therapy should not be undertaken in children. Previous studies have shown an increased platelet turnover in patients with mechanical heart valves, and therapy with platelet inhibitors has been recommended.[31] The complications already referred to that required reoperation are acceptable in the light of the total patient population and the congenital heart defects that were certainly complex in the majority of cases.

On catheterization, three other patients were discovered by angiography to have small ventricular septal defects (which were hemodynamically insignifcant), and mild aortic regurgitation due to the prosthetic valve was found in six more patients; there was no indication for reoperation on any of these cases.

The actuarial curve for survival in our patients since 1977 is the same as that for normal aortic valve replacement in children. The same is true for the event-free actuarial curve (Fig. 5.5). A 13-year-old boy with valvular and

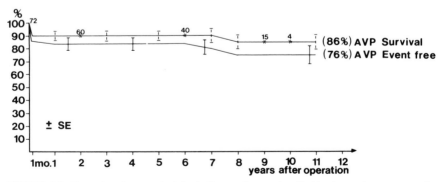

FIGURE 5.5 Plots showing survival, including patients who died in the early postoperative period *(upper curve)*. The lower curve shows freedom from reoperation among patients surviving the aortoventriculoplasty.

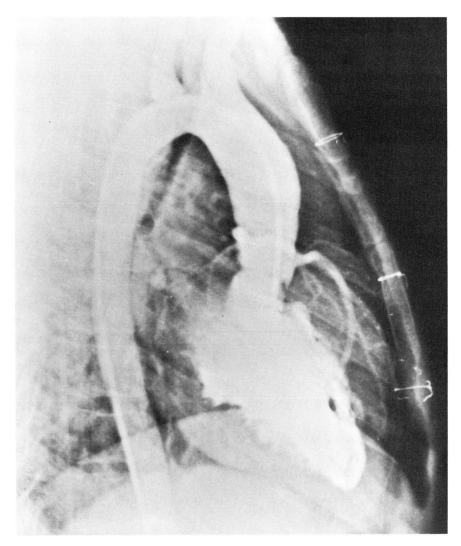

FIGURE 5.6 Preoperative left ventricular angiogram in lateral position. A 13-year-old boy with valvular and subvalvular aortic stenosis after commissurotomy in the first year of life.

subvalvular aortic stenosis demonstrates a typical case. The child had undergone commissurotomy in the first year of life. Figure 5.6 shows the preoperative angiogram 12 years after the first operation. After AVP the valvular and subvalvular stenosis could be enlarged, as illustrated in Figure 5.7.

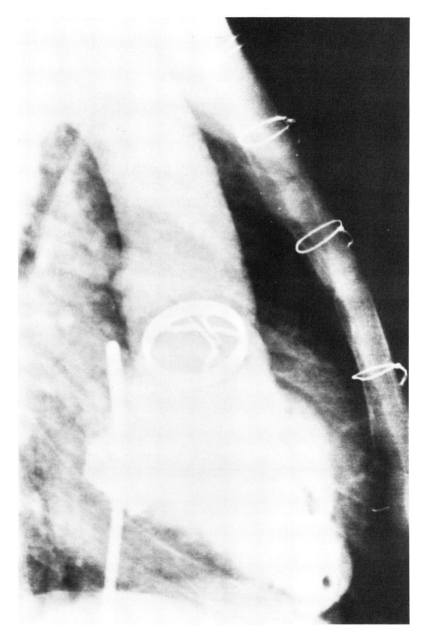

FIGURE 5.7 Postoperative left ventricular angiogram in lateral position after aortoventriculoplasty.

DISCUSSION

Aortoventriculoplasty for the enlargement of a small aortic annulus and left ventricular outflow tract stenosis has proved to be an operative method during an observation period of more than 10 years[24-27]; this surgical procedure has been successfully employed by several groups.[3,28] The risk of an iatrogenic aortoventricular block in cases with a normal course of the His bundle is seen as slight. An evaluation of the anatomic situation in patients who have undergone several previous operations is more difficult. The incision into the septum is analogous to Bigelow's incision[15,16] and is therefore regarded as without danger. Using this method, the small aortic annulus can be enlarged to twice its size compared with the so-called dorsal annuloplasty of Manouguian and Seybold-Epting, in which the incision is made through the noncoronary sinus into the anterior mitral valve of the small aortic annulus and is therefore limited.[23]

In the literature, excellent results are reported for other operative techniques for the enlargement of the left ventricular outflow tract.[2-4,7,22,29-31] Ross and Somerville[22,30] resected the small aortic annulus together with the whole aortic root and implanted a homograft. The advantage of this method lies in avoiding the use of prosthetic material, which makes it unnecessary to administer anticoagulants. The indication for this method is limited in cases of the elimination of long tunnel-shaped subaortic stenoses.

The apicoaortal conduit method used by Cooley and Norman[4] and Bernhard et al[2] involves a double cavity intervention.[2,4] The degeneration of the biological valve in the conduit and the two-directional hemodynamic and physiologic flow are critical disadvantages of this method. Most of the patients had sinusoidal rhythm after AVP, and three patients required implantation of a pacemaker for a permanent aortoventricular block. Our study, however, shows that the hemodynamic results obtained after AVP have been promising during a 10-year follow-up period. We believe AVP is indicated particularly in tunnel-type subaortic stenosis, severe multilevel stenosis, and small aortic ring in infancy.

CONCLUSION

It can be stated that aortoventriculoplasty is a surgical procedure for the enlargement of various stenoses of the left ventricular outflow tract, especially of small aortic annuli. Technically the method can be carried out easily and makes physiologic hemodynamics possible. Bioprostheses should be avoided in AVP, as early valve degeneration can be expected, making reoperation necessary. In cases of small aortic annulus in the first year of life, conservative surgical possibilities should take precedence as palliative measures. Aortoventriculoplasty in patients younger than age 5 years can only be recommended in exceptional cases.

REFERENCES

1. Bernhard WF, Keane JF, Fellow KE, Litwin SB, Gross RE. Progress and problems in the surgical management of congenital aortic stenosis. J Thorac Cardiovasc Surg 1973;66:404.
2. Bernhard WF, Poirier V, La Farge CG. Relief of congenital obstruction to left ventricular outflow with a ventricular aortic prosthesis. J Thorac Cardiovasc Surg 1975;69:223.
3. Blank RH, Pupello DF, Bessone LF, Harrison EE, Sbar SS. Method of managing the small aortic annulus during valve replacement. Ann Thorac Surg 1976;22:356.
4. Cooley DA, Norman JC. Apical left ventricular-abdominal aortic composite conduits for left ventricular outflow obstructions. Cardiovasc Dis Bull Tex Heart 1975;5:112.
5. Edwards JE. Pathology of left ventricular outflow tract obstruction. Circulation 1965;31:586.
6. Hossack KF, Neutze JM, Lowe JB, Barratt-Boyes BG. Congenital valvar aortic stenosis. Natural history and assessment for operation. Br Heart J 1980;43:561.
7. Jones EL, Craver JM, Morris DC, King SB III, Douglas JS Jr, Franch RH, Hatcher CR, Norgan EA. Hemodynamic and clinical evaluation of the Hancock xenograft bioprothesis for aortic valve replacement (with emphasis on management of the small aortic root). J Thorac Cardiovasc Surg 1978;75:300.
8. Krueger SK, French JW, Forker AD, Caudill CC, Popp RL. Echocardiography in discrete subaortic stenosis. Circulation 1979;59:506.
9. Keane JF, Fellows KE, La Farge CG, Nadas AS, Bernhard WF. The surgical management of discrete and diffuse supravalvular aortic stenosis. Circulation 1976;54:112.
10. Newfeld EA, Muster AJ, Paul MH, Idriss FS, Riker WL. Discrete subvalvular aortic stenosis in childhood. Study of 51 patients. Am J Cardiol 1976;38:53.
11. Vogt J, Rupprath G, de Vivie ER, Beuren AJ. Hemodynamic findings before and after aortoventriculoplasty. J Thorac Cardiovasc Surg 1981;29:381.
12. Maron BJ, Redwood DR, Roberts WC, Henry WL, Morrow AG, Epstein SE. Tunnel subaortic stenosis. Left ventricular outflow tract obstruction produced by fibromuscular tubular narrowing. Circulation 1976;54:404.
13. Nicks R, Cartmill T, Bernstein L. Hypoplasia of the aortic root. Thorax 1970;25:339.
14. Sommerville J, Stone S, Ross D. Fate of patients with fixed subaortic stenosis after surgical removal. Br Heart J 1980;43:629.
15. Bigelow WG, Trimble AS, Auger P, Marquis J, Wigle ED. The ventriculomyotomy operation for muscular Subaortic stenosis. J Thorac Cardiovasc Surg 1966;52:514.
16. Bigelow WG, Trimble AS, Wigle ED, Adelman AG, Felderhof CH. The treatment of muscular subaortic stenosis. J Thorac Cardiovasc Surg 1974;68:384.
17. Morrow AG, Brockenbrough EC. Surgical treatment of idiopathic hypertrophic subaortic stenosis; technique and hemodynamic results of subaortic ventriculomyotomy. Ann Surg 1961;154:181.
18. Morrow AG, Fogarty TJ, Hamah H, Braunwald E. Operative treatment in idiopathic hypertrophic subaortic stenosis: techniques and the results of preoperative and postoperative clinical and hemodynamic assessments. Circulation 1968;37:589.
19. Kono S, Imai Y, Iida Y, Nakajima M, Tetsuno KA. New method for prosthetic valve replacement in congenital aortic stenosis associated with hypoplasia of the aortic valve ring. J Thorac Cardiovasc Surg 1975;70:909.

20. Rastan H, Koncz J. Plastische Erweiterung der linken Ausfluβbahn. Eine neue Operations-methode. Thoraxchirur 1975;23:169.
21. Rastan H, Koncz J. Aortoventriculoplasty, a new technique for the treatment of left ventricular outflow tract obstructions. J Thorac Cardiovasc Surg 1976;71:920.
22. Ross D, Sommerville J. Total aortic valve and root replacement with aortic homograft and reimplantation of the coronary arteries for diffuse left ventricular outflow tract obstructions (abstr 313). First World Congress of Pediatric Cardiology, London, 1980.
23. Manouguian S, Seybold-Epting W. Patch enlargement of the aortic valve ring by extending the aortic incision into the anterior mitral leaflet. J Thorac Cardiovasc Surg 1979;78:402.
24. Björnstad PF, Rastan H, Keutel J, Beuren AJ, Koncz J. Aortoventriculoplasty for tunnel subaortic stenosis and other obstructions of left ventricular outflow tract. Circulation 1979;60:59.
25. de Vivie ER, Hellberg K, Heisig K, Rupprath G, Vogt J, Beuren AJ. Surgical treatment of various types of left ventricular outflow tract stenosis by aortoventriculoplasty—clinical results. J Thorac Cardiovasc Surg 1981;29:266.
26. de Vivie ER, Koncz, J, Rupprath G, Vogt J, Beuren AJ. Aortoventriculoplasty for different types of left ventricular outflow tract obstructions. J Cardiovasc Surg 1982;23:6.
27. Vogt J, Rupprath G, de Vivie ER, Koncz J, Beuren AJ. Aortoventriculoplasty (AVP) as an alternative second surgical procedure in the treatment of hypertrophic obstructive cardio-myopathie in childhood—hemidynamic and echocardiographic findings. Z Kardiol 1983;72:99.
28. Symbas PN, Ware RE, Hatcher CR, Temesy-Armos PN. An operation for relief of severe left ventricular outflow tract obstruction. J Thorac Cardiovasc Surg 1976;71:245.
29. Saggau W, Hatipoglu Ö, Kussäther E, Schmitz W, Zebe H. Die chirurgische Bahandlung supravalvulärer Aorten-stenosen mit hypoplastischer aszendierender Aorta durch einen apiko-aortalen Konduit. Herz 1981;6:185.
30. Sommerville J, Ross D. Homograft replacement of aortic root with reimplantation of coronary arteries. Br Heart J 1982;47:473.
31. Williams WG, Pollock JC, Geiss DM, Trusler GA, Fowler RS. Experience with aortic and mitral valve replacement in children. J Thorac Cardiovasc Surg 1981;81:326.

CHAPTER 6

Apicoaortic Conduits for Complex Left Ventricular Outflow Obstruction in Children

John W. Brown, MD, Donald A. Girod, MD, Roger A. Hurwitz, MD, and Randall L. Caldwell, MD

Congenital left ventricular outflow tract obstruction can usually be relieved by conventional surgical techniques with good short- and medium-term results, although late problems are not uncommon. Complex multilevel outflow obstruction presents a substantial surgical challenge that usually is not improved by standard single-level approaches. Insertion of a second outflow tract from the left ventricle in the form of an apicoaortic conduit has proven a valuable alternative in this complex group of children. This report summarizes the laboratory and clinical experience of the authors with apicoaortic conduits in children with emphasis on technique, hemodynamic results, and long-term follow-up.

The surgical indications, technique, clinical follow-up, and hemodynamic data in 24 children (aged 4 months to 19 years) who underwent insertion of an apicoaortic valve conduit by the author between December 1976, and June 1986, are reviewed. All children had complex forms of congenital left ventricular outflow obstructions. All were symptomatic, and 18 had 23 prior attempts at surgical relief of their obstruction. There were four early deaths in the series (16.6%) and three late deaths (12.5%). Four of the six deaths were in children who presented with profound cardiac decompensation, and three required emergency surgery. Three of the deaths were in children with complex congenital cardiac malformations in addition to their complex aortic stenosis. Twenty-one children survived the perioperative period and improved, and 17 have had one or more cardiac catheterizations from 1 to 7.5 years (mean 3.3 yr) after the initial operation. A demonstrated reduction or resolution of their resting left ventricular-to-aortic gradient from 91 ± 30 to 13 ± 8 mm Hg was demonstrated ($P < 0.001$). Two patients who have mechanical valves are taking anticoagulants, and no thromboembolic events have occurred. Four of the 19 survivors have undergone subsequent procedures from 1.5 months to 4.0 years postoperatively: two patients underwent conduit removal, two underwent aortoventriculoplasty, and two underwent conduit valve replacement. These data demonstrated that the apicoaortic conduit is effective in relieving complex left ventricular outflow obstruction and improvement in left ventricular performance with acceptable long-term results. Improvements in conduit valve durability will greatly improve the late results with this technique.

METHODS

Between December 1976 and June 1986, 24 children underwent insertion of an apicoaortic conduit for complex forms of left ventricular outflow obstruction. The patients ranged in age from 4 months to 19 years (mean, 10 years) and in weight from 2.3 to 70 kg; there were 13 males and 11 females. All children were symptomatic (syncope in one, angina in seven, and congestive heart failure in 24); four were admitted with pulmonary edema and were gravely ill; all had complex forms of aortic stenosis not amenable to repair by conventional methods (such as valve repair or replacement, resection of discrete subvalvular ring or simple prosthetic patch enlargement). The location of the major obstruction is shown in Table 6.1. Nineteen of the 24 children had undergone a total of 23 previous operations to relieve left ventricular outflow obstruction, as shown in Table 6.2. The mean preoperative gradient was 91 ± 30 mm Hg. The gradient exceeded 100 mm Hg in seven patients. Thirty-three associated lesions were present in the group, and are ennumerated in Table 6.3.

The Prosthesis

Twenty-two of the 24 conduits were commercially available woven Dacron grafts containing a gluteraldehyde sterilized porcine valve (Hancock-John-

TABLE 6.1 Site of Left Ventricular Outflow Obstruction in Twenty-Four Children Undergoing Apicoaortic Conduit Insertion

Tunnel aortic stenosis	10
Residual valvular and annular stenosis	8
Subvalvular	3
Supravalvular and IHSS	3

TABLE 6.2 Prior Surgery on the Left Ventricular Outflow Tract in Twenty-Four Patients Receiving Apicoaortic Conduits

Aortic valvotomy	8
Subvalvular resection	8
Coarctation repair	2
Valve replacement	1
Repair supravalvular aortic stenosis	4
None	5

son & Johnson Cardiovascular Model 100, King of Prussia, PA). One Shiley Bovine Pericardial valved conduit and one St. Jude valve containing a Dacron conduit were used in two additional patients. Conduit size varied from 12 to 20 mm: 12-mm conduits were used for infants and small children (aged less than 3 years), and 14–20-mm conduits were used for children aged 7–19 years. Because the conduit is a second avenue for left ventricular outflow, we believe that a conduit smaller than that generally used for the right ventricle is both acceptable and, in most instances, desirable. The valve in the conduit was positioned halfway between the stent and the aortic anastomosis. The position allows ample room for vascular clamp placement when and if conduit valve replacement becomes necessary.

More than ample graft material is supplied with the conduit as it comes from the manufacturer; the stent is packaged and sold separately. Several centimeters of graft were excised, leaving 4–6 cm of graft material proximal to the valve. Most, if not all, of the graft material was excised from the stent. Generally, a conduit 2–4 mm larger in diameter than the stent was selected in order to minimize the gradient across the porcine valve. When using the St. Jude conduit, the sewing ring of a 19-mm aortic valve was removed and the valve was inserted into an 18-mm Dacron graft. The valve was held in place by wrapping heavy suture around the graft over the middle of the valve annulus.

The conduit graft was then sutured to the external rim of the Dacron stent. The conduit with attached stent was brought into the wound to mea-

TABLE 6.3 Associated Cardiac Lesions in Twenty-Four Patients Receiving Apicoaortic Conduits for Complex Left Ventricular Outflow Obstruction

Mild aortic regurgitation	18
Severe aortic regurgitation	4
Mitral regurgitation	4
Complex intracardiac	4
Coarctation of aorta or interrupted arch	3

sure overall length, taking into consideration the elongation that will occur when the crimp in the graft straightens out under systemic pressure. Excess graft material distal to the valve was excised.

The conduit woven graft as sold by the manufacturer (Hancock–Johnson & Johnson Cardiovascular, King of Prussia, PA) comes in two woven graft porosities. We have generally used the conduit with standard porosity (Model 100) because of its superior handling and suturing characteristics and its theoretically more adherent neointima. The manufacturer also makes a low-porosity woven conduit for left ventricular application (Model 105), which would theoretically minimize bleeding through the graft during prolonged cardiopulmonary bypass, it may also be particularly useful in patients with altered coagulation states. It has the theoretical disadvantage of a poorer neointimal healing and it is less malleable when attached to the child's aorta. The Model 105 Hancock–Johnson & Johnson conduit has standard woven graft porosity, but it contains the modified-orifice porcine valve.

The Stent

A curved left ventricular stent was attached to the conduit and used in all 24 children. Work on animal models demonstrated that an apical left ventriculotomy would narrow over several months and produce obstruction unless a rigid stent was added to maintain this orifice[1]; the stent should project 3–8 mm into the cavity of the ventricle. We prefer the cloth-covered and -lined stent with a polypropylene framework (Hancock–Johnson & Johnson) because it permits neointimal ingrowth and more secure fixation to the ventricular myocardium. The 90-degree angle in the curved rigid stent prevents kinking of the conduit as it negotiates the acute angle from the left ventricular apex to the descending thoracic aorta. Straight stents for conduits attached to the abdominal aorta are also available from the manufacturer.

Aortic Anastomosis

The technique for insertion of apicoaortic conduit has been described in an earlier publication.[2,23] The approach through a left thoracotomy, fifth interspace, was used in 20/24 children and is our favored approach in most instances (Fig. 6.1). This transthoracic approach *(a)* gives direct access to the descending thoracic aorta without encroachment of the abdominal viscera; *(b)* avoids an additional sternotomy inasmuch as most of the children had undergone one or more sternotomies during prior attempts to correct left ventricular outflow obstruction; and *(c)* could usually be performed without

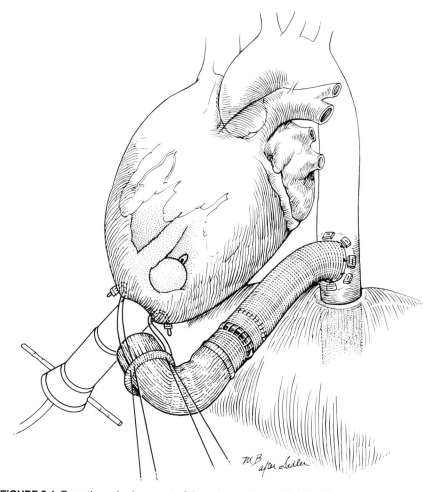

FIGURE 6.1 Transthoracic placement of the apicoaortic conduit (18 of 24 children). The aortic anastomosis is performed using a partial occluding clamp and interrupted pledgeted sutures. The apical ventriculotomy is made with a Foley catheter and cork borer.

the necessity of cardiopulmonary bypass (20/21 of those patients in whom a left thoracotomy was used did not require c/p bypass).

A transsternal approach was used in four children. The distal end of the conduit inserted into the ascending aorta in two patients (Fig. 6.2), into the supraceliac abdominal aorta in one patient, and into the descending thoracic aorta through a posterior pericardial incision in one patient (Fig. 6.3).

In each instance where a transsternal approach was used, repair of associated cardiac malformations was required or a direct attack on the left ventricular outflow tract was attempted. Two patients had severe associated aortic valve regurgitation in addition to obstruction and a smaller than desirable prosthetic valve was inserted to correct the regurgitation and the apicoaortic conduit was inserted to bypass their tunnel aortic obstruction. In both patients, the distal conduit was sutured to the oblique ascending aortomy through which the aortic valve replacement was performed (Fig. 6.2).

In two patients the supraceliac abdominal aorta was used as the site of the distal anastomosis. In one of these patients, a cardiopulmonary bypass was necessary to correct an associated incomplete atrioventricular (AV) canal. The abdominal aortic portion of the conduit was wrapped with

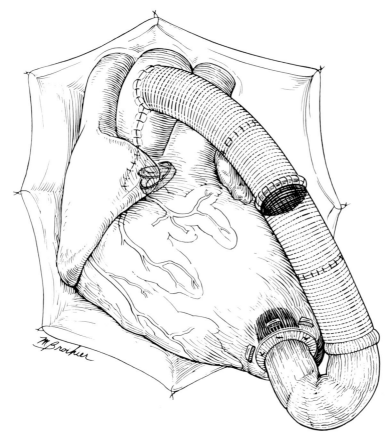

FIGURE 6.2 Apicoaortic conduit placed to the ascending aorta. Note that native aortic valve has been replaced with a prosthetic valve.

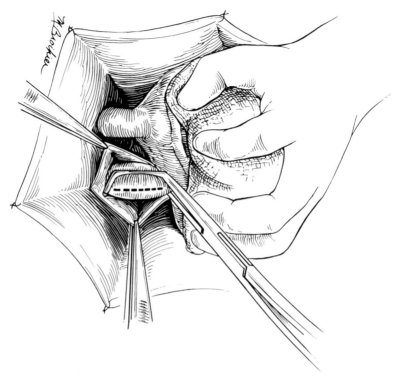

FIGURE 6.3 Transpericardial access to the descending thoracic aorta for insertion of apicoartic conduit.

omentum to prevent erosion of the graft into a hollow abdominal viscera; erosion of the conduit into the stomach has been reported by others when the omental wrap is omitted.[3] In one child with supravalvular aortic stenosis and idiopathic hypertrophic stenosis (IHSS), the distal conduit was sewn to the descending thoracic aorta through the posterior pericardium. This approach was surprisingly easy, but it required elevation of the heart during cardiopulmonary bypass (Fig. 6.3).

Regardless of the approach, a secure distal anastomosis was performed, using interrupted mattress sutures with pledgets along a vertical aortotomy; a partially occluding vascular clamp facilitates this anastomosis and avoids distal ischemia because bypass is not necessary for this anastomosis. Heparin was administered (3 mg/kg body wt) before releasing the aortic clamp and allowing blood to enter the distal half of the conduit to the level of the valve.

The aortic anastomosis was inspected and hemostasis obtained before proceeding.

Ventricular Anastomosis

A Foley catheter (16 French) and a standard brass laboratory cork borer were used to make the circular ventriculotomy (Fig. 6.1); it should be noted that the cork borer should have the same external diameter as the of the stent. Four double-armed sutures of 2-0 braided Dacron were placed at four equidistant points parallel to the proposed site of the apical ventriculotomy and were threaded through the sewing ring of the apical stent. The 5-mL balloon on the Foley catheter was distended with 8–12 mL of sterile saline so that the balloon was slightly larger than the cork borer and could not be pulled back through it; this volume of saline was aspirated back into the syringe and saved. (The standard cork border is sharp enough to cut through myocardium but will not cut and rupture the Foley balloon). A small stab wound was made in the left ventricular apex and dilated with a clamp to accept the catheter and deflated balloon. The predetermined amount of saline was injected into the balloon of the Foley inside the left ventricular cavity. Traction was placed on the catheter while the cork borer, threaded over the Foley catheter, was used to excise a circular piece of myocardium. The inflated catheter, core of muscle, and cork borer were withdrawn simultaneously and the apical stent lowered into position by applying traction on the mattress sutures. The traction sutures were tied, and additional pledgeted sutures were placed as needed for hemostasis. Air, which may become trapped in the conduit, was removed by inserting a 20-gauge needle into the prosthesis before inserting the ventricular end. The pericardium was drawn back and sutured to the sewing ring of the stent for additional support.

The Foley balloon serves to flatten the left ventricular apex as traction is applied and acts as a backstop to prevent the cork borer from injuring papillary muscles and cordal structures. The balloon also traps the ventricular core of muscle inside the cork borer. The cork borer cuts a precise hole and does not denude excess endocardium, which could serve as a site of thrombus formation. The ventricular punch produced by Hancock–Johnson & Johnson cannot be recommended for this procedure because it requires a relatively larger apical incision for insertion and the stainless steel blade will easily cut through the Foley balloon.

Although cardiopulmonary bypass was not required for insertion of the apicoaortic conduit in 20 of our 24 children, we have made it a practice to cannulate the left femoral artery and vein for bypass support should any problem arise during insertion of the conduit through the left thoracotomy.

RESULTS

The hospital records, catheterization data and arteriograms were reviewed on all children. All 18 long-term survivors underwent clinical follow-ups and and 16 of these underwent postoperative catheterization and angiography 12–17 months (mean, 15 months) postoperatively. Portions of the clinical and catheterization data have been published in earlier reports.[4,23]

The seven deaths in the series are summarized in Table 6.4. The first death was a 2-year old child with an incomplete AV canal and subvalvular aortic stenosis in whom the primum atrial septal defect had been closed. The child died 3 days after operation of low cardiac output and pulmonary congestion. Autopsy revealed unrecognized but severe cor triatriatum.

The second death was partially the result of severe intraoperative hemorrhagic diathesis with marked bleeding through the standard porosity woven graft (Model 100). The child experienced severe congestive heart failure with pulmonary edema and liver failure as well as severe aortic regurgitation due to acute bacterial endocarditis. His preoperative coagulation studies had been markedly abnormal. The rather prolonged perfusion necessary to replace the infected aortic valve and insert the conduit resulted in a severe bleeding diathesis. Although he survived the operation, he died of multisystem failure 8 days after operation. Use of lower porosity conduit (Model 105) might have reduced the bleeding problem in this patient had it been available at operation.

The third death was a patient with preoperative uremia and cardiogenic shock who had also experienced multiple cardiac arrests. He had an uneventful operation, but he died as a result of a mechanical airway obstruction on the second day after operation. Autopsy confirmed excellent placement of the conduit.

The fourth death was a 4-month-old infant (2.3 kg) with extremely complex cardiac anatomy including transposition of the great arteries, single ventricle, interrupted aortic arch, and subvalvular aortic stenosis, he had undergone repair of the interrupted arch and pulmonary artery banding at age 6 weeks. He improved greatly following conduit insertion but eventually died of *Pseudomonas* pneumonia and sepsis. Autopsy revealed thrombosis of two of the three cusps of the porcine valve. The 12-mm conduit was twice the size of his aorta and we presumed that cusp thrombosis was related to inability of his small left ventricular stroke volume to open all three cusps.

One of the three late deaths was a 13-year-old boy with residual supravalvular and tunnel subaortic stenosis who had undergone an uneventful conduit insertion and hospital course. He was discharged after operation 14 days but returned 3 weeks later with fever and left pleural effusion. Although the pleural fluid was initially sterile, it became secondarily infected and led to a staphylococcal empyema. His secondarily infected conduit was removed and aortoventriculoplasty (Konno) was performed 6 weeks after conduit insertion. The patient died 2 weeks after this second operation of renal failure and continued sepsis.

The second late death was a 24-year-old woman who had had a conduit inserted 5 years earlier for recurrent subvalvular stenosis. She had been asymptomatic for 5 years, and then presented with hemoptysis. Diagnostic evaluation included an aortogram, pulmonary arteriogram and cardiac catheterization, and bronchoscopy; all failed to show the source of bleeding. While under observation in the hospital, she had massive hemoptysis and died. The only pathologic finding at autopsy was lobar pulmonary hypertension.

The third late death was an 18-month-old child with diffuse subvalvular aortic stenosis and large VSD who had pulmonary artery banding in early infancy. She was readmitted while in extremis and underwent recatheterization and dopamine support therapy before an emergency operation. Her VSD was repaired, her PA band removed, and an apicoaortic conduit was inserted. Her postoperative course was stormy but she gradually improved. She developed a cardiac arrhythmia 2 months postoperatively and expired suddenly. Autopsy showed apparent good function of the conduit and an intact intracardiac repair.

The current clinical status of the 24 children in the series is shown in Table 6.5 at a mean follow-up period of 44.6 months (range, 15–77 months). Two of the 17 surviving patients are receiving anticoagulation therapy because of a mechanical valve in the conduit or native aortic position. Only one is taking a cardiac medication. All patients are clinically evaluated two or more times annually. Auscultation reveals a soft systolic and/or diastolic murmur across the native left ventricular outflow tract. A 2–3/6 systolic murmur is heared over all conduit valves in the midaxillary line. The ECGs of several patients have continued to show left ventricular hypertrophy. Chest x-rays continue to show relatively normal heart size with no evidence of calcification of the porcine valve or conduit, or both.

Sixteen of the 19 early survivors underwent cardiac catheterization from 1 to 1.5 years after the initial operation (mean 1.2 years); 14 patients underwent a second postoperative catheterization at an average of 44 months postoperatively. Figure 6.4 shows the change in the left ventricular to aortic gradient of the 16 patients with catheterization data. The reduction from 91 ± 30 mm Hg to 13 ± 8.5 mm Hg is highly significant ($P < 0.001$). The minimal residual gradient is more or less equally divided across the stent, the valve, and the distal aortic anastomosis. In addition to gradient reduction, the apicoaortic conduit has resulted in a reduction of the left ventricular end diastolic pressure from 14 ± 10 to 12 ± 6 mm Hg ($P > 0.5$)

TABLE 6.4 Early and Late Deaths in Seven Children After Apicoaortic Conduit Insertion

Age	Diagnosis	Days P.O. to Death	Cause of Death
2 years	Incomplete AV canal Subvalvular aortic stenosis Cortriatriatum	3 days	Congestive heart failure secondary to unrecognized cortriatriatum
17 years	Residual subvalvular aortic stenosis Acute bacterial endocarditis Severe aortic regurgitation Preoperative pulmonary edema Preoperative liver failure Intraoperative hemorrhagic diathesis	8 days	Cerebral edema (no evidence of emboli)
3 years	Tunnel aortic stenosis Preoperative cardiogenic shock Preoperative anuria Multiple preoperative cardiac arrests	2 days	Multisystem failure following an arrest caused by obstruction of an endotracheal tube
4 months[a]	Transposition Single ventricle Severe hypoplasia of transverse aortic arch Subvalvular aortic stenosis	42 days	*Pseudomonas* pneumonia (sepsis)

13 years	Residual supravalvular aortic stenosis Uneventful postoperative course Discharged 14 days after operation Admitted 3 weeks after operation with fever and left pleural effusion Developed staphlococcal empyema Conduit removed and aortoventriculoplasty 6 weeks after operation	2 months	Sepsis, renal failure
24 years	Insertion of apicoaortic for diffuse subvalvular AS 5 years after operation Asymptomatic for 5 years after operation Autopsy showed intact conduit	5 years	Massive hemoptysis 2° to lobal pulmonary hypertension
18 months	Tunnel aortic stenosis, VSD with PA band Admitted with hypotension and oliguria Taken urgently to or on dopamine drip	2 months	Cardiac arrhythmia

*Patient weighed 2.3 kg at time of operation.

TABLE 6.5 Current Status of Twenty-Four Children Receiving an Apicoaortic Conduit

Status	No. of Patients	Percent
Alive—no subsequent surgery (class 1)	13	54
Alive—subsequent surgery (class 1)	4	17
Early deaths	4	17
Late deaths	3	12
Total	24	100

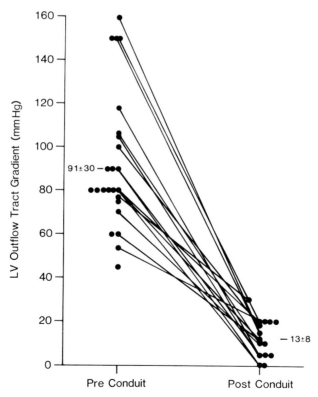

FIGURE 6.4 Pre- and postoperative left ventricular-to-aortic gradient in patients receiving apicoaortic conduits.

and an increase in cardiac index from 3.6 ± 1.2 to 4.15 ± 1 mm Hg ($P >$ 0.46). The favorable hemodynamic response to exercise was shown in our earlier report.[4]

Nine late postoperative problems have occurred in seven patients during the follow-up period and are shown in Table 6.6. A ventricular anastomotic aneurysm occurred in the first patient in the series 18 months after operation. The conduit was removed, the apex closed, and a successful direct reconstruction of the left ventricular outflow tract was accomplished. The cause for the aneurysm was secondary to inadequate reinforcement of the apical stent. In subsequent patients the pericardium was sutured around the stent. We have not encountered another problem involving left ventricular anastomotis since pericardial reinforcement has been used.

Gram-negative bacteremia has occurred in two patients. One patient developed a hemophylus influenza bacteremia and mild conduit valve regurgitation 19 months after conduit insertion; the infection was treated with 6 weeks of intravenous ampicillin therapy, which ended after clinical and bacteriologic resolution. This patient died of massive hemoptysis from lobar pulmonary hypertension 5 years after operation. No evidence of infection was found at autopsy.

The other patient developed bacteremia secondary to *Pseudomonas* pneumonia 2 months after operation and was treated with intravenous aminoglyceride with clinical and bacteriologic resolution. This patient has remained well 76 months after treatment, and repeat catheterization 45 months postoperatively shows good conduit function with trivial conduit valve regurgitation.

One patient developed empyema 3 months postoperatively. The patient underwent empycectomy with irrigation of the conduit with dilute (Betadine) solution for 4 days. No organism was grown from the empyema fluid. She was treated with intravenous antibiotics for 6 weeks and oral antibiotics for 3 months. This patient remained well 5 years after operation but she eventually died of hemoptysis from lobar pulmonary hypertension.

TABLE 6.6 Late Postoperative Problems in Children Receiving Apicoaortic Conduits

Complication	No. of Patients	Mortality
Ventricular anastomotic aneurysm	1	0
Gram-negative bacteremia	3	1
Empyema	2	1
Conduit valve regurgitation	5	0
Gastric erosion	0	0
Systemic emboli	0	0

Conduit valve regurgitation has developed in five patients at an average of 36 months postoperatively. In two, the regurgitation was severe enough that symptoms recurred 12 and 30 months postoperatively and the conduit valve was electively replaced with a second tissue valve. One patient, who died 5 years postoperatively of hemoptysis and lobar pulmonary hypertension, had moderate regurgitation and would have likely required conduit valve replacement in another year or two. In the other two patients, the regurgitation has remained mild and has not yet progressed. Twelve patients have shown no evidence of regurgitation from 6 months to 8 years after operation.

Gastric errosion or systembolic emboli have not occurred in our patients. As noted above, only two of the 24 conduits have been placed in the abdomen and in both the conduit was wrapped with omentum. The only patients in the series receiving postoperative anticoagulation therapy were those with mechanical valves: a 17-mm Björk-Shiley in the native aortic position and St. Jude valve in the apicoaortic conduit.

DISCUSSION

Conventional surgical techniques, including patch reconstruction of the aortic root for supravalvular stenosis, valvotomy for bicuspid valvular stenosis, and myotomy and myectomy for obstructive cardiomyopathy, are highly successful in treating most forms of left ventricular outflow obstructions in children. There are, however, a significant number of patients (primarily children) in whom there is diffuse hypoplasia and/or multilevel obstruction that is not adequately treated by these techniques. Aortoventriculoplasty and/or apicoaortic conduits provide alternatives for this complex group of patients.

Aortoventriculoplasty, a complex gusset technique for enlarging the annulus, replacment of the aortic valve, and enlargement of the aortic root as described by Konno,[5] Rastan,[6] and Symbus,[7] has been used in children, but it seems more radical because it involves incising and patching the ventricular septum, right ventricular outflow tract and aortic root. It allows insertion of an "adult size" prosthetic valve in adolescent patients, but it has been infrequently applied in children less than 5 years of age and the long-term results are unknown. Operative complications include a mortality of 12%–25%, acquired VSD, heart block, persistent or recurrent obstruction, moderately long operative ischemic period, coronary artery injury leading to infarction, and tricuspid valve insufficiency.[8,9] Anticoagulation therapy is obligatory because mechanical valves are used.

The concept of an apicoaortic valve conduit to bypass valvular aortic stenosis was conceived by Carrel in 1910,[10] performed experimentally by Sarnoff in 1955,[11] and performed clinically by Templeton in 1962.[12] This technique did not gain popularity early on because of problems related to the conduit components (such as hemolysis and emboli) and because direct aortic valve resection and replacement became quite successful in the early 1960s. The technique received little attention until we and others developed renewed interest in the concept for complex forms of left ventricular outflow obstruction. The woven Dacron graft containing a gluteraldehyde sterilized porcine heterograft (Hancock, King of Prussia, PA) was introduced in the early 1970s for right heart reconstruction.[13] We used the Hancock conduit and conduits containing mechanical valves, applied a rigid left ventricular stent, and showed experimentally that these conduits placed in the apicoaortic position functioned well to bypass the left ventricular outflow tract.[1]

Late follow-up studies in animal models and isolated clinical trials by other investigators[14,15,16] prompted us to extend this technique to a limited group of children.

Apicoaortic conduit insertion in contrast to aortoventriculoplasty is simple to perform, requires minimal to no cardiac ischemia for its insertion, and has no age or heart size restriction. It adds an additional outflow tract to the left ventricle and thus does not require as large a prosthetic valve because there are two avenues for egress of blood from the left ventricle. It does not violate unrelated cardiac structures, which can cause coronary artery injury, conduction disturbances, or tricuspid regurgitation. This and other reports support that conduit insertion relieves left ventricular obstruction, reduces left ventricular–end diastolic pressure, improves cardiac output, and permits a normal hemodynamic response to exercise.[4,23]

The reported long-term complications of apicoaortic conduits are left ventricular anastomotic aneurysms, erosion of the conduit into the esophagus or stomach, emboli, and tissue valve dysfunction.[3,4,16,17,18,19,20,23] A left ventricular anastomotic aneurysm seen in our first patient has been eliminated by use of a cloth-covered and -lined left ventricular stent and pericardial reinforcement of the stent. Systembolic emboli have not been encountered in our patients, and only two patients who received mechanical valves have undergone anticoagulation therapy. Systemic emboli reported by Stanzel et al[20] have not been encountered in other series and may be attributed to excessively denuded endocardium when the apical ventriculotomy was made or to irregularities in the suture line between the stent and the conduit. Erosion of the conduit into the esophagus or abdominal viscus[3] has not been encountered in our series. We believe that it can be prevented by placing omentum about the conduit in the abdomen, or by placing the conduit in the retroperitoneum as suggested by Ergin et al,[19] or by placing the entire conduit in the left chest, which is our preference.

The infrequent technical problem of bleeding through the woven graft may be reduced or eliminated by using a low-porosity woven graft, fibrin glue, or an alternate graft material such as expanded Teflon.

In the past, the major limitation of currently available apicoaortic conduits appears to be the limited durability of the porcine valve. Conduit valve regurgitation has occurred in five of our patients; in two, conduit valve replacement was necessary. Given the current status of porcine valves in children, it is likely that all porcine valves will eventually need to be changed.[21] Low-pressure gluteraldehyde fixation of tissue valves and/or anticalcification additives to the porcine valve may improve their durability. Use of a more durable mechanical valve in the conduit is an alternative, and our preliminary laboratory experience with several mechanical valves in apicoaortic conduits is quite promising, even without Coumadin anticoagulation therapy.[22] We have used a St. Jude valve in one conduit in a child and have seen an excellent result over the first 8 months. Unlike aortoventriculoplasty, the extracardiac location of the valve in apicoaortic conduits make it ideal for reoperation on malfunctioning prosthetic valves, and it permits a future primary attack on the left ventricular outflow tract. It is also apparent that the porcine heterograft has greater durability in the extracardiac conduit than it has in an intracardiac location.

Like many surgical procedures for congenital heart disease, insertion of an apicoaortic conduit is not a curative procedure. The apicoaortic conduit relieves left ventricular obstruction and permits a normal hemodynamic response to exercise. The technique is simple to perform, and it does not compromise major coronary arteries, the conduction system, or other valves.

Although the combined early and late mortality in the series is substantial 7/24 (29%), it must be remembered that four of the seven deaths occurred in critically ill children in whom operation was performed as a recessitative measure. Only one operative death occurred in a patient presenting for elective operation: the child had an additional unrecognized complex cardiac anomaly.

We believe that improvements in conduit composition, tissue valve durability, or mechanical valve substitutes will eliminate many of the late problems with this technique and make it the procedure of choice for complex forms of left ventricular outflow obstruction.

ACKNOWLEDGMENT
The authors wish to acknowledge the skilled secretarial assistance of Ms. Geri French.

REFERENCES

1. Brown JW, Myerowitz PD, Cann MS, et al. Apicol–aortic anastomosis: a method for relief of diffuse left ventricular outflow obstruction. Surgical Forum 1974;25:147.

2. Brown JW, Kirsh MM. Technique for insertion of apico–aortic conduit. J Thorac Cardiovasc Surg 1978;76:90.

3. Berry BE, Quaid TP. Left ventricular abdominal aortic conduit complicated by late gastric erosion. J Thorac Cardiovasc Surg 1981;82:147.

4. Rocchini AP, Brown JW, Crowley DE, et al. Clinical and hemodynamic follow-up of left ventricular to aortic conduits in patients with aortic stenosis. J Am Coll Cardiol 1983;1(4):1135.

5. Konno, S, Yasuharu I, Iida Y, et al. A new method for prosthetic valve replacement in congenital aortic stenosis associated with hypoplasia of the aortic valve ring. J Thorac Cardiovasc Surg 1975;70:909.

6. Rastan H, Koncz J. Aortoventriculoplasty: a new technique for the treatment of left ventricular outflow tract obstruction. J Thorac Cardiovasc Surg 1976;71:920.

7. Symbus PN, Ware RE, Hatcher CR, et al. An operation for relief of severe left ventricular outflow tract obstruction. J Thorac Cardiovasc Surg 1976;71:245.

8. Björnstad PG, Rastan H, Keutel J, et al. Aortoventriculoplasty for tunnel subaortic stenosis and other obstructions of the left ventricular outflow tract. Circulation 1979;60:59.

9. DeVivie ER, Koncz J, Ruggroth G, et al. Aortoventriculoplasty for different types of left ventricular outflow tract obstructions. J Cardiovasc Surg 1982;23:6.

10. Carrel A. Experimental surgery of the aorta and heart. Ann Surg 1910;52:83.

11. Sarnoff SJ, Donovan TJ, Core RB. The surgical relief of aortic stenosis by means of apical aortic valved anastomosis. Circulation 1955;11:564.

12. Templeton JY. Unpublished data.

13. Bowman FO Jr, Hancock WD, Malin JR. A valve-containing Dacron prosthesis. Its use in restoring pulmonary artery–right ventricular continuity. Arch Surg 1973;107:724.

14. Bernhard WF, Poeries V, LaForge CG. Relief of congenital obstruction to left ventricular outflow with a ventricular–aortic prosthesis. J Thorac Cardiovasc Surg 1975;69:223.

15. Cooley DA, Norman JC, Mullins CE, et al. Left ventricle to abdominal aorta conduits for relief of aortic stenosis. Cardiovascular Diseases. Bull Tex Heart Inst 1975;2:376.

16. Dembitsky WP, Weldon CS. Clinical experience with the use of a valve-bearing conduit to construct a second left ventricular outflow in cases of unresectable intraventricular obstruction. Ann Surg 1976;184:317.

17. Norman JC, Nihill MR, Cooley DA. Valved apico–aortic composite conduits for left ventricular outflow tract obstructions. Am J Cardiol 1980;45:1265.

18. Brown, JW, Rocchini A, Behrendt D. Follow-up after use of left ventricular to aortic conduit in patients with aortic stenosis. Abstract 312. First World Congress of Pediatric Cardiol, London, 1980.

19. Ergin MA, Cooper R, LaCante M, et al. Experience with left ventricular apicoaortic conduits for complicated left ventricular outflow obstruction in children and young adults. Ann Thorac Surg 1981;32:369.

20. Stansel HC, Tabry II, Hellenbrand WE, et al. Aprico–aortic shunts in children. Am J Surg 1978;135:547.

21. Dunn JM. Porcine valve durability in children. Ann Thorac Surg 1981;32:357.

22. Brown JW, Fiore A. Mechanical valve function in aprico-aortic conduits: experimental evaluations without Coumadin anticoagulation, abstracted. Submitted to the 64th Annual Meeting of the Association of Thoracic Surgeons, New York, May 1984.

23. Brown JW, Girod DA, Hurwitz RA, Caldwell RL, Rocchini AP, Behrendt DM, Kirsh MM. Apicoaortic valved conduits for complex left ventricular outflow obstruction: technical consideration and current status. Ann Thorac Surg 1984;38:162–168.

CHAPTER 7

Palliation for Hypoplastic Left Heart Syndrome

William I. Norwood, MD, PhD

Hypoplastic left heart syndrome is a term used to describe varying degrees of underdevelopment of the structures in the left side of the heart — most particularly, the left ventricle. Aortic valve atresia or stenosis, atresia or interruption of the aortic arch, and severe stenosis or atresia of the mitral valve in combination with severe hypoplasia of the left ventricle all compose a constellation of defects called "hypoplastic left heart syndrome" by Noonan and Nadas.[1] The most complex and common form is atresia of the aortic valve. As a result of the atresia, the ascending aorta generally measures between 2 and 3 mm in diameter as it carries only retrograde flow to the coronary circulation. In more than 90% of patients with aortic atresia, there is coexisting atresia or severe hypoplasia of the mitral valve and a diminutive or absent left ventricle.[2] Therefore, perinatal survival is dependent on maintenance of the systemic circulation through the ductus arteriosus and on adequate pulmonary venous return to the right ventricle — most commonly through a patent foramen ovale. Neonatal death usually results from inadequate coronary and systemic perfusion secondary to the combination of physiologic closure of the ductus arteriosus and high pulmonary-to-systemic flow ratio as the pulmonary vasculature resistance physiologically decreases in the early neonatal period.

Hypoplastic left heart syndrome is not rare. It is the fourth most common cardiac defect reported in the New England Regional Infant Cardiac Program, and it accounts for nearly 25% of cardiac deaths during the first week of life.[3] Between 1969 and 1979, there were 223 infants reported to the New England Regional Infant Cardiac Program with hypoplastic left heart syndrome of the aortic atresia type. None survived 1 year.

With the ever-increasing prospect of significant physiologic improve-

78

ment of patients with all forms of single ventricle using surgical techniques originally introduced clinically by Fontan, there has been an increasing interest in establishing surgical repair of hypoplastic left ventricular syndrome.

However, the pulmonary vascular resistance of the newborn infant is physiologically high; therefore, a staged surgical approach is necessary for definitive treatment. Initial palliation must establish permanent unobstructed communication between the right ventricle and the aorta, limit the pulmonary blood flow and pressue to near-normal levels, and assure a large interatrial communication. The first objective is necessary for adequate systemic perfusion and for preserving ventricular function, while the second two objectives are essential for normal development of the pulmonary vasculature to establish low pulmonary resistance in preparation for a modified Fontan procedure.[4-6]

Most patients present in the first week of life with cyanosis that is usually mild and with tachypnea. More than one-half will have decreased peripheral pulses and mild-to-severe metabolic acidosis from reduced systemic blood flow as the ductus arteriosus narrows. Resuscitation of these neonates can almost always be achieved by constant infusion of prostaglandin E_1 (0.1 mg/kg per minute) in a peripheral vein for maintenance of ductal patency and by administration of sodium bicarbonate to reverse the acidosis.

The diagnosis is easily established by electrocardiography. Angiographic study may discern the coexistence of tricuspid regurgitation or coarctation of the aorta.

In our experience, the objectives of palliation have been accomplished recently by anastomosis of the proximal main pulmonary artery to the ascending aorta. A patch is used to further augment the aortic arch and thoracic aorta just beyond the level of the ductus arteriosus, which has been divided. Pulmonary atresia is created and a modified Blalock-Taussig shunt provides appropriate pulmonary blood flow.

From January 1984 through May 1985, 42 neonates with aortic valve atresia or stenosis have undergone palliation by anastomosis of the main pulmonary artery to the ascending aorta and arch, atrial septectomy, and creation of a modified Blalock-Taussig shunt. There were 14 early deaths and seven late deaths. Two patients developed late interatrial obstruction, treated by repeat septotomy, and four developed late coarctation of the aorta, treated by either balloon dilatation or patch aortoplasty.

REFERENCES

1. Noonan JA, Nadas AS. The hypoplastic left heart syndrome: an analysis of 101 cases. Pediatr Clin North Am 1958;5:1029.

2. Moodie DS, Gallen WJ, Friedberg DZ. Congenital aortic atresia: report of long survival and some speculations about surgical approaches. J Thorac Cardiovasc Surg 1976;63:726.
3. Flyer DC. Report of the New England Regional Infant Cardiac Program. Pediatrics 1980;65:376.
4. Norwood WI, Lang P, Castaneda AR, Campbell DN. Experience with operations for hypoplastic left heart syndrome. J Thorac Cardiovasc Surg 1981;82:511.
5. Norwood WI, Lang P, Hansen D. Physiologic repair or aortic atresia – hypoplastic left heart syndrome. N Engl J Med 1983;308:23.
6. Norwood WI. Technics of palliative and reparative surgery for hypoplastic left heart syndrome. Modern Techn Surg 1983;59:1 – 8.

CHAPTER 8

Truncal Valve Insufficiency and Persistent Truncus Arteriosus

Paul A. Ebert, MD

The incidence of truncal valve insufficiency may be in the range of 25% of all babies born with truncus arteriosus. Thus, there may not be much interest in a subject that has a probability of less than 1% occurrence. It is certainly a difficult subject to approach, especially with such minimum experience. Most of what I am going to say about truncal valve incompetence has been gathered from our own experience with truncus and specifically, the first 106 babies operated upon up until 1982.

Of these initial 106 infants with truncus arteriosus, six were treated medically, while 100 underwent repair. Twenty-nine patients demonstrated the presence of truncal valve insufficiency (Table 8.1). All six of the medically treated infants died. Thus, I believe all infants in heart failure require surgical intervention.[1,2]

Five of the six deaths in the medically treated infants had truncal insufficiency, while eight of the eleven operative deaths were in patients also with truncal insufficiency. The operative deaths in the surgical group were equally distributed by age (Fig. 8.1). Two patients had truncal valve replacement with total correction. One of these two children died, I believe, because the disc became caught on the prosthetic VSD patch. This particular child demonstrated moderate overriding of the truncus on to the right ventricle. In addition, two infants had replacement of regurgitant truncal valve within the first 30 days after initial repair. In each case, they never did well in the intensive care unit after the initial procedure. The ventricular septal defect was closed and it seemed like their only problem was that of residual truncal valve incompetence. We chose to return these children to the operating room and replace the truncal valve. Both these children did well. Six patients had truncal valve replacements three to four years after the initial procedure,

TABLE 8.1 Truncal Valve Insufficiency in 100 Infants with Truncus Arteriosus

	No. of Patients	Deaths	TI Present	Deaths in TI Patients
Medical management only	6	6	5	5
Surgical correction without truncal valve replacement	98	11	24	8
Surgical correction with truncal valve replacement	2	1	2	1

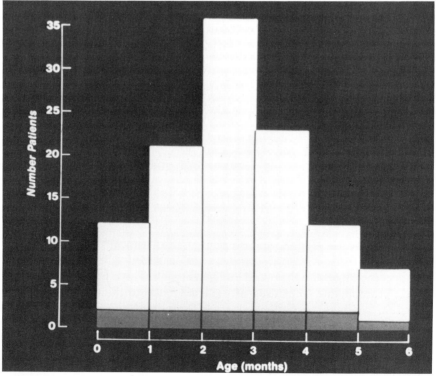

FIGURE 8.1 Depicts age distribution of 100 operated cases of truncus arteriosus during the first 6 months of life. *Shaded area* represents operative deaths.

at the time of replacement of the pulmonary conduit (Table 8.2). Thus, I think that there is no question that truncal valve incompetence is one of the major causes of failure in infants with truncus.[3,4]

It is very difficult to tell preoperatively what the degree of truncal valve insufficiency is in these infants.[5] Most truncus babies are in high cardiac output with large left-to-right shunts and left ventricular failure.[6] When coupled with truncal valve incompetence, the quantity of insufficiency is almost impossible to estimate. The cardiac x-ray is not much help because most of these babies are already in left ventricular failure and have significant cardiomegaly. The presence or absence of a diastolic murmur is only suggestive of truncal valve insufficiency.

From a diagnostic viewpoint, the single most important diagnostic test is the aortogram because it does tell you whether or not the child has truncal valve insufficiency. It will also tell you the size and give you some idea of the take-off of the pulmonary arteries. One aspect of truncus that we have been interested in is the morphology of the ascending trunk and its role in truncal valve insufficiencies. Many times, we see a fairly large trunk with a large diameter at its base, and perhaps three to four truncal cusps that you are unable to distinguish because these cusps are rudimentary. This is the kind of aorta that usually has insufficiency (Fig. 8.2).

The truncus with what looks like a perfect aorta coming directly off the left ventricle and with a fairly small ventricular septal defect is a group in which I have not seen truncal valve insufficiency.

Although the preoperative aortogram is probably the best method of assessing truncal valve insufficiency, it remains difficult to assess the importance of this insufficiency because the regurgitation and regurgitant volume is distributed to both ventricles. After repair, when the ventricular septal defect has been closed, the same amount of regurgitant volume enters the left ventricle only. Thus, the regurgitant fraction for the left ventricle increases once the ventricular septal defect is closed.

TABLE 8.2 Truncal Valve Replacement

	No. of Patients	Deaths
At time of initial truncal repair	2	1
Less than 30 days after truncal repair	2	—
More than 3 years after truncal repair	6	—

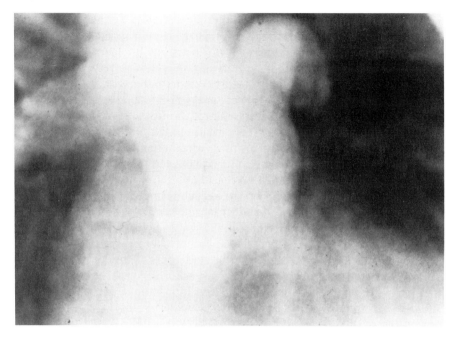

FIGURE 8.2 Characteristic truncus with truncal valve insufficiency. The trunk is fairly large at its base.

OPERATIVE CONSIDERATIONS

During the operation, the most important diagnostic tool is evaluation of the truncal valve before closing the ventricular septal defect. We perform these procedures with continuous perfusion and single venous canulae drainage with moderate hypothermia of 25–27°C. If the heart keeps beating during the period of cooling, there is little chance of ventricular distension. We have not found ventricular venting through the atrium or ventricle to be helpful in these infants so we usually cool them as quickly as possible with the pump until the ventricles stop beating. At this point, the aortic cross clamp is applied.

The pulmonary trunks are removed from the aorta and the aortic defect is closed. It is usually a good idea at this time to perform the ventriculotomy. Then the aortic cross clamp can be removed and the amount of truncal valve leaking can be assessed. If the defect is approximately the size of an 18 guage needle, and through the center of the valve, it is probably not going to be of great significance. If however, regurgitation is enough, even at low perfusion pressure, to obscure the ventricular septal defect, then the regurgitation is going to cause difficulty. It is in this setting today that I believe we should be fairly aggressive and that we are better off to replace the truncal valve. The nice thing about replacement of the truncal valve is that the right ventriculotomy can be extended up the aorta across the truncal valve so that a larger prosthesis can be emplaced. The left coronary artery and the right coronary artery are usually off to the side and thus this transannual ventriculotomy is quite analogous to pulmonary outflow patch in tetralogy of Fallot.[7] In two children, we extended the ventriculotomy across the anulus and put a patch over the top to be able to place a larger prosthesis. However, even in the smallest of infants, one can usually place a 17- to 21-mm valve without anular enlargement. We have always used the Björk-Shiley valve because it has a low profile, it is easy to insert, it comes in small sizes, and it is a quick, easy valve to replace.

SUMMARY

Our total experience today with truncus is about 134 infants. We have now replaced the truncal valve primarily in three of these patients with a single mortality.

It is most important to be aware of the child with truncal valve insufficiency as I suspect that much of the failure in treatment of truncus has been mainly due to insufficiency that may look modest when it regurgitates into the right and left ventricle preoperatively, but becomes quite significant when it is isolated to the left ventricle alone after VSD closure. Our approach today has been more aggressive because, I believe, it adds little to replace the truncal valve at the time of the truncal repair. With the ventriculotomy open, one can assess the truncal valve and in most cases the valve can be placed directly through the ventriculotomy and the VSD without extending the ventriculotomy across the annulus. If the incision does have to be extended, however, it does not cross any critical territory, and one is able to place a slightly larger valve with a transannular patch. If we have erred in the past it is been that we have not been aggressive enough with babies with insufficiency of the truncal valve.

REFERENCES

1. Applebaum A, Bargeon LM Jr, Pacifico AD, Kirkland JW. Surgical treatment of truncus arteriosus with emphasis on infants and small children. J Thorac Cardiovasc Surg 1976;71:936.

2. Ebert PA. Truncus arteriosus. In Wil GW (ed): Thoracic and Cardiovascular Surgery, 4th ed. Appleton–Century–Crofts, Norwalk, Conn, 1983, pp 785–793.
3. Deely WJ, Hagstrom JW, Engle MA. Truncus insufficiency: Common truncus arteriosus with regurgitant truncus valve; report of four cases. Am Heart J 1963;65:542.
4. Gelband H, Van Meter S, Gersony WM. Truncal valve abnormalities in infants with persistent truncus arteriosus: a clinical pathologic study. Circ 1972;45:397.
5. de Leval MR, McGoon DC, Wallace RB, Danielson GK, Mair DD. Management of truncal valve. Ann Surg 1974;180:427–432.
6. Kidd BSL. Persistent truncus arteriosus. In Keith JD, Rowe RD, Vlad P (eds): Heart Disease in Infancy and Childhood, 3rd ed. Macmillan, New York, 1978, p 457.
7. Shrivastara S, Edwards JE. Coronary arterial origin in persistent truncus arteriosus. Circ 1977;55:551–554.

CHAPTER 9

Aortic Insufficiency Associated with Ventricular Septal Defect

Rohinton K. Balsara, MBBS, FACS, FCCP

The syndrome of ventricular septal defect (VSD) and aortic incompetence (AI) is of congenital origin, usually secondary to cusp prolapse or a bicuspid aortic valve. This syndrome is related to congenital aneurysm of the sinus of Valsalva and tetralogy of Fallot with aortic valve incompetence.

HISTORICAL

The early description of VSD and AI with prolapsed aortic cusp was by Laubry and Pezzi[1] in 1921. In 1960, Garamella et al[2] and Starr et al[3] reported early attempts at operative repair by shortening the free margin of the prolapsed cusp. Historically, operative correction of this syndrome was delayed beyond childhood whenever possible in order to avoid valve replacement at a young age. In 1973, Spencer et al[4] and Trusler et al[5] separately introduced the concept of aortic valvuloplasty for repair of aortic insufficiency. The work by Sakakibara et al[6] in Japan has done much not only to elucidate the morphology, but also to suggest a classification and surgical management of this lesion.

The exact incidence of aortic valve incompetence among patients with VSD is uncertain. It is estimated that the incidence in the Western Hemisphere[7] is about 3%–5% where infracristal VSDs are most commonly seen. In Japan, where the occurrence of supracristal VSD is higher, the incidence of VSD and AI is likewise higher, about 8%–10%.

Anatomically this lesion can be classified by the location of the VSD and the presence of stenosis of the right ventricular outflow tract:[8]

Type I: Supracristal VSD and AI

Type II: Infracristal VSD and AI

Type III: Infracristal VSD and AI with infundibular pulmonic stenosis (IPS)

Type IV: Supracristal VSD and AI with infundibular pulmonic stenosis (IPS)

MORPHOLOGY

In isolated or uncomplicated VSD, the sinus of Valsalva and the aortic valve annulus are supported by thick conal septum issuing from the right ventricular septal components even in the presence of most VSDs. Anatomically, VSD and AI is characterized by a high VSD with little or no supporting tissue separating the septal defect from the right sinus of the aortic valve.[9] Aortic incompetence is thus most frequently associated with a subaortic VSD where no muscular support is present in the superior margin of the defect. The right coronary cusp and, occasionally, the noncoronary cusp is thus exposed and unsupported. The prolapsed cusp may be dilated and pouch-like, sagging into the right ventricular outflow tract adjacent to the VSD. The leaflet margin is usually thickened. The VSD is characteristically oval with its long axis parallel to the aortic ring, and it is usually moderate to large in size. Occasionally the infundibular septum may be underdeveloped and displaced anteriorly and leftwards (as in tetralogy of Fallot) a feature responsible for the infundibular stenosis seen occasionally in these cases. Less common is a perimembranous VSD near the anteroseptal commissure of the tricuspid valve (the so-called infracristal variety). In patients with infracristal VSD,[6] two anatomic anomalies are felt to contribute to the aortic valve prolapse into the VSD. One is the same muscular defect observed as in subaortic VSD although the deficient portion of the conal septum is slightly lower. The second factor is an abnormal development of the sinus of Valsalva especially the lower margins of the right and noncoronary sinuses.

The aortic valve and root exhibit a variety of anomalies.[10] Aortic incompetence may be due to *(a)* anomalies of cusp, *(b)* a deformed bicuspid valve, or *(c)* abnormal commissural attachments and/or a dilated annulus. It is usually secondary to cusp prolapse, in which case the right aortic cusp, occasionally the noncoronary cusp, and, rarely, both cusps, are elongated and enlarged along the free margin and in the body of the leaflet. Hemodynamically the blood shunting through the VSD during early systole prolapses the aortic valve by a Bernouli effect. Early in systole, a small amount of blood from the left ventricle shunts through the VSD into the right ventricle.

As the valve sags over and through the VSD—thus reducing the effective size of the VSD—the velocity of the shunting blood is increased, thus further drawing the aortic cusp through the defect and into the right ventricle. In some cases, the prolapse of the aortic cusp through the VSD may plug up the defect and decrease the shunt significantly (Fig. 9.1). The influence of left-to-right shunt is greater during early stages of the disease before aortic prolapse decreases the VSD effective size. Extensive cusp proplapse through a large VSD may also produce some obstruction to the right ventricle outflow tract. The effect of the shunting and insufficiency is to produce not only dilatation, but also hypertrophy of the left ventricle and right ventricle also. The defect may also become a suitable site for development of bacterial endocarditis.

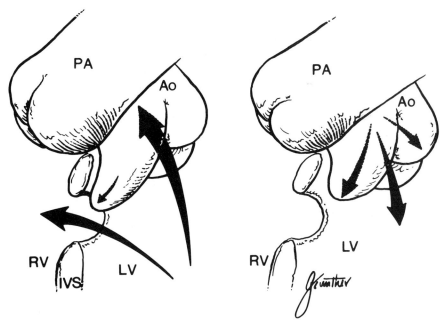

FIGURE 9.1 Illustrations showing the hemodynamic action causing prolapse of the aortic valve and the sinus, and regurgitation. *Left:* Early systolic phase: the anatomically unsupported aortic valve and sinus are drawn into the right ventricular cavity by the action of shunting blood through the VSD. *Right:* diastolic phase: The free margins of the leaflets of the aortic cusp close and establish competency as a result of the intraaortic pressure. This results in less prominence of the prolapsed leaflet, but eventually the sagging leaflet separated from the other two leaflets results in incompetence. Abbreviations: PA = pulmonary artery; Ao = aorta; RV = right ventricle; LV = left ventricle; IVS = interventricular septum.

CLINICAL PRESENTATION

The onset and severity of the AI can alter the clinical course of the disease. The murmur of AI appears between the ages of 2 and 8 years, and rarely after 8 years. Aneurysms of the sinus of Valsalva also may develop as part of the natural history of patients with subpulmonic VSD, but this is a slower process than the progression of the AI.[11] Obstruction of the right ventricular outflow tract is not uncommon in this anomaly, and it is due to valvular or infundibular stenosis or to prolapse of the aortic valve leaflets through the VSD. The additional burden of the AI may precipitate congestive heart failure or aggravate an existing one. With small defects in the infracristal position, however, there may be no change even if the valvular lesion is moderately severe. The usual course is a worsening of the aortic insufficiency, and the prolapsing leaflet may partially or completely occlude the VSD and thereby help reduce a left to right shunt. The prolapsed leaflet may give rise to subpulmonic obstruction. The incidence of endocarditis has been reported between 15%–25%.[12]

These patients characteristically have a to-and-fro murmur that may simulate a continuous murmur of patent ductus arteriosus. Occasionally the murmur can be mistaken for combined aortic incompetence and stenosis, coronary artery fistula, arteriovenous malformation, or sinus of Valsalva aneurysm with rupture.

Chest x-ray may demonstrate increased pulmonary vascularity and left ventricular enlargement. Electrocardiogram characteristically shows left ventricular hypertrophy with deep S-waves in V_1 or tall R-waves in V_6 and this is frequently associated with an increased depth of the Q in V_6. Occasionally the T-wave in V_6 is depressed. Echocardiography will assess the location and size of the VSD, and identify the aortic valve morphology and prolapse. Doppler studies will demonstrate the aortic incompetence.

A right- and left-sided heart catheterization should also be done in all these cases. The right heart study will help shunt calculations, record pulmonary artery pressures, and elicit any subpulmonic gradient if present. The left heart study will help identify the size and location of the septal defects and the aortography will estimate the magnitude of the AI and size of the aortic root (Fig. 9.2).

The aortic valve prolapse may be angiographically graded by the criteria used by Menahen et al,[13] as follows:

*Grade 1:*Mild aortic valve deformity with a nipplelike protrusion of part of a cusp or slight prolapse of the leaflet into the VSD. No AI present (Fig. 9.3).

*Grade 2a:*Moderate deformity of one or more cusps with further prolapse

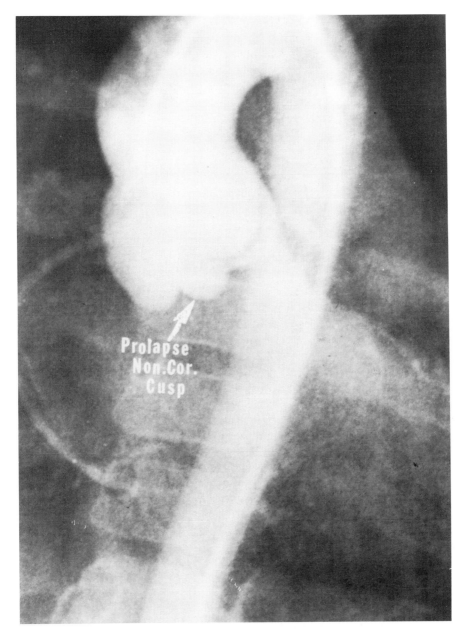

FIGURE 9.2 Aortogram (*anteroposterior view*) showing prolapse of noncoronary cusp with associated aortic valve regurgitation.

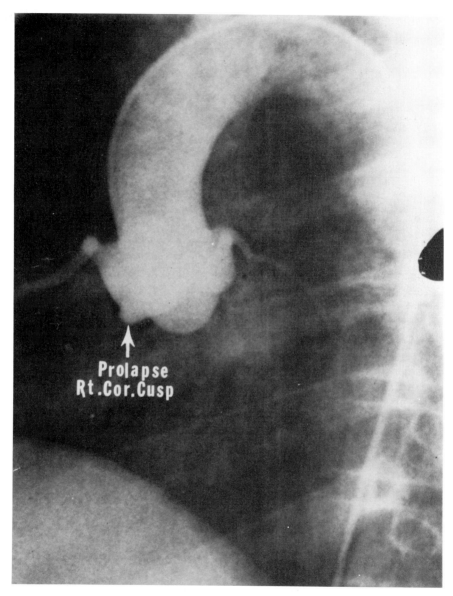

FIGURE 9.3 Aortogram (*lateral view*) showing early prolapse of right conary cusp. No AI present.

into the ventricular septal defect with resultant abnormal opening of the involved leaflets. No AI present.

*Grade 2b:*As in Grade 2(a) but with associated AI.

*Grade 3:*Severe aortic valve deformity with one or more cusps tethered to the margin of the VSD with resultant AI.

The severity of the AI can be quantitated usually by noting *(a)* widening of the pulse pressure to more than 50 mm Hg, *(b)* degree of opacification of the body of the left ventricle (LV) after aortic root contrast injection, *(c)* failure of clearing of contrast from LV after one or two systolic beats, and *(d)* increased LV end-diastolic volume in the absence of left to right shunt of greater than 35%.

SURGICAL CONSIDERATIONS

Early experience at repair of aortic valve was by Garamella et al[2] and Starr et al[3] in 1960; each of whom reported a single case that survived following shortening of the free margin of the prolapsed cusp. In 1963, Ellis et al[14] reported 19 cases with repair of VSD and AI of whom 13 required cusp reconstruction; of these, 10 patients were left with moderate to severe insufficiency. Plauth et al[15] reviewed the total experience until 1965 finding that only six of 17 patients treated by cusp plication had satisfactory result. These discouraging results lead to an increased utilization of aortic valve replacement. In 1969, Gonzalez-Levin and Barratt-Boyes[16] reported improved results in seven patients in whom the prolapsed cusp was used to close the VSD after which an aortic homograft was inserted. Similarly, in 1970 Somerville et al[17] reported their experience with 20 patients. In six patients, the aortic valve was repaired, while in 14 a prosthetic valve was inserted. Aortic competence was achieved in only one of the patients with valvuloplasty. Subsequently, Trusler et al[5] and Spencer et al[4] have reported improved results with aortic valvuloplasty.

There have been varying opinions as to the best timing and types of repair for this combined anomaly. In patients with VSD and aortic valve prolapse without AI some, authors have suggested a delay in repair.[18] They follow-up these patients until the onset of AI when the VSD is small or insignificant. Considering the difficulty of repairing the insufficient valve and the probable irreversible pathologic valve changes that occur, we advocate early repair of the VSD with progressive aortic valve prolapse before the development of AI. There is a general agreement, however, that the presence of aortic insufficiency complicating an otherwise hemodynamically insignificant VSD is an indication for surgery. In patients in whom AI is trivial or mild, VSD closure (patch or suture) alone is adequate; arresting the progression of AI and often reversing it. When the AI is significant (moderate or severe), the aortic valve will require repair or replacement.

Without significant AI, routine open heart surgical technique is employed. When aortic valve incompetence is significant, cardiopulmonary pulmonary bypass is instituted, the patient is cooled, and the aorta is cross clamped before left ventricular distention occurs. The aorta is opened by a curved transverse incision, and cold cardioplegia solution is administered by cannulation of both the coronary ostia under direct vision. The aortic valve is inspected to assess the feasibility of the repair. If the leaflet edges are thickened and retracted or the valve bicuspid, the repair may not be possible; in such cases, aortic valve replacement using a prosthetic valve is required. When the leaflets are pliable and coapt readily, the repair is performed as reported by Trusler et al.[5] The prolapsed leaflet, usually the right, is inspected and measured with particular attention to the length and appearance of the free margin and the formation and competence of each commissure. If the prolapse is severe and the free margin is severely elongated, the valve leaflet is plicated at both commissures. If, however, the prolapse is less severe and the free edge only slightly elongated, then plication at one commissure will suffice (usually at the shallow and less formed commissure). Plication at this site will deepen the commissure and eliminate the weak portion of the leaflet. The pulmonary artery is dissected free from the aorta when the commissure between the right and left leaflets is repaired to facilitate the repair and protect the pulmonary artery and the pulmonic valve. A 5.0 stay suture is placed through the corpora arantii of the two normal leaflets and the future central point of the redundant leaflet. This stitch (Frater stitch)[19] helps align the central point of the leaflets. The length of the free margin of the redundant leaflet is then easily adjusted to mimic that of the two normal leaflets. The excess amount of the leaflet is tacked to the adjacent leaflet at the commissure with fine, nonabsorbable sutures. The excess leaflet tissue is folded or plicated, and the commissure is then secured to the aortic wall with one or two permanent mattress sutures bolstered with Teflon felt pledgets (Fig. 9.4). Adequacy of the repair is ascertained by irrigating the valve with saline under direct vision. Final evaluation is not feasible until after aortotomy closure and unclamping the aorta in the beating heart. After closure of the aortotomy, the aortic clamp is temporarily released and the valve repair is inspected through the VSD (via right ventriculotomy) for any residual aortic incompetence. When necessary, an identical plication is performed at the second commissure. The VSD is closed by using a Dacron patch for further annular support.

An alternate technique of aortic valvuloplasty is described by Spencer et al.[4] This technique differs by plicating the excessive right cusp length into the commissure rather than through the adjacent aortic wall (Fig. 9.5). Simple

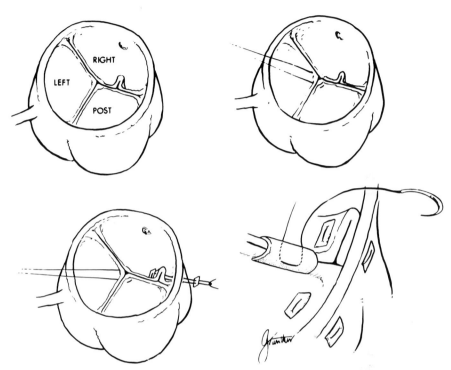

FIGURE 9.4 Diagram of aortic valve. The Trusler repair. *Top left:* Elongated free margin of the prolapsed leaflet. *Top right:* Sutures in the corpora arantii allowing accurate coaptation of the leaflets. *Bottom left:* The excess valve leaflet sandwiched against aortic wall by pledgetted mattress sutures. *Bottom right:* Commissure reinforced with hood of fine Dacron.

plication of the free margin of the redundant leaflet to form a pleat has also been tried with success. In general, shortening of the cusp free margin is adequate and tailoring of the body of the prolapsed leaflet is not necessary.

Van Praagh and McNamara[20] have reported abnormal commissures to be common, especially with infracristal septal defects. These changes include a widened commissure, an abnormally low cusp attachment, or commissural adhesions restricting mobility. Correction of such abnormalities must be entertained as part of the valvuloplasty. Partly obliterating the commissure by pledget reinforced sutures at the cusp margins has been successful.

The success of repair can be assessed by comparing the severity of the aortic diastolic murmur, pulse pressure, heart size (cardiothoracic ratio), aortography, and doppler echocardiography with that prior to surgery. Stress testing in the older patients will also help assess improvement in cardiac function and exercise tolerance.

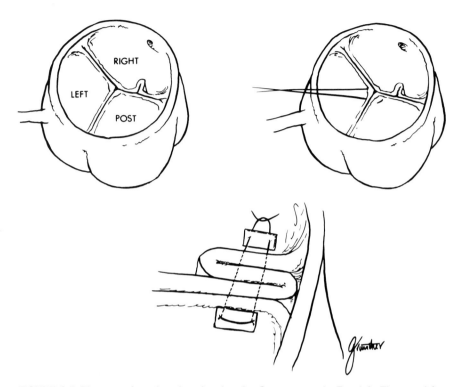

FIGURE 9.5 Diagram of aortic valve showing the Spencer repair. *Top left:* Elongated free margin of the prolapsed leaflet. *Top right:* Sutures in corpora arantii allowing for accurate coaptation of the central point of the leaflets. *Bottom:* Horizontal pledgetted mattress sutures placed through plicated redundant leaflet and adjoining normal leaflet.

ST. CHRISTOPHER'S HOSPITAL FOR CHILDREN EXPERIENCE

Seventeen children have undergone repair of VSD with aortic valve incompetence at our institution. This group includes 10 males and seven females ranging in age from 18 months to 14 years. Thirteen patients (76%) had supracristal VSDs while four (24%) had infracristal VSDs. In general, the supracristal VSDs were larger in size, averaging 12–15 mm in diameter; the infracristal VSDs were about 5–7 mm in diameter. The aortic valve insufficiency was assessed before operation as mild in six patients, moderate in nine, and severe in one. While one patient had no valvular insufficiency in spite of significant valve leaflet prolapse.

Right coronary cusp prolapse was the most common, being noted in 14 of 17 patients, while three patients had prolapse of their noncoronary cusp. Six of the 17 patients had additionally infundibular pulmonic stenosis of the mild to moderate severity present.

Thirteen patients (76%) required no aortic valve repair and after operation their AI has not progressed; in three patients their AI even reduced in magnitude. Four others underwent aortic valvuloplasty for aortic incompetence. Two of these four patients underwent subsequent aortic valve replacement at 4 months and 13 years after operation, respectively, for progression of their aortic insufficiencies. All but two patients had their VSD closed with a Dacron patch.

Our follow-up observations, which ranged from 3 months to 180 months, showed 15 of the 17 patients (88%) to have good results. Chest x-rays of these patients showed cardiomegaly to regress to the extent that heart size was normal in all but the two patients who still had mild cardiomegaly. The two patients with Björk-Shiley prosthesis remain on anticoagulation therapy and have shown no hemodynamic deterioration.

REFERENCES

1. Laubry C, Pezzi C. Traite des maladies carpentales du cocur. In Laubrey C, Routier D, Soulie P (eds): Les souffles de (a maladie de Roger). Rev Med Paris 1933;50:439.
2. Garamella JJ, Cruz AB, Heupel WH, et al. Ventricular septal defect with aortic insufficiency: successful surgical correction of both defects by transaortic approach. Am J Cardiol 1960;5:266.
3. Starr A, Menasche V, Dotter D. Surgical correction of aortic insufficiency associated with ventricular septal defect. Surg Gynecol Obstet 1960;111:71.
4. Spencer FC, Doyle EF, Danielowicz DA, et al. Long-term evaluation of aortic valvuloplasty for aortic insufficiency and ventricular septal defect. J Thorac Cardiovasc Surg 1973;65:15.
5. Trusler GA, Moes CAF, Kidd BSL. Repair of ventricular septal defect with aortic insufficiency. J Thorac Cardiovasc Surg 1973;66:394.
6. Tatsuno K, Konno S, Ando M, Sakakibara S. Pathogenetic mechanisms of prolapsing aortic valve and aortic regurgitation associated with ventricular septal defect. Circulation 1973;48:1028.
7. Chung KJ, Manning JA. Ventricular septal defect associated with aortic insufficiency: medical and surgical management. Am Heart J 1974;87:435.
8. Kawashima Y, Danno M, Shimizu Y, et al. Ventricular septal defect associated with aortic insufficiency: Anatomic classification and method of operation. Circulation 1973;47:1057.
9. Kirklin J, Barratt-Boyes B. Cardiac Surgery. John Wiley & Sons, New York, 1986, pp 65.
10. Edwards JE, Burchell HB. The pathologic anatomy of deficiencies between aortic root and the heart including aortic sinus aneurysm. Thorax 1957;12:125.
11. Momma K, Toyama K, Takao A, et al. Natural history of subarterial infundibular ventricular septal defect. Am Heart J 1984;108:1312.
12. Hallidie-Smith KA, Hollman A, Cleland WP, et al. Effects of surgical closure of ventricular septal defects upon pulmonary vascular disease. Br Heart J 1969;31:246.

13. Menahen S, Johns JA, Del Torso S, et al. Evaluation of aortic valve prolapse in ventricular septal defect. Br Heart J 1986;56:242.

14. Ellis FH Jr, Ongley PA, Kirklin JW. Ventricular septal defect with aortic valvular incompetence: Surgical considerations. Circulation 1963;27:789.

15. Plauth WH Jr, Braunwald E, Rockoff SD, et al. Ventricular septal defect and aortic regurgitation: clinical, haemodynamic and surgical considerations. Am J Med 1965;39:552.

16. Gonzalez-Levin L, Barrett-Boyes BG. Surgical considerations in the treatment of ventricular septal defect associated with aortic valvular incompetence. J Thorac Cardiovasc Surg 1969;57:422.

17. Somerville J, Brandao A, Ross DN. Aortic regurgitation with ventricular septal defect: surgical management and clinical features. Circulation 1970;41:317.

18. Karpawich PP, Duff DF, Cooley DA, et al. Ventricular septal defect with associated aortic valve insufficiency: progression of insufficiency and operative results in young children. J Thorac Cardiovasc Surg 1981;82:182.

19. Frater RWM. The prolapsing aortic cusp: Experimental and clinical observations. Ann Thor Surg 1967;(Jan)3:63.

20. Van Praagh R, McNamara JJ. Anatomic types of ventricular septal defect with aortic insufficiency: diagnostic and surgical considerations. Am Heart J 1968;75:604.

Section II

THE PULMONARY VALVE

CHAPTER 10

Pulmonary and Subpulmonary Stenosis — An Anatomic Approach

Robert H. Anderson, MD, FRC Path,
Simcha Milo, MD,
James R. Zuberbuhler, MD, FACC, and
Siew Yen Ho, PhD

SUMMARY

In this chapter we discuss the anatomic substrates for so-called isolated pulmonary stenosis and then consider the morphology of subpulmonary stenosis in the setting of tetralogy of Fallot. To set the scene, we commence with an account of the normal valve, emphasizing the semilunar attachments of its leaflets and the presence of the commissural ring between the pulmonary sinuses and the tubular trunk. Isolated stenosis can occur within the apical trabecular component of the right ventricle, at the muscular infundibulum, within the valve complex or at supravalvar level. Valve stenosis is by far the commonest. Most usually it is of domed variety produced by commissural fusion. The other well-recognized variant is dysplasia of the valve leaflets. We describe a third and less recognized variant, namely an hour-glass constriction at the commissural ring with dilation of the valve sinuses.

Tetralogy of Fallot is produced because of anterocephalad deviation of the outlet septum so that it is attached above and beyond the extensive septomarginal trabeculation. We define precisely our understanding of these muscle structures along with the ventriculo-infundibular fold. The subpulmonary stenosis, which is an integral part of the lesion, exists primarily because of the displacement of the outlet septum. This is exacerbated by hypertrophy of the septoparietal trabeculations. We discuss the notion that the subpulmonary infundibulum is "too short, too narrow and too shallow," and we show that this is not the case. Valve lesions usually coexist with the subpulmonary obstruction. In this respect we focus attention upon valve stenosis and so-called absence of the leaflets.

INTRODUCTION

In this chapter we will discuss stenosis of the pulmonary outflow tract in the usually constructed heart along with subpulmonary stenosis in the setting of tetralogy of Fallot. To set the scene for understanding the morphology of all these lesions, we must first discuss the anatomy of the normal valve, which is not as simple as it might seem. It is fallacious to consider the valve as possessing an annulus or ring in the sense of a collagenous structure encircling the right ventricular outflow tract in a single plane. Instead, the pulmonary valve leaflets are supported from beneath by the complete muscular cone of the right ventricular outflow tract and from above by the fibrous sinuses of Valsalva in the pulmonary trunk. It is more appropriate, therefore, to think of the pulmonary valve as a complex arrangement of rings and triangles (Fig. 10.1).

The leaflets are attached in scalloped fashion to the ventricular muscle

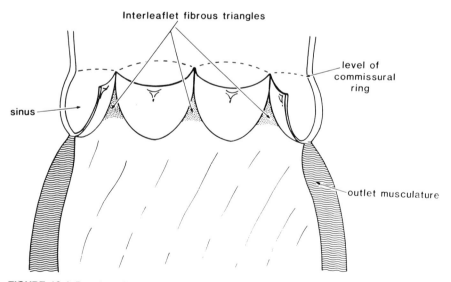

FIGURE 10.1 Drawing showing the complex arrangement of the pulmonary valve with the semilunar attachments of the leaflets to the outlet musculature of the right ventricle. Note the site of the interleaflet triangles and the position of the intercommissural ring.

in their proximal part but to the arterial wall at their commissural zenith. Three contoured triangles are therefore found between the nadir of each leaflet attachment extending up to the commissural zenith. The proximal parts of these triangles are all made of muscle, but the commissural tip extends out onto the fibrous arterial wall. Virtually all of the inferior support mechanism is a free-standing tube which is potentially in communication with the pericardial cavity. All of this area can be removed without entering the left ventricle. In the normal heart it is incorrect to think of the outlet component of the muscular septum extending out to support and separate the pulmonary and aortic valve leaflets (Fig. 10.2; see also Chapter 1).

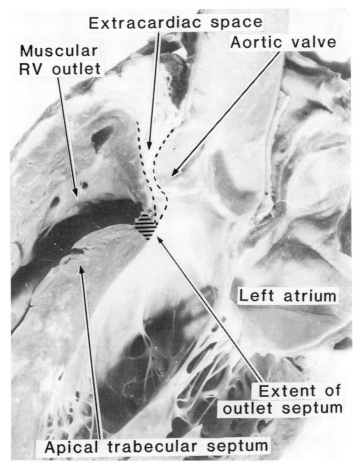

FIGURE 10.2 A cross-section showing the tissue plane separating the muscular outlet component of the right ventricle from the subaortic outflow tract. Very little of the septum is a true "outlet septum."

The sinuses of the pulmonary trunk support the leaflets in reciprocal fashion, rising to the commissures where they constrict at the pulmonary bar. The bar is the most obvious annular formation in the valve complex, linking as it does the three triangularly spaced commissures (Fig. 10.3). The opening area of the leaflets is also triangular when at the half-open point. Because the free edges of the leaflets are longer than the intercommissural segments of the circumference of the pulmonary trunk, however, the normal leaflets are able to open fully to the periphery and approximate to the commissural ring.

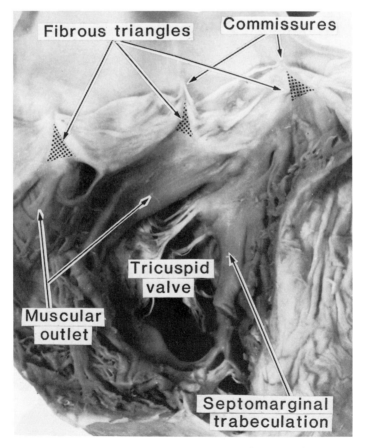

FIGURE 10.3 The outflow tract of the right ventricle opened to show the complex arrangement of the pulmonary valve, illustrated diagramatically in Figure 1.

"ISOLATED" PULMONARY STENOSIS

We use the term "isolated" in the sense that these lesions can be found as isolated lesions. They can also be found in association with other malformations that do not affect the stenotic lesion itself, and the remainder of the heart may be and usually is abnormal even when the lesion does exist in "isolation." The term must therefore be used cautiously in a clinical setting while remaining appropriate in this anatomic setting. Isolated lesions can be found at various levels within the usually constructed outflow tract of the right ventricle. They may occur within the apical trabecular component; at the level of the muscular outflow component or may be due to lesions of the valve leaflets. Stenosis can also exist within the pulmonary trunk and its branches ("supravalve" stenosis). The more peripheral of the supravalvar lesions have been extensively studied by Gay et al[1]; we will not discuss them further.

Stenosis within the Apical Trabecular Component

This is the substrate of the so-called "two-chamber right ventricle." Usually the obstruction coexists with a ventricular septal defect, but it can occur in isolation. There are two anatomic potentials that produce potential obstruction. It is always difficult when examining autopsy specimens to be sure if the potentially obstructive lesion had produced an hemodynamic disturbance in life, hence the use of the term potentially obstructive. The more frequent lesion observed anatomically is a thick and prominent septoparietal trabeculation that spans the junction of the apical trabecular and outlet components (Fig. 10.4). Previously this anomalous muscle bundle (a better term than two-chambered ventricle) has been described as a free-standing septal or moderator band. If so, it would be expected to carry the right bundle branch.

The studies of Byrum et al[2] militate against this possibility. In most instances, therefore, the hypertrophied muscle is likely to be one of the series of septoparietal trabeculations[3] that are always found in the normal heart. The obstruction produced by such an hypertrophied trabeculation is unlikely to be great. Stenosis is more severe when the effect of the trabeculation is excacerbated by formation of an apical muscle shelf. It is the presence of the shelf together with an anomalous muscle bundle that produces the more obvious two-chambered right ventricle.[4,5] The anatomic feature of most concern to the surgeon is the possibility that the tension apparatus of the tricuspid valve takes origin from the inlet aspect of the muscle shelf. If this is the case, then great care is needed if the shelf is to be excised.

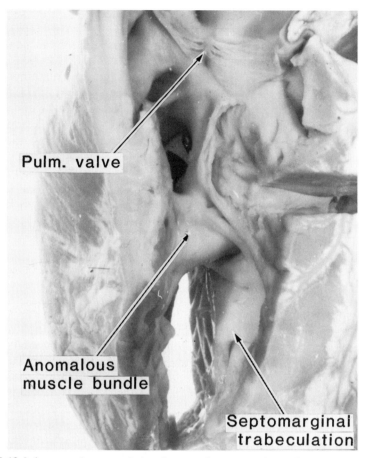

Pulm. valve

Anomalous muscle bundle

Septomarginal trabeculation

FIGURE 10.4 An anomalous muscle bundle extending across the outflow tract of the right ventricle and potentially producing obstruction. The bundle is a hypertrophied septoparietal trabeculation.

Muscular Infundibular Obstruction

Isolated obstruction in the immediate subvalvar area of the right ventricle is more usually found in the setting of a ventricular septal defect. As discussed in the introduction, when the septum is normally formed the outlet septum is an insignificant structure. Infundibular obstruction is then most usually seen in association with valve stenosis. In presence of a septal defect, however, the outlet septum achieves its own identity; this is even more pronounced in the setting of tetralogy of Fallot (see below). With a septal defect, therefore, the outlet septum is more likely to become hypertrophied and contribute to tubular outflow tract obstruction. Should the septal defect then become closed, the tubular muscular obstruction will seem to be isolated. In the extensive experience of Rowe,[6] most examples of such "isolated" obstruction were considered to be existing in the setting of a closed ventricular septal defect, and our experience endorses his.

Valvar Pulmonary Stenosis

Unlike the aortic valve, significant pulmonary stenosis occurs most usually with a trifoliate arrangement. Bifoliate valves can become stenotic (Fig. 10.5) and are frequent in the setting of tetralogy of Fallot (see below). Isolated bifoliate stenosis, however, is rare in pulmonary position; also rare is the unicuspid, unicommissural variety found with some frequency in the aorta. Of more significance in the pulmonary valve is the precise morphology of the stenotic leaflets. Dome-shaped stenosis[7,8] and dysplastic leaflets[9,10] are well recognized variants. More recently, Milo et al[11] have highlighted a further type that they term the hour-glass deformity with bottle-shaped sinuses.

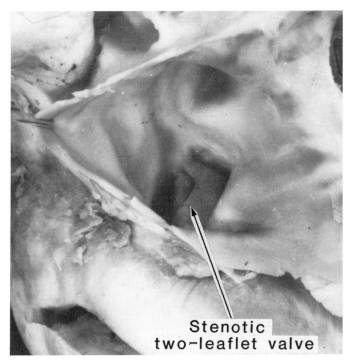

Stenotic
two-leaflet valve

FIGURE 10.5 The rare finding of an obstructive bifoliate valve in pulmonary position in an otherwise normal heart.

The dome-shaped variant is the commonest. This results from fusion of the leaflets; initially at the commissures. As the leaflet fusion extends centripetally, the initially triangular opening becomes converted into a stenotic circle that protrudes superiorly into the pulmonary trunk. In most valves it is possible to recognize evidence of the initial commissural sites (Fig. 10.6). In some hearts, however (particularly those presenting with pin-hole openings in the neonatal period), the surface of the dome is smoother with little evidence of the initial commissures. The sinuses are of normal size and the commissural ring is of normal diameter. It is usually an easy matter to divide the commissures at surgery (Fig. 10.7). This is also the variety of valve stenosis that lends itself most readily to balloon dilatation (Fig. 10.8).

Stenosis due to dysplastic leaflets is now well recognized. It occurs most frequently in Noonan's syndrome but the association is not complete. The leaflets are thickened by cauliflowerlike excresences on their surfaces composed of firm myxomatous material (Fig. 10.9). Unlike in the dome-shaped valve, the dysplastic valve is not characterized by commissural fusion. It is usually necessary to remove part or all of the dysplastic valve tissue so as to achieve an unobstructed outflow into the pulmonary trunk. Dyplastic valves are often accompanied by secondary hypertrophy of the muscular outflow tract that may require surgical excision.[11]

The third variety of valve stenosis is less well-recognized, but was

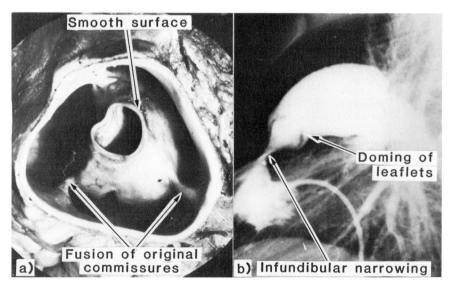

FIGURE 10.6 The more usual anatomy of pulmonary valve stenosis is found in the setting of a domed trifoliate valve. The angiogram in **b** is from a different patient.

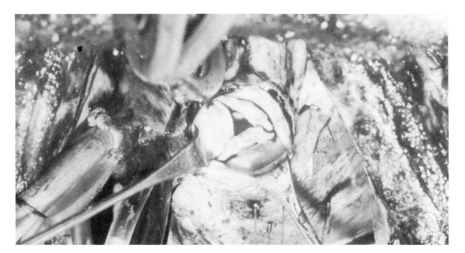

FIGURE 10.7 Division of the commissures of an initially domed and stenotic pulmonary valve at the conclusion of successful surgery. (Reproduced by kind permission of Dr. Benson R. Wilcox, University of North Carolina, Chapel Hill.)

present in seven of the 39 patients recently studied by Milo et al.[11] The essential anatomic feature was an hour-glass constriction at the level of the commissural ring (Fig. 10.10). This effectively narrows down the distal openings of the sinuses of Valsalva to the pulmonary trunk. The sinuses themselves are dilated and bottle-shaped, while poststenotic dilation of the pulmonary trunk itself further enhances the hour-glass effect (Fig. 10.11). The thickening of the commissural bar also extends onto the free edge of the leaflets, which are considerably shorter than normal. The leaflets themselves are thickened. Angiographic recognition of this variety and distinction from the other types was an easy matter (Fig. 10.12).[11] Although not described as a separate entity prior to the account of Milo et al,[11] cases have been illustrated that correspond to this hour glass variant.[10,12] The previous cases have been said to have supravalve stenosis, but anatomically the commissural bar is an integral part of the valve complex. Recognition is important because excision of the shortened free edges of the leaflets permits the commissural area to dilate to its usual size.[11]

SUBPULMONARY STENOSIS IN TETRALOGY OF FALLOT

The essence of the subpulmonary stenosis that is the hallmark of tetralogy of Fallot is anterocephalad deviation of the septal insertion of the outlet septum such that it is attached above and in front of the septomarginal trabecula-

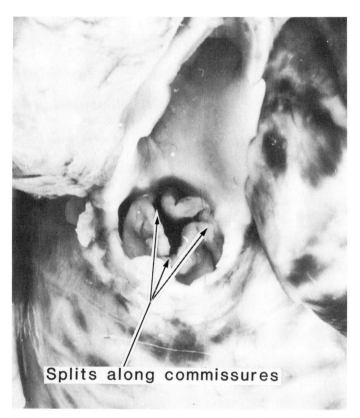

Splits along commissures

FIGURE 10.8 Similar division of the commissures of an initially stenotic pulmonary valve, produced in this example by balloon valvoplasty. The patient died from causes unrelated to the valvar procedure.

tion.[13,14] To be sure of precision in making this description, we must first define exactly what we mean by the outlet septum, the septomarginal trabe-culation, and so on. Previously, considerable confusion has arisen from the failure to define precisely the muscular boundaries of the ventricular septal defect and the subpulmonary outflow tract. By the *outlet septum*, we mean the extensive muscular structure that, in tetralogy of Fallot, divides the subpulmonary and subaortic outflow tracts of the right ventricle and that supports the facing leaflets of the arterial valves (Figs. 10.13 and 10.14). Previously we suggested that the outlet septum formed an integral part of the subpulmonary infundibulum in the normal right ventricle.[13]

Careful dissection (see Fig. 10.2) indicates this not to be the case. The so-called supraventricular crest of the normal right ventricle forms the floor

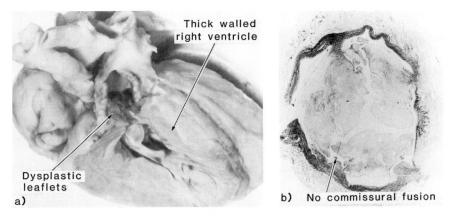

FIGURE 10.9 A dysplastic (**a**) and stenotic (**b**) pulmonary valve. Note the lack of commissural fusion.

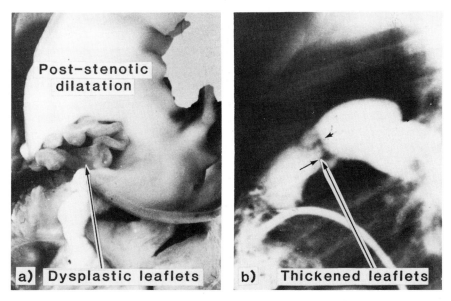

FIGURE 10.10 A further example of a dysplastic pulmonary valve (**a**) together with a typical angiogram (**b**) from a different patient.

112

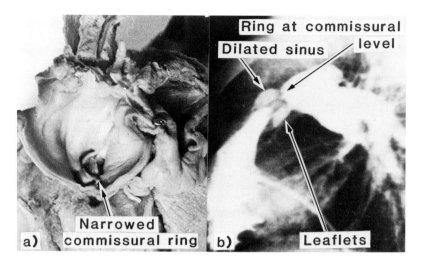

FIGURE 10.11 Photographs of an autopsy example (**a**) and an angiogram (**b**) showing hourglass stenosis at the level of the commissures of the pulmonary valve with dilation of the sinuses.

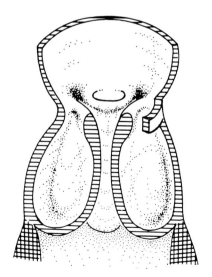

FIGURE 10.12 A drawing showing the basic arrangement of hour-glass pulmonary stenosis with dilation of the sinuses.

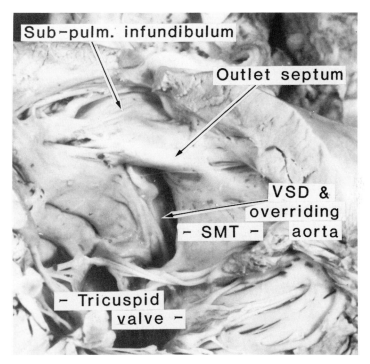

Sub-pulm. infundibulum

Outlet septum

VSD &
overriding
- SMT -   aorta

- Tricuspid
valve -

FIGURE 10.13 The extensive outlet septum found in tetralogy of Fallot as seen in a specimen opened through the parietal wall of the right ventricle.

of the transverse sinus of the pericardium. The subpulmonary infundibulum can be completely removed from the remainder of the right ventricle without entering the cavity of the left ventricle. The muscular structure forming the supraventricular crest, which separates the tricuspid and pulmonary valves, is the ventriculo-infundibular fold.[15] The morphology of this fold is disturbed in tetralogy because the aortic valve has (to greater or lesser extent) a right ventricular origin in addition to its usual left ventricular connection.

In tetralogy, therefore, the ventriculo-infundibular fold separates the tricuspid valve from the right ventricular segment of the aortic valve circumferential and provides the anchor for the parietal attachment of the outlet septum (Figs. 10.13 and 10.14). The septomarginal trabeculation, or septal band, is extensive septal trabeculation of the normal right ventricle that extends towards the apex, supports the anterior papillary muscle of the tricuspid valve, and spans the ventricular cavity as the moderator band. In tetralogy, the septomarginal trabeculation cradles in its limbs the floor of the

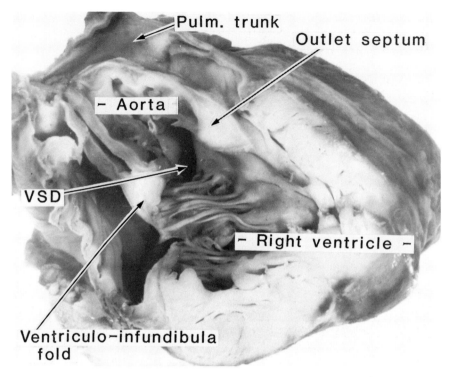

FIGURE 10.14 The morphology of subpulmonary obstruction is tetralogy of Fallot, as shown in a section that replicates an oblique subcostal echocardiographic cut (the right anterior oblique equivalent).

ventricular septal defect. The precise morphology of the postero-inferior rim of the defect depends on the extent of the posterior limb of the septomarginal trabeculation. If this limb fuses with the ventriculo-infundibular fold, the septal defect has a muscular postero-inferior rim. This is unusual, however, occurring in only about one-fifth of cases. More usually the muscular structures fall short of each other and the posterior corner is formed by tricuspid – aortic mitral valve fibrous continuity; in other words the defect is perimembranous.

It follows from the above description that the septomarginal trabeculation has minimal relationship to the subpulmonary outflow tract in tetralogy. This is a possible source of confusion because the "septal band" is often said to be an integral part of the stenotic subpulmonary area. The septal band is this location, however, is not the septomarginal trabeculation, which is nonetheless described in this fashion by Van Praagh[16] and others. The name "septal band" in this position derives from the convention of the Swedish group[17] who defined the outlet septum as the "crista" and then described its septal and parietal extensions. Careful analysis of the subpulmonary muscle bundles in tetralogy, however, shows that the so-called septal band defined angiocardiographically (Fig. 10.15) has nothing to do with either the outlet septum or its attachments. The more anterior of the obstructing muscles is one of a series of hypertrophied septoparietal trabeculations (Fig. 10.16). Thus, the tight ring of subpulmonary obstruction that is the hallmark of tetralogy is formed posteriorly by the outlet septum and its attachments and anteriorly by the parietal ventricular wall buttressed by the hypertrophied septoparietal trabeculations.

It has been claimed that the subpulmonary infundibulum in tetralogy is "too short, too narrow and too shallow."[18] There is no question concerning its narrow width. There is no evidence, however, to support the notion that it

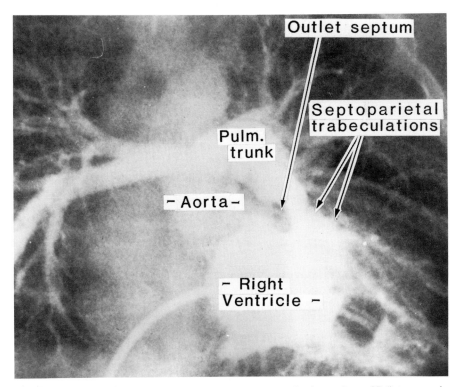

FIGURE 10.15 The morphology of the outflow tract obstruction in tetralogy of Fallot as seen in an oblique right anterior projection of a right ventricular angiogram. (Reproduced by kind permission of Dr. Michael Rigby, Brompton Hospital, London.)

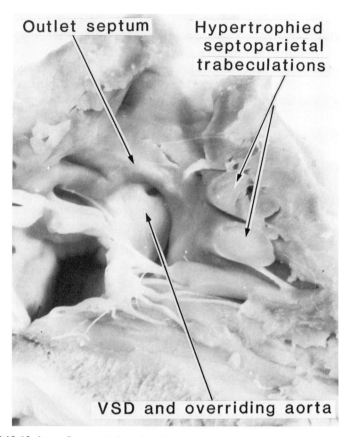

Outlet septum   Hypertrophied
                 septoparietal
                 trabeculations

VSD and overriding aorta

FIGURE 10.16 An outflow tract view showing how a good part of the subpulmonary muscular obstruction found in tetralogy of Fallot is produced by hypertrophy of septoparietal trabeculations.

is too short. Measurements comparing tetralogy with the normal heart showed that the subpulmonary infundibulum was significantly longer in the malformed heart.[13] Sometimes the outlet septum itself may seem short in tetralogy, but most times it is an extensive structure (Fig. 10.17). This variability must then be set against the fact that the outlet septum is virtually indistinguishable from the rest of the septum in the normal heart and plays little part if any in producing the subpulmonary infundibulum.

The subpulmonary stenosis in tetralogy can often be accentuated by hypertrophy of apical trabeculations, including the body of the septomarginal trabeculation. In its extreme form this arrangement can produce a "two-chambered right ventricle." Exacerbation of the stenosis, however, occurs more usually at valvar level. Deformities of the pulmonary valve itself are frequent, often in the setting of a bifoliate valve. A further lesion of the valve leaflets of major significance is their so-called absence. In most cases the leaflets are represented by verrucous rudiments that form a stenotic ring (Fig. 10.18). The major problem is the severe dilation of the pulmonary trunk and its branches. It is the extent of this process of dilation into the lung parenchyma that probably determines the clinical outcome.[19]

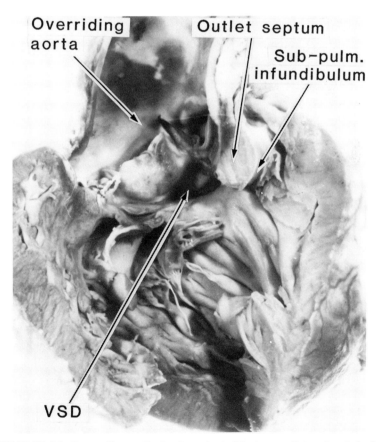

FIGURE 10.17 A further section confirming the extent of the large outlet septum to be found in tetralogy of Fallot.

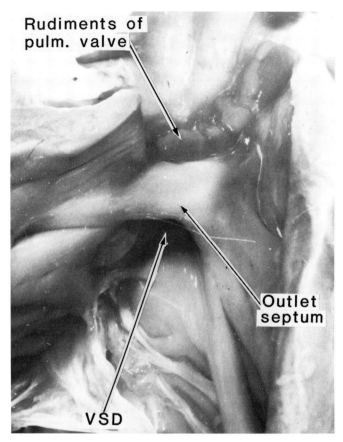

FIGURE 10.18 The rudimentary tissue tags at the anticipated site of attachment of the valve leaflets, which are the anatomic features of so-called absence of the pulmonary valve.

REFERENCES

1. Gay BB, Franch RH, Shuford WH, et al. Roentgenologic features of simple and multiple coarctations of the pulmonary artery and branches. Am J Roentgenol 1963;90:599–613.
2. Byrum CJ, Dick II M, Behrendt DM et al. Excitation of the double chamber right ventricle: electrophysiologic and anatomic correlation. Am J Cardiol 1982;49:1254–1258.
3. Goor DA, Lillehei CW. The anatomy of the heart. In: Congenital Malformations of the Heart. Grune and Stratton, New York, 1975, pp 1–37.
4. Rowland JW, Rosenthal AR, Castenada AR. Double chamber right ventricle: experience with 17 cases. Am Heart J 1975;89;455–462.
5. Restivo A, Cameron AH, Anderson RH, et al. Divided right ventricle: A review of its anatomical varieties. Pediatr Cardiol 1984;5:197–204.

6. Rowe RD. Pulmonary stenosis with normal aortic root. In: Keith JD, Rowe RD, Vlad RD (eds): Heart Disease in Infancy and Childhood. Macmillan, New York, 1978, pp 761–788.

7. Brock R. The Anatomy of Congenital Pulmonary Stenosis. Cassell, London, 1957, pp 114.

8. Castaneda-Zuniga ET, Formanek A, Amplatz K. Radiologic diagnosis of different types of pulmonic stenosis. Cardiovasc Intervent Radiol 1978;1:24–33.

9. Koretzky ED, Moller JH, Korns ME, et al. Congenital pulmonary stenosis resulting from dysplasia of valve. Circulation 1969;40:43–53.

10. Jeffrey RF, Moller JH, Amplatz K. The dysplastic pulmonary valve: a new roentgenographic entity. With discussion of the anatomy and radiology of other types of valvular pulmonary stenosis. Am J Roentgenol Radium Therap Nucl Med 1972;114:322–331.

11. Milo S, Fiegel A, Shem-Tov A, et al. Isolated pulmonic stenosis: anatomical aspects and surgical implications. Br Heart J (submitted for publication).

12. Utley JR, Roe BB. Surgical considerations in obstruction of the right ventricular outflow tract. J Thorac Cardiovasc Surg 1973;65:391–398.

13. Becker AE, Connor M, Anderson RH. Tetralogy of Fallot: a morphometric and geometric study. Am J Cardiol 1975;35:402–412.

14. Anderson RH, Allwork SP, Ho SY, et al. Surgical anatomy of tetralogy of Fallot. J Thor Cardiol Surg 1981;81:887–896.

15. Anderson RH, Becker AE, Van Mierop LHS. What should we call the "crista"?. Br Heart J 1977;39:856–859.

16. Van Praagh R. What is the Taussig-Bing malformation. Circulation 1968;38:445–449.

17. Kjellberg SR, Mannheimer E, Rudhe U, et al. Diagnosis of Congenital Heart Disease, 2nd ed. Year Book Medical Publishers, Chicago. 1959.

18. Van Praagh R, Van Praagh S, Nebesar RA, et al. Tetralogy of Fallot: Underdevelopment of the pulmonary infundibulum and its sequelae. Am J Cardiol 1970;26:25–33.

19. Rabinovitch M, Grady S, David I, et al. Compression of intrapulmonary bronchi by abnormally branching pulmonary arteries associated with absent pulmonary valves. Am J Cardiol 1982;50:804–813.

CHAPTER 11

Evaluation of the Severity of Pulmonary Stenosis and Results of Pulmonary Valve Balloon Angioplasty in Children

Robert M. Freedom, MD, FRCP(C), FACC,
Jeffrey F. Smallhorn, MD, FRACP, FRCP(C),
and Lee N. Benson, MD, FRCP(C), FACC

Obstruction to pulmonary blood flow can occur within the morphologically right ventricle, at pulmonary valve (or annulus) level, or within the pulmonary arterial vascular bed (Fig. 11.1).[1] There is now an extensive literature addressing the morphological nature of these various types of obstruction, and considerable emphasis has been placed on their characteristic angiocardiographic features.[2,3] We will only address, in this chapter, the evolution in our assessment of the severity of valvular pulmonary stenosis (Fig. 11.2) and our preliminary results in percutaneous pulmonary valve balloon angioplasty in children.

Beyond the neonatal period and early infancy, the clinical assessment and electrocardiographic findings may be helpful in the assessment of the severity of isolated pulmonary valvular stenosis. Obvious features of severe pulmonary stenosis are cyanosis indicative of right-to-left shunting at the atrial level, congestive heart failure, or progressive cardiomegaly with tricuspid regurgitation.

In the absence of these parameters of clinically severe pulmonary stenosis, the intensity and length of the systolic ejection murmur, the increasing A_2-P_2 interval, the progressive diminution in the intensity of the pulmonary closure sound, and the shortening of the S_1 click interval are all findings that may be used to predict the severity of right ventricular outflow obstruction.[4-6]

120

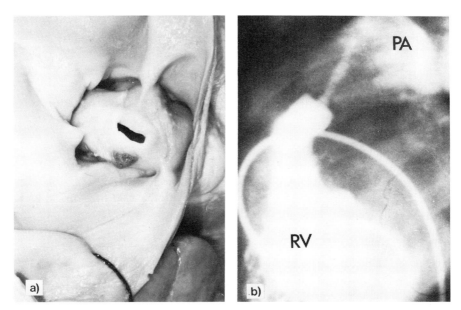

FIGURE 11.1 (a) Appearance of the pulmonary valve from an infant succumbing with critical pulmonary stenosis. **(b)** Lateral right ventriculogram (RV) from an infant with severe pulmonary stenosis. The pulmonary artery (PA) is dilated. Note the jet of contrast medium *(arrow)*.

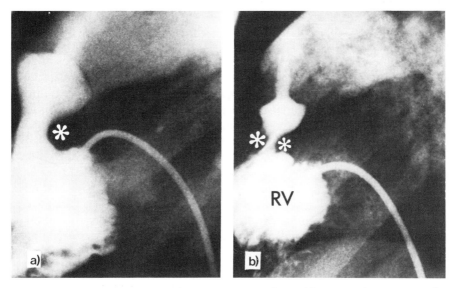

FIGURE 11.2 Lateral right ventriculograms from two patients with severe pulmonary stenosis. Infundibular (*) narrowing is relatively mild in one patient **(a)**, whereas in the other **(b)**, dynamic subpulmonary stenosis is quite severe.

Certain features of the electrocardiogram have also been utilized in the assessment of the severity of isolated valvular pulmonary stenosis.[7-9] These include the magnitude of R wave in V_1 (in millimeters), RV_1 and SV_6, T-wave changes, a wave in V_1, etc. But it is clear from the U.S. Natural History Study that electrocardiographic evidence of right ventricular hypertrophy may not discriminate mild from severe right ventricular hypertrophy.[10] Data derived from the U.S. Natural History Study has been integrated into a multivariant analysis in order to provide better discrimination between mild and severe disease. Several equations were obtained, one using items from the scalar electrocardiogram alone, and one using a combination of clinical and electrocardiographic items to estimate the pressure gradient across the stenotic pulmonary valve. The equation based on clinical and electrocardiographic data obtained from 443 patients (between 2 and 21 years of age) provided reasonable correlation with an R value of 0.83. From the regression equation derived from electrocardiographic items alone, and based on data from 457 patients between 2 and 21 years of age, the correlation between estimated and measured pressure gradient was somewhat poorer, with an R value of 0.77.

Perhaps the newest noninvasive modality in estimating the severity of valvular pulmonary stenosis is the application of pulsed Doppler ultrasound to quantitate transventricular pressure difference.[11-15] There is currently an ample literature validating this technique.

The transventricular pressure difference (P) can be calculated according to a simplified Bernoulli equation: $P = 4 (V_{max})^2$, where V_{max} (in meters per second) is the maximal velocity in the jet. Vasko et al[14] have studied those factors influencing accuracy of in vitro valvular pressure gradient estimates by Doppler ultrasound. Those factors include (*a*) flow rate, (*b*) viscosity, and (*c*) orifice size and shape. Good correlations were obtained between measured and Doppler ultrasound-predicted gradients for triangular orifices of area as small as 78.5 mm, and for circular and elliptical orifices as small as 50.2 mm^2; a poor correlation was found with smaller orifices. No observable differences were found in this study between high and low flow rates; similarly, viscosity had no effect on correlation with Doppler ultrasound-predicted gradient over a wide range of viscosities. Many investigators have stressed the importance of correct alignment of the Doppler ultrasound sample with the poststenotic flow jet. Incorrect measurement of maximal poststenotic flow velocity will, of course, lead to serious underestimation of the transventricular pressure gradient.

Until recently, in most institutions the gold standard for the determination of the severity of pulmonary valvular stenosis has been the invasive recording of the transpulmonary valvular pressure gradient on withdrawal of a catheter (usually fluid filled) from the pulmonary artery to the right ventricle with the patient in a so-called steady state. Cardiac output can be measured using any of a variety of techniques, and then a pulmonary valve area can be calculated and indexed to body surface area.

We validated the utility of Doppler ultrasound-derived transpulmonary valve-pressure gradients in our institution by measuring the Doppler ultrasound-derived pressure gradient in the cardiac catheterization laboratory and then immediately performing a catheter-withdrawal pressure tracing from pulmonary artery to right ventricle. As shown in Figure 11.2, there is an excellent correlation between the invasive and noninvasive techniques ($r = 0.951$). Based on these observations, we are quite confident, then, in the Doppler ultrasound-determination of the pressure gradient across a stenotic pulmonary valve, and based on such a methodology, we are comfortable in recommending intervention to ameliorate the severity of the obstruction.

Since the initial 1980 report by Kan et al[16] on the feasibility and efficacy of percutaneous transluminal balloon angioplasty (BA) in the setting of pulmonary valve stenosis, a number of publications have appeared that reproduce these observations, improve our technical information, and expand on the patient population managed with this procedure.[17-19]

At The Hospital For Sick Children, Toronto, Canada, from January 1984 through April 1985, 14 patients (seven male, seven female) underwent BA for stenosis of the pulmonary valve. Two patients had dysplastic pulmonary valves, one patient had associated left ventricular outflow tract obstruction and had previously undergone a transventricular aortic dilation. The mean age was 5.0 ± 4.5 years (range, 1 month to 15 years) (Table 11.1). For the oldest patient, and first in our series, surgical relief of fixed right ventricular outflow tract obstruction after valvuloplasty was required. A bicuspid pulmonary valve was found, torn to the annulus along the commissure.[20] A second child died as the result of associated cardiac anomalies, despite adequate relief of the right ventricular–pulmonary artery gradient.

TABLE 11.1 Pulmonary Valve Stenosis: Patient Group[a]

Lesions	Number
Isolated pulmonary valve stenosis	11
Dysplastic pulmonary valve	2
Critical left ventricular outflow obstruction, pulmonary valve stenosis	1
Total	14

[a]Seven male, seven female, mean age, 5 ± 4.5 years (1 month–15 years).

TECHNIQUE

Sedation during the procedure was initially achieved with a mixture of demerol/phenergan/thorazine (CM3). In the last seven patients general anesthesia was electively initiated because of the often required additional sedation requirement for frequent catheter changes and patient discomfort. Before the procedure, an echocardiogram and Doppler flow study was performed in which pulmonary annulus size, valve morphology, and valve mobility was determined from short axis, long axis and "*en face*" views.[20] Additionally, the presence of an atrial septal defect and the morphology of the right ventricular outflow tract was outlined.

A 5F dilator is placed percutaneously in the left femoral artery and 7F NIH and end-hole catheters in the right and left femoral veins. Simultaneous right ventricular, pulmonary artery, and femoral artery pressures were recorded; dye curves were obtained (injection in the pulmonary artery and IVC), and oximetry were measured while the patient was breathing room air. An angiogram was performed in the right ventricle in the posterior–anterior/lateral projections, and the pulmonary annulus was measured by using catheter size to correct for magnification. A balloon dilation catheter with a 1-cm tip was chosen in order to not exceed 20%–30% of the annular diameter. A 0.034-in., Teflon-coated guide wire was placed in the left pulmonary artery using the end-hole catheter, placed as distally as possible. The balloon-dilating catheter was inserted over the wire and placed to straddle the pulmonary valve (Fig. 11.3). The balloon was inflated, monitoring developed pressure (in atmospheres) to its maximal tolerance. During the initial phase, one could see an indentation (waist) along the balloon from the stenotic valve; inflation–deflation cycles, lasting no more than 15 second, were repeated until no indentation was seen on the balloon. The right ventricular and femoral artery pressures were continually measured during the procedure (Fig. 11.4).

In patients without intraatrial communications, systemic blood pressure fell during the inflation–deflation cycle. Frequently, the right ventricular pressure remained elevated after the BA, while the deflated balloon catheter remained across the outflow tract. This reflects the often-observed hypercontractile nature of the infundibular after the procedure (Fig. 11.5) and the obstruction to outflow by the catheter. Upon removal of the balloon, with the wire in place, reduction in right ventricular pressures was then observed. If the right ventricular pressure was still elevated upon balloon withdrawal, a Doppler flow study was performed to determine if the pressure gradient was at valve or subvalvular level. If a gradient persisted across the valve, a larger balloon (again, not to exceed 30% of the diameter of the valve annulus) was placed across the valve and the dilatation repeated. A repeat

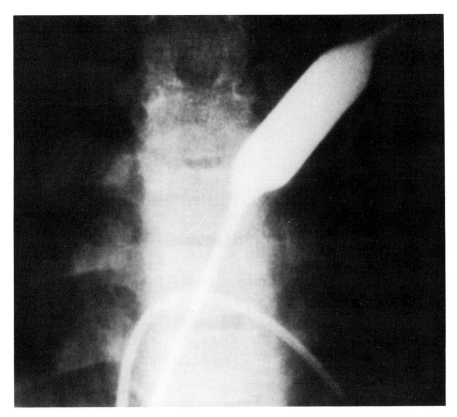

FIGURE 11.3 An 18-mm diameter balloon inflated while straddling the pulmonary valve. Note the guide wire projecting beyond the catheter tip into the left pulmonary artery.

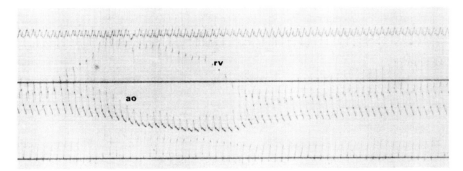

FIGURE 11.4 Simultaneous aortic (*ao*) and right ventricular (*rv*) pressures during a typical inflation-deflation cycle. Heart rate is not affected, and systemic pressure rapidly increases upon deflation of the balloon.

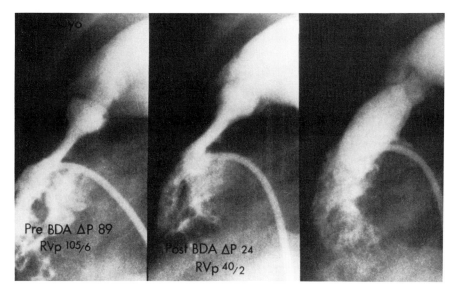

FIGURE 11.5 Predilatation and postdilatation right ventricular angiograms. A domed pulmonary valve is apparent with an 89-torr gradient. Systolic and diatolic frames after the procedure, gradient 24 torr. Note the hypercontractile right ventricular outflow tract.

right ventricular angiogram (Fig. 11.6) was performed in the posterior–anterior/lateral projections and cardiac output measured by dye curves from the pulmonary artery to aorta. Fluoroscopy time averaged 28.4 ± 13 minutes (range, 7–59 minutes).

In the patient group, managed in this manner, the mean right ventricular pressure was 93 ± 24 torr and fell acutely (60%) to 56 ± 22 torr ($P<0.05$). The pulmonary artery pressure remained unchanged, the gradient falling 46% from 75 ± 26 torr to 34 ± 20 torr ($P < 0.0005$) (Table 11.2 and Fig. 11.7).

COMMENTS

Clearly, a substantial reduction in pulmonary valve gradient is possible with this technique. It appears to be safe, provided simple precautions are taken. The pulmonary annulus is fairly resistent to distention and is damaged little.[21] The major damage appears in the right ventricular outflow tract where subendocardial hemorrhages occur, varying in severity with balloon size. Damage appears "minor" if balloon sizes no greater than 30% of the annulus diameter are used. Whether these minor areas of hemorrhage can become sites for dysrhythmias in the future has not become a clinically

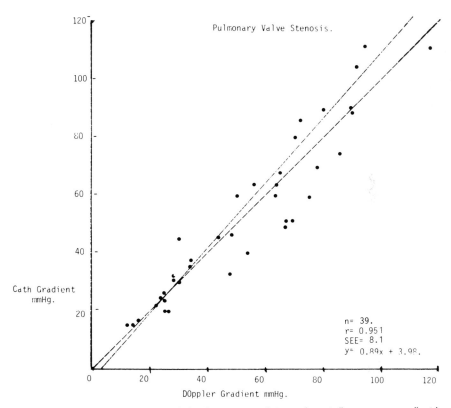

FIGURE 11.6 Graph showing correlation between peak to peak systolic pressure gradient in valvular pulmonary stenosis with Doppler derived gradient.

TABLE 11.2 Hemodynamic Data

	Predilatation (torr)	Postdilatation (torr)
Right ventricular systolic pressure[a]	93 ± 24	56 ± 22
Pulmonary artery systolic pressure	16 ± 5.5	21 ± 9.2
Gradient[b]	75 ± 26	34 ± 20

[a]Reduced 60% ($P < 0.05$).
[b]Reduced 46% ($P < 0.005$).

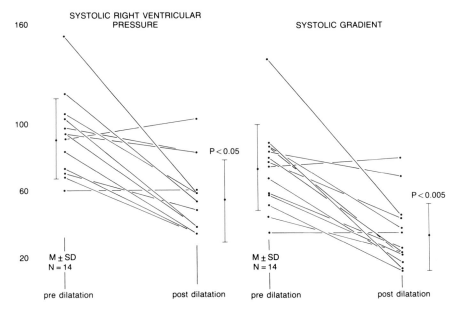

FIGURE 11.7 Graphs showing change in right ventricular pressure and systolic pressure gradient subsequent to pulmonary valve balloon angioplasty.

important issue in the patients having undergone valvuloplasty, although long-term studies are not available. From our echocardiographic studies, the mechanism of valve disruption in the majority of cases was rupture along the commissures toward the annulus. Two patients in our series had flail leaflets, both initially tricuspid. Pulmonary insufficiency has not been an important problem, most often only with Doppler evidence of its presence.

Development of severe infundibular obstruction was observed in one patient after a seemingly successful percutaneous pulmonary balloon valvuloplasty.[22] Prior to angioplasty, the patient, a 14-month-old infant, had a right ventricular pressure of 105 mm Hg, compared with a simultaneous peak systolic aortic pressure of 80 mm Hg. Immediately after the balloon angioplasty, the right ventricular pressure had increased to 180 mm Hg and to 214 mm Hg following day, coincident with angiographic evidence of progressively severe infundibular obstruction. This patient was taken to surgery where inspection of the pulmonary valve showed satisfactory valvuloplasty. Whether or not such severe postvalvuloplasty infundibular obstruction would regress without surgical intervention is unclear, but it is possible.[23,24]

In summary, early studies on the application of this technique in the setting of pulmonary valve stenosis appears efficacious and readily applicable. Although the youngest patient in our institution to undergo pulmonary balloon angioplasty was 1 month old, others have applied this technique to the younger neonate.[25] This approach in the critically ill neonate certainly warrants critical study. The impact of this technique on the severity of this lesion in which it is applied will stimulate considerable debate. At present, surgical candidates have been primarily the population to undergo valvuloplasty. What would be the clinical course of those patients with resting gradients in the mild to moderate range is an area for further thought.

ADDENDUM

Since preparation of this manuscript, more than 100 infants and children have undergone percutaneous pulmonary valve angioplasty. Among those older children with larger pulmonary valve annuli, we performed the dilatation procedure with two dilating catheters. More than 95% have had a good clinical response.

REFERENCES

1. Emmanouilides GC, Baylen BG. Pulmonary stenosis. In, Adams FH, Emmanouilides GC (eds): Moss' Heart Disease in Infants, Children, and Adolescents, 3rd ed. Williams & Wilkins, Baltimore, 1983, pp 234–250.
2. Freedom RM, Culham JAG, Moes CAF. Angiocardiography in Congenital Heart Disease. MacMillan New York, 1984, p 222–230.
3. Restivo A, Cameron AH, Anderson RH, Allwork SP. Divided right ventricle: a review of it's anatomical varieties. Pediatr Cardiol 1984;5:197–204.
4. Perloff JK. The clinical recognition of congenital heart disease. WB Saunders, Philadelphia, 1978, p 185–221.
5. Leatham A, Weitzman D. Auscultatory and phonocardiographic signs of pulmonary stenosis. Br Heart J 1957;19:303–310.
6. Vogelpoel I, Schrire V. Auscultatory and phonocardiographic assessment of pulmonary stenosis with intact ventricular septum. Circulation 1960;22:55–72.
7. DePasquale N, Burch GE. The electrocardiogram and ventricular gradient in isolated congenital pulmonary stenosis. Circulation 1960;21:181–187.
8. Bassingthwaite JB, Parkin TW, Duschane JW, Wood EH, Burchell HB. The electrocardiographic and hemodynamic findings in pulmonary stenosis with intact ventricular septum. Circulation 1963;28:897–905.
9. Cayler GG, Ongley PA, Nadas AS. Relation of systolic pressure in right ventricle to the electrocardiogram. A study of patients with pulmonary stenosis and intact ventricular septum. N Engl J Med 1958;258:979–982.
10. Report from the Joint Study of the Natural History of Congenital Heart Defects. Nadas AS (ed). Circulation 1977;56:14–20.
11. Lima CO, Sahn DJ, Valdes-Cruz LM, Goldberg SJ, Barron JV, Allen HD, Grenadier E.

Non-invasive precution of transvalvular pressure gradient in patients with pulmonary stenosis by quantitative two-dimensional echocardiographic Doppler studies. Circulation 1983;67:866–871.

12. Stamm RB, Martin RP. 1983 Quantification of pressure gradients across stenotic valves by Doppler ultrasound. J Am Coll Cardiol 1983;2:707–718.

13. Kosturaksis D, Allen HD, Goldberg SJ, Sahn DJ, Valdes-Cruz LM. Non-invasive quantification of stenotic semilunar valve areas by Doppler echocardiography. J Am Coll Cardiol 1984;3:1256–1262.

14. Vasco SD, Goldberg SJ, Requarth JA, Allen HD. Factors affecting accuracy of in vitro valvar pressure gradient estimates by Doppler ultrasound. Am J Cardiol 1984;54:893–896.

15. Teien R, Eriksson P. Quantification of transvalvular pressure differences with aortic stenosis by Doppler ultrasound. Int J Cardiol 1985;7:121–126.

16. Kan JS, White RI Jr, Mitchell SE, Gardner TJ. Percutaneous balloon valvuloplasty: a new method for treating congnital pulmonary valve stenosis. N Engl J Med 1982;307:540–542.

17. Lababidi Z, Wu J. Percutaneous balloon valvuloplasty. Am J Cardiol 1983;52:560–562.

18. Pepine CJ, Gessner IH, Feldman RL. Percutaneous balloon valvuloplasty for pulmonic valve stenosis in the adult. Am J Cardiol 1982;50:1442–1445.

19. Kan JS, White RI, Mitchell SE, Anderson JH, Gardner TJ. Percutaneous transluminal balloon valvuloplasty for pulmonary stenosis. Circulation 1983;69:554–560.

20. Benson LN, Smallhorn JS, Freedom RM, Trusler GA, Rowe RD. Pulmonary valve morphology after balloon dilatation of pulmonary valve stenosis. Cath Cardiovasc Diagn 1985;11:161–166.

21. Ring JC, Kulik TJ, Burke BA, Lock JE. Morphological changes induced by dilatation of the pulmonary valve annulus with over-large balloon in normal newborn lambs. Am J Cardiol 1985;55:210–214.

22. Ben-Shachar G, Cohen MH, Sivakoff MC, Portman MA. Riemendchneider TA, Van Heeckeren DW. Development of infundibular obstruction after percutaneous pulmonary balloon valvuloplasty. J Am Coll Cardiol 1985;5:754–756.

23. Engle MA, Holswade GR, Goldberg HP, Lukas DS, Glenn F. Regression after open valvotomy of infundibular stenosis accompanying severe valvular pulmonic stenosis. Circulation 1958;17:862–873.

24. Shuck JW, McCormick DJ, Cohen IS, Oetgen WJ, Brinker JA. Percutaneous balloon valvuloplasty of the pulmonary valve. Role of right to left shunting through a patent foramen ovale. J Am Coll Cardiol 1984;4:132–135.

25. Tynan M, Jones O, Joseph MC, Deverall PB, Yates AK. Relief of pulmonary valve stenosis in first week of life by percutaneous balloon valvuloplasty. Lancet 1984;Feb4:273.

CHAPTER 12

Pulmonary Insufficiency After Repair of Tetralogy of Fallot
Early Results

Albert D. Pacifico, MD

Some patients with tetralogy of Fallot have a small pulmonary valve annulus. Classically, this has been managed at time of definitive repair by incision and enlargement with the placement of a transannular patch. For most patients, the transannular patch relieves the possibility of residual obstruction at the annulus level, but in exchange it leaves significant pulmonary incompetence. There are a few groups around the world who have recommended the placement of monocusps or other valve substitutes as a routine.[1] When enlargement of the pulmonary annulus valve is required, we have not subscribed to this policy. Among the reasons for our judgement are the poor durability of the available valve substitutes, the need for anticoagulation therapy, and the question of early and late function of monocusps. Here I would like to demonstrate early results with transannular patching, late results, and also review the selection of patients for the placement of a transannular patch at the University of Alabama. When looking at our data on tetralogy, it is important to realize that over the years we have used different policies for the management of these patients.[2-5] Between the years of 1967 and 1972, we performed an initial shunt and then later corrective repair when the patient was older than about 4 years. Between 1972 and 1978, we followed a policy of routine primary repair regardless of young age, small size, or intracardiac or pulmonary artery anatomy. From 1979 to the present we have followed a selective policy. The criteria of that policy have undergone some alteration over the years.

Eight hundred thirty-six patients with tetralogy of Fallot repair from 1967 to 1982 were reviewed to identify incremental risk factors for hospital

TABLE 12.1 Incremental Risk Factors for Repair of Tetralogy of Fallot

Factor	P Value
Pulmonary arterial problems	0.002
Multiple previous operations	0.0004
Small size of patient	0.02
High hematocrit	0.0003
Use of transannular patch	0.05
Earlier date of repair	0.08
Major associated anomalies	0.0001

death (Table 12.1). Significant factors included the presence of pulmonary arterial problems, multiple previous operations, small size of the patient, high hematocrit, and the use of transannular patch at the time of definitive repair. The P-valve (0.05) for transannular patch was collected from an analysis of 713 patient with pulmonary stenosis and 123 with pulmonary atresia. We can divide that experience from 1967 thru 1982 according to those who have uncomplicated tetralogy of Fallot, of which there were 531, and those who had tetralogy of Fallot complicated by associated pulmonary arterial problems, of which there were 94. When a transannular patch was not employed in the repair, the hospital mortality for 399 patients was 3.9% in the uncomplicated group as compared to 14% when pulmonary arterial problems were present. In the uncomplicated group, a transannular patch was required in 126, and the hospital mortality was higher at 8%, but the confidence limits are barely overlapping, indicating the marginal significance of the affect of transannular patching. On the other hand, when pulmonary arterial problems were present and the transannular patch was placed, the hospital mortality among 63 patients was 21%—quite significantly higher. So I suppose that an orthotopic pulmonary valve instead of a transannular patch would, perhaps, be beneficial in the subset of these patients with pulmonary arterial problems. However, there is no information to indicate that in fact the hospital mortality would be lower in this group if an orthotopic valve had been placed. We do know, however, that when pulmonary arterial problems are present, the postrepair ventricular pressure ratio is often higher, and this is of course related to hospital mortality.

Between 1979 and 1982, we used a selective policy. As part of that policy no patients under the age of 12 months received a transannular patch. Patients requiring a transannular patch received shunts in that age group. The hospital mortality was 1.8%; for the group of 69 who had a simple repair the risk was 1.4%, and for the 19 who had a transannular patch as part of the repair, the risk was 5%. These differences are not significant. Currently our policy does not select away patients under the age of 12 months as a routine for classical shunting, since the affect of transannular patching on hospital mortality has become weaker in more recent years.

Figure 12.1 is constructed from our overall experience from 1967 through 1982. It is an estimate of the probability of hospital death compared with the body surface. It segregates the patients according to those who would have received a transannular patch versus those who would not for the year 1982. This computer estimate of the probability of hospital death under these two surgical conditions demonstrates how close the mortality is. In fact, the 70% confidence limits overlap throughout, demonstrating the rather weak affect on hospital mortality of transannular patching. In summary, then the affect of transannular patching on hospital mortality is weak. It is somewhat increased by high hematocrit levels in the younger age groups. It seems more importantly increased by the presence of pulmonary arterial problems.

In addition, the presence of a transannular patch at the time of opera-

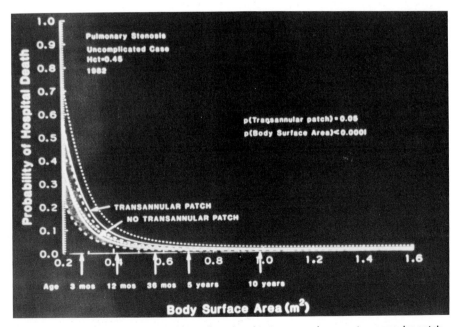

FIGURE 12.1 Probablity of hospital mortality related to transannular or no transannular patch. (From Kirklin JW, Blackstone EH, Pacifico AD, et al: Risk factors for early and late failure after repair of tetralogy of Fallot, and their neutralization. Thorac Cardiovasc Surg 1984;32:208–214. Reproduced with permission.)

tion had no affect on the survival over a 10 year follow-up. In contrast, the only data that we are aware of that indicates that transannular patching alters late survival comes from that of Klinner at al[6] in Munich who reported on more than 600 patients who were followed-up as long as 24 years (Fig. 12.2). Among their patients, the mean age of operation was 10 years, so they were considerably older than most other experiences. After about 8 years there was significant reduction in late survival among the group who received transannular patching.

Wessel and Paul[7] have reported on the exercise performance of patients after tetralogy repair. Comparing the 10 highest performers with the 10 lowest performers, it should be noticed that of the 10 lowest performers, the

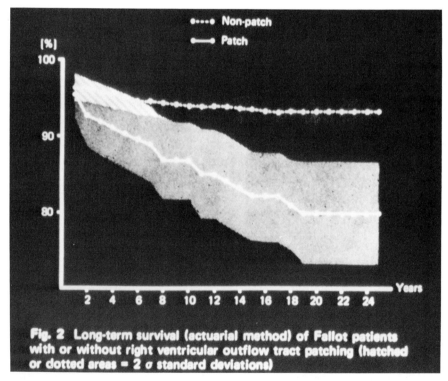

Fig. 2 Long-term survival (actuarial method) of Fallot patients with or without right ventricular outflow tract patching (hatched or dotted areas = 2 σ standard deviations)

FIGURE 12.2 Long-term survival after repair of tetralogy of Fallot, with or without a right ventricular outflow patch. *Hatched area* represents 2 standard deviations. (From Klinner W, Reichart B, Pfaller M, et al: Later results after correction of tetralogy of Fallot necessitating outflow tract reconstruction. Comparison with results after correction without outflow tract patch. Thorac Cardiovasc Surg 1984;32:244–247. Reproduced with permission.)

cardiothoracic ratio was larger, the postrepair right ventricular pressure was higher, the age at the time of repair was older, and eight of the 10 had pulmonary valve incompetence from transannular patching. In comparison none of the 10 highest performers had pulmonary valve incompetence. In addition, in patients who have a right ventricular pressure of less than 50 mm Hg, exercise duration was near normal when there was no pulmonary valve incompetence; exercise duration became significantly reduced — to 75% of normal — in the presence of pulmonary valve incompetence. The poorest performance group were patients with elevated right ventricular pressure and pulmonary incompetence. In this group, the exercise tolerance was only 51% of normal.

Over the intermediate term — considering this to describe the result out to about 20 years — the placement of a transannular patch at the time of repair probably does not affect survival. It does, however, result in reduced exercise capacity, larger right ventricular volume, and larger cardiothoracic ratio. This makes one wonder if over the long term — 30 to 50 years — this will not ultimately have a deleterious affect upon survival. We have shown previously that from angiocardiographic studies one can predict the postrepair right-to-left ventricular pressure ratio, with and without transannular patching, by making measurements of the diameter of the right and left pulmonary arteries before the upper lobe branches of the narrowest (Fig. 12.3) part of the pulmonary tree and of the pulmonary valve annulus and normalizing this for the cardiac catheterization and also including a measurement of the angiographic diameter of the descending aorta at the diaphragm and from this type of information one can predict the postrepair right ventricular – left ventricular pressure ratio using this normogram for these angiographic ratios (Fig. 12.4).

Just one comment about the placement of the patch across the annulus. Classically the transannular patch has been placed with the middle of the patch at the annulus. The reason why patients have reduced exercise tolerance after repair of the tetralogy of Fallot with a transannular patch may be complex, but it may include some degree of right ventricular dysfunction that results from the placement of the noncontractile patch over the ventricular body. Currently we try to minimize the extent of this incision. In fact, if one uses the transatrial and transpulmonary approach for repair of the tetralogy, one can make the pulmonary arteriotomy extend through the annulus only for the distance of about 10 mm and still significantly effect enlargement of the small pulmonary valve annulus in most patients. Whether or not this may have a late altered effect on the late exercise performance remains to be seen.

In conclusion, we believe that transannular patches should be used only when necessary at definitive repair. The necessity can be estimated from

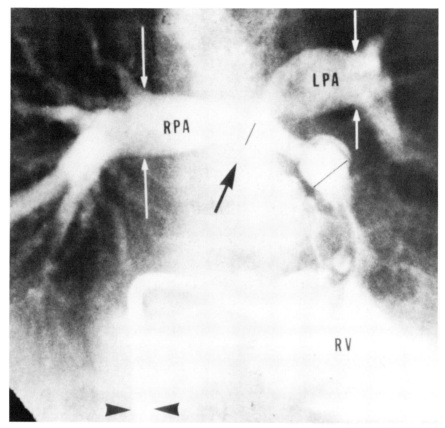

FIGURE 12.3 Angiogram demonstrated pulmonary arteries in tetralogy of Fallot. *White arrows* demonstrate measurement of right pulmonary artery (RPA), and left pulmonary artery (LPA) diameters. (From Blackstone EH, Bertranou EG, Labrosse CJ, et al: Preoperative prediction from cineangiograms of postrepair right ventricular pressure in tetralogy of Fallot. J Thorac Cardiovasc Surg 1979;78:542. Reproduced with permission.)

measurement of the pulmonary valve annulus in comparison with that of the normal heart. Orthotopic pulmonary valve replacement should be considered when a small annulus is associated with pulmonary arterial problems and one predicts a high postrepair right ventricular – left ventricular pressure ratio. After operation we would advise orthotopic pulmonary valve replacement when patients have important cardiomegaly, even in the absence of symptoms prior to the development of right ventricular cardiomyopathies.

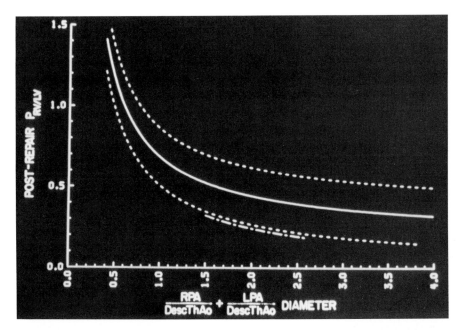

FIGURE 12.4 Pressure ratio of right to left ventricle related to pulmonary artery anatomy. Abbreviations: RPA = right pulmonary artery; LPA = left pulmonary artery; Desc Th Ao = descending thoracic aorta at level of the diaphragm. (From Blackstone EH, Bertranou EG, Labrosse CJ, et al: Preoperative prediction from cineangiograms of postrepair right ventricular pressure in tetralogy of Fallot. J Thorac Cardiovasc Surg 1979;78:542. Reproduced with permission.)

REFERENCES

1. Abdulah SA, Silverton NP, Yakirevich VS, Ionescu MI. Right ventricular outflow tract reconstruction with a bovine pericardial monocusp patch. Longer term clinical and hemodynamic evaluation. J Thorac Cardiovasc Surg 1985;89:764–771.
2. Blackstone EH, Kirklin JW, Pacifico AD. Decision-making in repair of Tetralogy of Fallot based on intraoperative measurement of pulmonary arterial outflow tract. J Thorac Cardiovasc Surg 1977;77:526–532.
3. Kirklin JW, Blackstone EH, Pacifico AD. Routine primary repair vs. two-stage repair of tetralogy of Fallot. Circulation 1979;60:373.
4. Kirklin JW, Blackstone EH, Kirklin JK, Pacifico AD, Aramendi J, Bargeron LM Jr. Surgical results and protocols in the spectrum of tetralogy of Fallot. Ann Surg 1983;198:251–265.
5. Pacifico AD, Kirklin JW, Blackstone EH. Surgical management of pulmonary stenosis in tetralogy of Fallot. J Thorac Cardiovasc Surg 1977;74:382–395.
6. Klinner W, Reichart B, Psaller M, Hatz R. Late results after correction of tetralogy of Fallot necessitating outflow tract reconstruction. Comparison with results after correction without outflow patch. J Thorac Cardiovasc Surg 1984;32:244–247.
7. Wessel HV, Cunningham WJ, Paul MH, Bastanier CK, Muster AJ, Idriss FS. Exercise performance in tetralogy of Fallot after intracardiac repair. J Thorac Cardiovasc Surg 1980;80:582–593.

CHAPTER 13

Pulmonary Insufficiency After Repair of Tetralogy of Fallot
Late Results

Edward L. Bove, MD, and
Rae-Ellen W. Kavey, MD

The anatomy of tetralogy of Fallot includes right ventricular outflow tract obstruction at both the infundibular and valvar levels due to anterior displacement of the infundibular septum and varying degrees of pulmonary valve hypoplasia. Surgical repair, therefore, requires resection of obstructing hypertrophied muscle and either pulmonary valvotomy or insertion of a patch across the pulmonary valve anulus. The need for transanular patching varies but ranged from 36% to 68% in recently reported series.[1-5] Thus, pulmonary insufficiency is a common postoperative effect, occurring in as many as 85% of cases.[6] Despite this, traditional assessment of the adequacy of repair has included no reference to pulmonary insufficiency. The standard criteria for an adequate postoperative result include: *(a)* elimination of intracardiac shunting; *(b)* right ventricular systolic pressure of less than or equal to 60 mm Hg; and *(c)* right ventricular outflow tract gradient less than or equal to 30 mm Hg. It has become increasingly appreciated that right ventricular dysfunction must also be considered, and that pulmonary insufficiency plays a major role in this dysfunction.

RIGHT VENTRICULAR FUNCTION AFTER REPAIR OF TETRALOGY OF FALLOT

What information is available concerning the evaluation of right ventricular function and the impact of pulmonary insufficiency after tetralogy of Fallot repair? Some reduction in right ventricular function after operation seems

138

unavoidable because repair itself includes ventriculotomy and outflow tract resection of hypertrophied ventricular muscle. Pathologic studies have demonstrated fibrotic change in right ventricular myocardium subjected to prolonged hypertension at systemic levels.[7,8] Postoperative exercise studies demonstrate that even when hemodynamics were considered satisfactory at rest, exercise performance was abnormal.[9] Importantly, Wessel et al[10] demonstrated that exercise performance was significantly worse in patients with pulmonary insufficiency, whether or not residual right ventricular hypertension was present. Angiographically, right ventricular volume and ejection fraction have been assessed after tetralogy repair by Graham et al.[11] Patients who did not require a transanular patch and clinically had mild or no pulmonary insufficiency had normal right ventricular end diastolic volumes and ejection fractions. In contrast, patients with a transanular patch and resultant significant pulmonary insufficiency had abnormally dilated right ventricles with low ejection fractions. Ventricular arrhythmias are common after tetralogy of Fallot repair and have been correlated with a significant risk for late sudden death.[12] Kavey et al[13] studied the association between pulmonary insufficiency, right ventricular function, and ventricular ectopy by using M-mode echocardiography and radionuclide ventriculography. A group of postoperative tetralogy patients, all with right ventricular pressures of less than 65 mm Hg, were classified by the intensity of their pulmonary insufficiency murmur. Patients with prominent murmurs of pulmonary insufficiency had significantly larger right ventricles on echocardiography, lower right ventricular ejection fractions on radionuclide ventriculography, and more high-grade ventricular ectopy than did those patients with minimal or no pulmonary insufficiency.

PULMONARY INSUFFICIENCY AS A RISK FACTOR

It is difficult to evaluate the impact of isolated pulmonary insufficiency in the postoperative tetralogy patient. Right ventricular hypertrophy, residual right ventricular outflow tract obstruction at any level, and conduction disturbances may coexist to some extent in any individual patient. Surgical repair itself alters the structure and function of the right ventricle and evaluation of any postoperative residual must be viewed in this context. Review of the natural history of isolated congenital pulmonary valve insufficiency is helpful in understanding the consequences of this lesion. Shimazaki, Blackstone, and Kirklin recently reviewed the world's literature and found 72 cases for evaluation.[14] They studied the time interval until the onset of symptoms or death. Seventeen patients developed symptoms and three of these died, all with markedly enlarged right ventricles. The probability of having symptoms was determined to be 6% at 20 years of age and 20% at 40 years of age. Further, the rate of development of symptoms increased with time. The probability of developing symptoms within 5 years was 3.7% at age 20 years and 9.2% at age 40 years. This study indicates that symptoms will develop with time as a consequence of pulmonary insufficiency even in otherwise normal hearts. In the postoperative tetralogy patient, the time interval to the development of symptoms would be anticipated to be considerably shorter.

In order to further examine the influence of pulmonary insufficiency on ventricular function specifically in the postrepair tetralogy patient, our group studied 20 patients at an average of 9 years after operation.[15] Only patients with excellent hemodynamic results were included: *(a)* no residual shunt; *(b)* right ventricular peak systolic pressure of ≤ 60 torr; *(c)* right ventricular pulmonary artery gradient of ≤ 30 torr; and *(d)* no tricuspid insufficiency. All the patients were New York Heart Association class 1. Evaluation was done with standard chest roentgenograms, M-mode echocardiograms, 24-hour Holter monitoring, and radionuclide ventriculography. The patients were divided into two groups based on the presence or absence of clinically significant pulmonary insufficiency. Group 1 consisted of eight patients with no pulmonary insufficiency, and group 2 consisted of 12 patients with moderate to severe pulmonary insufficiency. One-half of the patients in group 2 had transanular patches.

The age at operation (Table 13.1) was not different between the two groups, and the duration of follow-up observation until the time of study was 9 years for both. Seventy-five percent of group 1 patients and 42% or those in group 2 ($P =$ NS) required a systemic to pulmonary artery shunt procedure before complete repair.

Cardiac catheterization was done at a mean of 2.4 years (range, 1–6 years) after operation (Table 13.2). The hemodynamics were similar between groups with the pulmonary insufficiency patients having slightly higher right ventricular and pulmonary artery systolic pressures ($P =$ NS).

Overall cardiac size, as assessed by standard posteroanterior chest

TABLE 13.1 Late Effects of Pulmonary Insufficiency

	Age at Operation (years)	Follow-Up (years)	Patients with Previous Shunt (%)
No PI	6.4 ± 1.8	8.8 ± 3.1	75
PI	7.5 ± 3.0	9.0 ± 3.0	42

Abbreviation: PI = pulmonary insufficiency.

TABLE 13.2 Late Effects of Pulmonary Insufficiency on Hemodynamics

	RV Systolic (mm Hg)	PA Systolic (mm Hg)	Gradient (mm Hg)
No PI	37.0 ± 6.7	24.9 ± 7.5	12.1 ± 7.5
PI	45.0 ± 9.7	31.3 ± 8.7	13.7 ± 9.9

Abbreviations: PI = pulmonary insufficiency; RV = right ventricular; PA = pulmonary arterial.

roentgenograms, was slightly higher in the group with pulmonary insufficiency (0.53 ± 0.02 vs 0.48 ± 0.04; $P =$ NS) (Table 13.3). The six patients with a transanular patch had significantly greater cardiothoracic ratios (0.58 ± 0.03) when compared with those without pulmonary insufficiency (0.48 ± 0.04, $P < 0.01$) and with those with pulmonary insufficiency but without transanular patch (0.48 ± 0.08, $P < 0.01$). M-mode echocardiography demonstrated larger right-to-left ventricular diastolic ratios in the group with pulmonary insufficiency (0.83 ± 0.17 vs 0.55 ± 0.15, $P < 0.01$).

Although slightly more frequent in patients with pulmonary insufficiency, serious ventricular dysrhythmias consisting of grade 3 or 4 by Lown's criteria were not significantly different between the two groups (50% vs 38% for pulmonary insufficiency and no pulmonary insufficiency, respectively; $P =$ NS). Comparison of ventricular function by means of radionuclide ventriculography demonstrated better right and left ventricular ejection fractions in those patients without pulmonary insufficiency (Table 13.4). The right ventricular ejection fraction was 0.39 ± 0.08 in the patients without pulmonary insufficiency and 0.27 ± 0.07 in those with pulmonary insufficiency ($P < 0.01$). In addition, the left ventricular ejection fraction was 0.64 ± 0.12 vs 0.53 ± 0.07, $P < 0.24$, respectively.

It appears then, that in this small group of patients, all with excellent repairs by traditional criteria, the presence of significant pulmonary insufficiency was associated with impaired right and left ventricular function at rest. Early postrepair hemodynamics were not sensitive enough indicators to

TABLE 13.3 Late Effects of Pulmonary Insufficiency on Heart Size

	CT Ratio	RVED/LVED[a]
No PI	0.48 ± 0.04	0.55 ± 0.15
PI	0.53 ± 0.08	0.83 ± 0.17

[a]$P < 0.01$

Abbreviations: PI = pulmonary insufficiency; CT = cardiothoracic; RVED = right ventricular end diastolic; LVED = left ventricular end diastolic.

TABLE 13.4 Late Effects of Pulmonary Insufficiency on Radionuclide
Ventriculography

	RVEF[a]	LVEF[b]
No PI	0.39 ± 0.08	0.64 ± 0.12
PI	0.27 ± 0.07	0.53 ± 0.07

[a]$P < 0.01$.
[b]$P < 0.02$.
Abbreviations: PI = pulmonary insufficiency; RVEF = right ventricular ejection fraction; LVEF = left ventricular ejection fraction.

detect this. Despite this finding, these patients were asymptomatic and only continued follow up will determine if clinical deterioration occurs.

ROLE OF PULMONARY VALVE REPLACEMENT

When symptoms of congestive heart failure become evident after tetralogy repair and significant pulmonary insufficiency is present, a number of groups have reported small numbers of patients who have benefited from pulmonary valve replacement.[16-21] The indications for operation have been diverse, with a paucity of objective data relative to right ventricular function. We evaluated right and left ventricular function in 11 patients who underwent pulmonary valve replacement for a variety of indications (Table 13.5). Eight of these patients had predominant pulmonary insufficiency and were operated upon for progressive exercise intolerance (two patients), progressive cardiomegaly (three patients) and new onset of tricuspid insufficiency (three patients). The remaining three patients had predominant pulmonary stenosis secondary to obstructed previously placed valves or conduits. The age at the time of pulmonary valve replacement was 14.6 ± 1.5 years (range, 5–20 years), and the interval from initial repair to pulmonary valve replacement was 8 years (range, 1–12 years). Excluding the three patients with pulmonary stenosis, no patient with predominant pulmonary insufficiency

TABLE 13.5 Pulmonary Valve Replacement

Pulmonary insufficiency	8 patients
Progressive exercise intolerance	2
Progressive cardiomegaly	3
New onset tricuspid insufficiency	3
Pulmonary stenosis	3 patients

had a right ventricular outflow tract gradient greater than 25 mm Hg, although one did have an occluded left pulmonary artery. Only two of these patients had elevated pulmonary artery pressures. After pulmonary valve replacement, heart size, as judged by standard chest roentgenograms, was significantly reduced from a cardiothoracic ratio of 0.59 ± 0.02 to 0.55 ± 0.02 1 year after operation ($P < 0.01$). M-mode echocardiography demonstrated a significant reduction in right ventricular dilatation: right ventricular–left ventricular end diastolic dimension was reduced from a mean of 1.03 ± 0.30 to 0.73 ± 0.13 ($P < 0.01$) at an average of 10 months after operation. Radionuclide ventriculograms were done in all patients within 6 months prior to pulmonary valve replacement and within 11 months after valve insertion. Right ventricular ejection fraction (Table 13.6) was 0.29 ± 0.12 (range, 0.16–0.48) before operation and rose to 0.35 ± 0.10 (range, 0.19–0.48; $P < 0.05$). A significant change was defined as an increase or decrease of more than 0.05. Using this criterion, two out of three patients with pulmonary stenosis and five out of eight patients with pulmonary insufficiency improved after pulmonary valve replacement. The remaining four patients were unchanged, with no patient showing a decline. Left ventricular ejection fraction was unchanged for all 11 patients (0.55 ± 0.12 and 0.54 ± 0.66, before and after operation, respectively). It is difficult to correlate symptomatic status with ventricular function studies in this small group of patients. However, each of the seven patients with an increase in right ventricular ejection fraction felt improvement in exercise tolerance. Of the remaining four, one patient was too young to evaluate, while one was improved and two were unchanged.

Our data confirms the usefulness of pulmonary valve replacement in selected patients with significant right ventricular dysfunction associated with severe residual pulmonary insufficiency or stenosis. Further, we have shown that right ventricular function can improve after operation as it did in the majority of our patients. The indications for insertion of a pulmonary valve in the setting of residual pulmonary insufficiency remain difficult to define, particularly since the heterografts available for use carry their own risks and complications. We proceed with pulmonary valve replacement in the presence of two or more of the following criteria (Table 13.7): *(a)* symp-

TABLE 13.6 Effects of Pulmonary Valve Replacement on Right Ventricular Ejection Fraction[a]

Preoperative	0.29 ± 0.12
Postoperative	0.35 ± 0.10

[a]$P < 0.05$.

TABLE 13.7 Pulmonary Valve Replacement: Suggested Indications

Symptoms refractory to medical management
Progressive right ventricular enlargement[a]
Progressive decrease in right ventricular ejection fraction[b]
Progressive increase in heart size[c]
Peripheral pulmonary artery stenosis

[a]As measured by echocardiography.
[b]As measured by radionuclide studies.
[c]As shown by chest roentgenogram.

toms refractory to medical management; *(b)* progressive right ventricular enlargement as measured by echocardiography; *(c)* progressive decrease in right ventricular ejection fraction, as measured by radionuclide study, *(d)* progressive increase in heart size, as shown by standard chest roentgenogram; and *(e)* presence of significant peripheral pulmonary artery stenosis.

Studies such as those reviewed here have also led to modification of our initial surgical approach to tetralogy of Fallot repair.[23] The ventricular septal defect is closed through the tricuspid valve, obviating the need for exposure of the defect through the ventriculotomy. A limited incision can then be made high in the right ventricular outflow tract at the level of maximal obstruction and is closed with a patch to widen the diameter of the infundibulum; the patch is extended across the anulus when necessary. Muscle excision is minimized as much as possible, and it is often completely avoided. Since February 1982, this technique has been used in 28 patients, and nine have been evaluated 1–2.5 years after operation by catheterization, M-mode echocardiography, and radionuclide ventriculography. The results in these nine patients (group 1) were compared with those of all patients studied in our division who had undergone tetralogy of Fallot repair by the traditional approach and who had been evaluated in the same fashion within 3 years of surgery (group 2: n = 14). Mean age at surgery was 3.1 years for group 1 and 3.8 years for group 2. When postoperative catheterization results were compared (Table 13.8), group 1 patients had significantly lower right ventricular systolic pressures (35 ± 4.7 mm Hg) than did those in group 2 (54 ± 5.1 mm Hg; $P < 0.005$). Right ventricular end diastolic pressures were also significantly lower. The M-mode echocardiographic right-to-left ventricular end diastolic ratio was used as an index of right ventricular dilatation, with normal being less than 0.45. Patients with the modified surgical approach had significantly lower ratios (0.57 ± 0.10 vs 0.79 ± 0.17; $P < 0.005$). Right ventricular ejection fractions determined by radionuclide ventriculography were normal in group 1 patients (0.44 ± 0.05) and were significantly higher than those in group 2 patients (0.32 ± 0.08; $P < 0.005$). These results demonstrate that in tetralogy of Fallot, right ventricular outflow tract obstruction

TABLE 13.8 Minimal Outflow Tract Excision

	Modified Approach (n = 9)	Standard Approach (n = 14)	P Value
RV pressure (mm Hg)			
Systolic	35.0 ± 4.7	54.0 ± 5.1	0.005
Diastolic	7.4 ± 1.4	10.1 ± 2.6	0.01
RVED/LVED	0.57 ± 0.10	0.79 ± 0.17	0.005
RVEF	0.44 ± 0.05	0.32 ± 0.08	0.005
LVEF	0.55 ± 0.07	0.54 ± 0.08	NS

Abbreviations: RV = right ventricular; RVED = right ventricular end diastolic; LVED = left ventricular end diastolic; RVEF = right ventricular ejection fraction; LVEF = left ventricular ejection fraction.

can be effectively relieved with a less aggressive approach. Early postoperative assessment by cardiac catheterization, M-mode echocardiography, and nuclear ventriculography suggests that there is less right ventricular dilatation and better preservation of right ventricular function with this technique.

In conclusion, considerable information has now accumulated to indicate that pulmonary insufficiency is one risk factor in the development of progressive right ventricular dysfunction after tetralogy of Fallot repair. A small percentage of patients with otherwise excellent repairs but with residual significant pulmonary insufficiency will eventually develop symptoms, cardiomegaly and right ventricular dysfunction. Long-term follow-up after tetralogy repair should include serial M-mode echocardiography and radionuclide ventriculography to aid in early detection of these patients. These results suggest that such children are benefited by pulmonary valve replacement, both subjectively and objectively. Although the indications are not entirely certain, continued observation is necessary to identify those patients at risk before irreversible right ventricular failure develops. Additionally, modification of the initial surgical approach to the outflow tract obstruction should allow better long-term preservation of right ventricular function in patients with tetralogy of Fallot.

REFERENCES

1. Fuster V, McGoon DC, Kennedy MA, Ritter DG, Kirklin JW. Long-term evaluation (12 to 22 years) of open heart surgery for tetralogy of Fallot. Am J Cardiol 1980;46:635–642.
2. Piccoli GP, Dickinson DF, Musumeci F, Hamilton DI. A changing policy for the surgical treatment of tetralogy of Fallot: early and late results in 235 consecutive patients. Ann Thorac Surg 1981;33:365–373.
3. Yankah AC, Sievers HH, Lange PE, Regensburger D, Bernhard A. Surgical repair of tetralogy of Fallot in adolescents and adults. Thorac Cardiovasc Surg 1982;30:69–74.
4. Calder AL, Barratt-Boyes BG, Brandt PWT, Neutze JM. Postoperative evaluation of patients with tetralogy of Fallot repaired in infancy. J Thorac Cardiovasc Surg 1979;77:704–720.

5. Arciniegas E, Farooke ZQ, Hakimi M, Perry BL, Green EW. Early and late results of total correction of tetralogy of Fallot. J Thorac Cardiovasc Surg 1980;80:770–778.
6. Garson A Jr, Nihill MR, McNamara DG, Cooley DA. Status of the adult and adolescent after repair of tetralogy of Fallot. Circulation 1979;59:1232–1240.
7. Jones M, Ferrans VJ. Myocardial degeneration in congenital heart disease: Comparison of morphologic findings in young and old patients with congenital heart disease associated with muscular obstruction to right ventricular outflow. Am J Cardiol 1977;39:1051–1063.
8. Shakibi JG, Aryanpur I, Nazarian I. The anatomic correlate of ventricular dysfunction in tetralogy of Fallot (abstr). Proceedings of the 47th Scientific Sessions of the American Academy of Pediatrics, Chicago, 1978, p 15.
9. Hirschfeld S, Tuboku-Metzger AJ, Borkat G, Ankeney J, Clayman J, Liebman J. Comparison of exercise and catheterization results following total surgical correction of tetralogy of Fallot. J Thorac Cardiovasc Surg 1978;75:446–451.
10. Wessel HU, Cunningham WJ, Paul MH, Bastanier CK, Muster AJ, Idriss FS. Exercise performance in tetralogy of Fallot after intracardiac repair. J Thorac Cardiovasc Surg 1980;80:582–593.
11. Graham TP, Cordell D, Atwood GF, Boucek RJ, Boerth RC, Bender HW, Nelson JH, Vaughn WK. Right ventricular volume characteristics before and after palliative and reparative operation in tetralogy of Fallot. Circulation 1976;54:417–423.
12. Kavey REW, Blackman MS, Sondheimer HM: Incidence and severity of chronic ventricular dysrhythmias after repair of tetralogy of Fallot. Am Heart J 1982;103:342–350.
13. Kavey REW, Byrum CJ, Blackman MS, Sondheimer HM, Bove EL. Pulmonary insufficiency, ventricular arrhythmias and ventricular dysfunction after tetralogy of Fallot repair (abstr). Circulation 1983;68:(III)268.
14. Shimazaki Y, Blackstone EH, Kirklin JW. The natural history of isolated congenital pulmonary valve incompetence: surgical implications. Thorac Cardiovasc Surg 1984;32:257–259.
15. Bove EL, Byrum CJ, Thomas FD, Kavey REW, Sondheimer HM, Blackman MS, Parker FB Jr. The influence of pulmonary insufficiency on ventricular function following repair of tetralogy of Fallot. J Thorac Cardiovasc Surg 1983;85:691–696.
16. Misbach GA, Turley K, Ebert PA. Pulmonary valve replacement for regurgitation after repair of tetralogy of Fallot. Ann Thorac Surg 1983;36:684–691.
17. Shaher RM, Foster E, Farina M, Spooner E, Sheikh F, Alley R. Right heart reconstruction following repair of tetralogy of Fallot. Ann Thorac Surg 1983;35:421–426.
18. Laks H, Hellenbrand WE, Kleinman CS, Stansel HC Jr, Talner NS. Patch reconstruction of the right ventricular outflow tract with pulmonary valve insertion. Circulation 1981;64(suppl II):II154–II161.
19. Idriss FS, Markowitz A, Nikaidoh H, Muster AJ, Paul MH. Insertion of Hancock valve for pulmonary valve insufficiency in previously repair tetralogy of Fallot (abstr). Circulation 1976;53,54(suppl II):II100.
20. Miller DC, Rossiter SJ, Stinson EB, Oyer PE, Reitz BA, Shumway NE. Late right heart reconstruction following repair of tetralogy of Fallot. Ann Thorac Surg 1979;28:239–261.
21. Uretzky G, Puga FJ, Danielson GK, Hagler DJ, McGoon DC. Reoperation after correction of tetralogy of Fallot. Circulation 1982;66(supplI):I202–I208.
22. Bove EL, Kavey REW, Byrum CJ, Sondheimer HM, Blackman MS, Thomas FD. Improved right ventricular function following late pulmonary valve replacement for residual pulmonary insufficiency or stenosis. J Thor Cardiovasc Surg 1985;90:50–55.
23. Kavey REW, Bove EL, Sondheimer HM, Byrum CJ, Blackman MS, Pottenat J. Postoperative assessment of modified surgical approach to repair of tetralogy of Fallot. J Thorac Cardiovasc Surg 1987;93:533–538.

CHAPTER 14

The Role of Valves in Pulmonary Conduits

Paul A. Ebert, MD

It is very difficult to separate valved and nonvalved conduits. There is no single direction that one should take in patients such as this, and I think that you probably want to keep your options open and use a valve conduit in situations where you believe it is necessary. We have swung the entire spectrum as others have that if it is possible to obtain a homograft for long-term use in a reasonably sized child, then I think that clearly is the conduit of choice. The biggest advantage of the Dacron heterograft conduits is the availability of them and the small size availability when you use such a conduit in infants.

I would like to emphasize a couple of areas when working with valves. Basically, the main reason for using a valved conduit is either pulmonary hypertension or a small child with unstable pulmonary vascular resistance.

This can be best demonstrated by a representative case of a three month old infant with truncus arteriosus in the immediate postoperative period (Fig. 14.1), which demonstrates the unstable pulmonary artery pressure. What are the biggest problems in the management of such an infant? One is just getting through the operation. Then it is that postoperative period when they awaken, and when they come off the ventilator. During these periods there is a tremendous swing in pulmonary artery pressure. Many times it exceeds aortic pressure. It is at this point that the child looks grayish, becomes acidotic, and if something is not done, you end up with a bradycardic child in whom resuscitation often is impossible to accomplish. These swings in pressure due to the unstable pulmonary vasculature are where most of the babies with truncus have difficulty in the postoperative period. You can minimize these episodes by keeping the patient sedated longer, because there is no question that over a period of days the pulmonary vascular reactivity

147

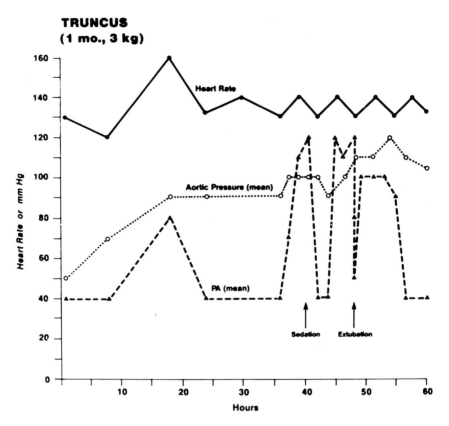

FIGURE 14.1 Postoperative hemodynamics of a 3-month-old infant with persistant truncus arteriosus. PA (mean) = mean pulmonary artery pressure.

becomes less. However to have a right ventricle with a 12-mm conduit exposed to wide open pulmonary regurgitation does not make much sense in this setting. If you evaluate the Michigan experience in the babies with nonvalved conduits, you find that the conduits used have been small, 8 or 10 mm in diameter. So there is a degree of stenosis through the conduit, and you have to remember that if there is a degree of stenosis in one direction there is also a degree of stenosis in the other direction. Thus a small conduit does decrease the incidence and the amount of pulmonary regurgitation. I think to argue the point of valved versus nonvalved conduits in small babies is not logical because these high-risk patients need all the benefits they can get. I would much rather have a valve here and worry about what you do with them at a later time. In small children it does not matter whether you enplace a nonvalved conduit or a valved conduit of the same size. You are going to change it at approximately the same time simply because of the age and growth of the patient.

If you do choose to use a heterograft valved conduit, we are aware that the rigid ring has two distinct disadvantages: often times it pushes on the sternum and can push on the left coronary artery. It is probably of benefit to have this ring as far out to the distal anastomosis as possible and parallel to the sternum as demonstrated on the angiogram in Figure 14.2. In this position, there is unlikely to be any major compression.

In the first year of life, we would also sway towards the valved rather than the nonvalved conduit. Of course the larger the pulmonary arteries and the lower the pulmonary resistance, the less the need in the acute phase for a valved conduit. We still do not know, over the longrun, the effects of valved or nonvalved conduits on right ventricular performance.

HOW LONG DO THESE CONDUITS LAST?

In our experience, the valved conduits have a durability of 2 – 6 years. Often the truncus babies are re-studied at an early age. It looks like an intimal peel is layed down in the conduit fairly early (Fig. 14.3). They often have elevated

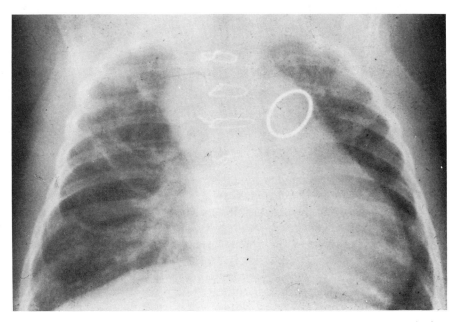

FIGURE 14.2 Chest roentgenogram of valved conduit in the correct position. The ringed valve is placed distally and parallel to the sternum.

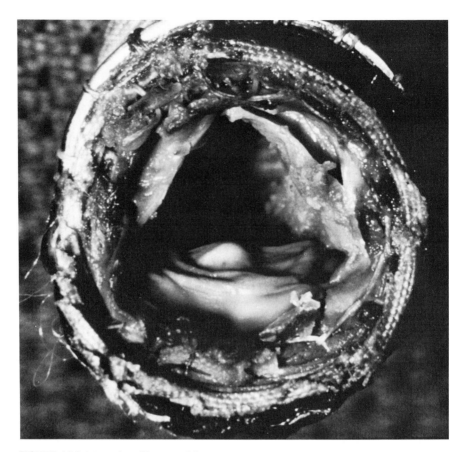

FIGURE 14.3 Internal peel in a conduit.

right ventricular pressure sometimes by 6 months or a year, which then stabilizes. The right ventricular hypertension does not seem to be as devastating as one often sees in pulmonary stenosis. I do not know whether that is because they do not have an infundibular component to the obstruction or because of different ventricle anatomically, or because the muscle performs better. Thus, we have tried to extend the period as long as the child is growing and no overt sign of right heart failure. Obviously the later in life that a conduit is placed, the longer the time span between replacements. It is still fairly hard to say whether the conduits are outgrown strictly from ingrowth of neointima or from patient growth as well.

Table 14.1 demonstrates that there has been a very small number of conduits replaced in the older age patients, although these are few patients.

TABLE 14.1 Conduits Replaced

Age	No. Replaced	Durability Mean (years)
0–6/12	94/110	2–6 (3.2)
6–1	24/31	3–8 (5.4)
1–2	19/25	3–8 (5.8)
2–6	12/32	6–9 (7.3)
6–4	4/23	6–14 (7.1)

More of the valved conduits have been replaced than the nonvalved conduits. When they have been changed, most have had a nonvalved conduit placed (Table 14.2). We have had only one patient who had poor right ventricular performance following implantation of a valveless conduit. This was a child with transposition of the great arteries who did not tolerate the pulmonary regurgitation, and thus we placed a valved conduit at the time of that change. But the swing certainly has been to the use of a nonvalved conduit for replacement.

I do not think any of us know really what is the optimum material because even though we all have these terrible-looking pseudointima ingrowths in Dacron grafts, it also makes the Dacron almost entirely extracorporeal in its location. I think the incidence of infection will be less yet with Dacron than it is likely to be with some of the surfaces that do not have the endothelial lining on it. We will discuss infections below. We are concerned as to the advantages and disadvantages of using a material that is less likely to be obstructive but may be more susceptible to endocarditis.

Any child that has a piece of plastic in its bloodstream is at a greater risk for infection than those that do not. This may be the biggest reason in the long run as to the choice of a homograft that does seem to have a lower incidence of infection or to some type of autologous or other tissue that is different from plastic. We have had eight patients with early positive blood cultures during their initial hospitalization. They have all been successfully treated with antibiotics. We have not had to operate on any patients and have

TABLE 14.2 Conduit Replacement—A Comparison of Valved versus Nonvalved Conduits

	Number	Replaced with Valved Conduit	Replaced without Valved Conduit
Valved	106	32	76
Nonvalved	12	1	11

not removed the conduit during their initial hospitalization. This is the case even in two patients with *Monilia* fungus infections, probably secondary to over treatment with antibiotics. When the patients have had good hemodynamics, we have been able to ride them out and get them through irrespective of what one might see.

Two patients with late infections were treated with antibiotics and were successfully sterilized, at least clinically. Two late infections were treated with antibiotics and surgical removal: one patient had severe stenosis of the conduit at about the time that he had his episode of sepsis and we thus elected to treat him for 10 days and then remove the conduit. The other patient's conduit was demonstrated by echo to have a loose floating neointima attached only at the distal suture line. As in the Mayo Clinic experience, we have found that conduit replacements—at least on the first time around—have been without mortality and have been a considerably easier procedure than what we had anticipated. Generally speaking, one does not know whether the second, third, or fourth replacements will also be easy and without significant risk.

SUMMARY

Most infants, certainly in the first year of life, have a degree of pulmonary vasculature instability or pulmonary hypertension such that I would still choose to put in a conduit that has a valve. I do not see that there is any great loss to the patient and probably you shorten the lifespan of that conduit very little by having a valve in place at that time. The big decision is what to do at the time of the conduit replacement. Should one place a homograft knowing that it has a limited lifespan? If the size of the homograft is large enough, we do not know how long the homograft valve will last. The disadvantage initially with the homograft has simply been that of size. I think it has been a mistake to put in a very large homograft in a small infant because it acts like a ventricular aneurysm. Although the very first truncus we did was on a baby, who is now about 14 years old and still has the original homograft in place, I must say she was awfully ill for a long time in the postoperative period. This homograft is totally calcified but the leaflets still function and she still has a low pulmonary artery pressure. So, I think the real decision making has to be done on the 4-, 5-, or 7-year-old child as to what one chooses at that point. I am not certain that the nonvalved conduit is the ideal choice and it may be another 10 years before we see how much right ventricular dysfunction is present secondary to pulmonary insufficiency. I am glad to see a revival in interest in the homograft. I think that when one listens to this type of session 3–4 years from now, there will probably be a lot less Dacron at least present in the second operation as compared to the present.

CHAPTER 15

Use of Nonvalved Conduits to Establish Pulmonary Ventricle-to-Pulmonary Artery Continuity

Hartzell V. Schaff, MD, and
Gordon K. Danielson, MD

A variety of biologic and synthetic materials have been utilized to establish continuity between the pulmonary ventricle (PV) and the pulmonary artery (PA). The earliest successful PV – PA conduit operation appears to have been that reported by Klinner and Zenker in 1963.[1] In their patient with pulmonary atresia and a hypoplastic pulmonary artery, a woven Teflon graft was interposed between the pulmonary artery and the right ventriculotomy as a palliative procedure. At the Mayo Clinic, the first successful congenital heart repair using an extracardiac PV – PA conduit was performed by Kirklin in 1964 and was reported by Rastelli et al 1 year later; this was also a nonvalved graft, one constructed from pericardium.[2] Ross and Somerville developed the use of aortic homografts with integral valves for reconstruction of the right ventricular outflow tract.[3]

Variations of these earlier methods have been used to correct a wide variety of lesions, including transposition of the great arteries with ventricular septal defect and pulmonary stenosis, pulmonary atresia with ventricular septal defect, truncus arteriosus, double-outlet right ventricle, double-outlet left ventricle, and more complex anomalies with a single pumping chamber.[4-8] At the Mayo Clinic, more than 1100 operations employing extracardiac PV – PA conduits have been performed (Table 15.1).

Choice of a prosthesis for PV – PA reconstruction involves several considerations, including the size of the patient, the anticipated route and length of the conduit, and the expected hemodynamic result after repair. Aortic homografts with integral valves are advantageous because of ease of han-

TABLE 15.1 Conduit Operations for Congenital Heart Disease Performed at the Mayo Clinic From 1964 Through 1984

Primary Patient Diagnosis	No. of Patients
Pulmonary atresia with ventricular septal defect	346
Transposition of the great arteries	218
Truncus arteriosus	188
Double outlet right ventricle	86
Univentricular heart	65
Tetralogy of Fallot	60
Corrected transposition of the great arteries	43
Other	94
Total	**1100**

dling, but limited length is a disadvantage in some cases. Late durability of these grafts appears to be related to the method of sterilization and preservation. Aortic homografts sterilized by radiation or chemical methods and preserved by freezing have shown a propensity for late calcific obstruction. During 10-year follow-up, more than 50% of patients with this type of conduit used for a PV–PA reconstruction required reoperation.[8,9] These results contrast with the reports of good long-term conduit function in fresh antibiotic-sterilized homografts.[10-13]

Currently we have resumed use of both homograft aorta with integral valve and pulmonary artery with valve prepared with the antibiotic sterilization method.[14] Modern techniques of cryopreservation may extend the potential for storage of these grafts, although additional follow-up is necessary to determine whether late results match those of "fresh" homografts.

Dacron grafts containing glutaraldehyde-preserved porcine valves have been used at our institution since 1972. These conduits have the advantages of ready availability in a wide variety of sizes and longer length for complex reconstructions. The early hemodynamic results are satisfactory, but in many patients late progressive obstruction of the PV–PA conduit develops because of calcification and stiffening of the heterograft valve and/or accumulation of exuberant fibrous peel within the conduit proximal and distal to the valve. The pathological features of obstructed PV-PA porcine-valved Dacron conduits have been studied extensively.[15-17]

Calcification of the heterograft valve caused the principal stenosis in 46% of explanted conduits studied by Edwards et al,[15] and in 30% of specimens the major obstruction was caused by thick fibrous neointima (peel); in 16% it was caused by both stenosis of the valve and fibrous peel. In the remaining 8% of patients, obstruction was due to extrinsic compression by the sternum and/or anastomotic problems. The precise incidence of conduit obstruction is not known, but in our experience, approximately 6% of patients will require reoperation during the first 5 years postoperatively.[8] Thereafter, the risk of conduit obstruction may increase. Results in other series suggest that the risk of Hancock obstruction is progressive and may exceed 30% by 10 years postoperatively.[18-20]

To avoid late complications of valved conduits, some surgeons have proposed valveless PV–PA connections. Experience after repair of tetralogy of Fallot in which the pulmonary valve is either absent, removed, or rendered incompetent by valvotomy, has shown that most patients tolerate pulmonary insufficiency well.[21] Although there is some experimental evidence that peel formation within a Dacron PV–PA conduit is less when the valve is not present,[22] it should be recalled that such a nonvalved prosthetic graft would not completely prevent all future possibility of conduit obstruction.

NONVALVED CONDUIT FOR PALLIATIVE RIGHT VENTRICULAR OUTFLOW RECONSTRUCTION

Right ventricular outflow reconstruction for patients with pulmonary atresia, ventricular septal defect, and hypoplastic confluent pulmonary arteries is useful both for improving arterial oxygen saturation and for enlarging central pulmonary arteries.[23] Previously, pericardial patches were used for outflow reconstruction,[24] but, with time, some of these patches developed aneurysmal dilatation under the stress of systemic right ventricular pressure. Currently, we prefer nonvalved conduits for right ventricular outflow reconstruction and have used a variety of materials, including Dacron and polytetrafluoroethylene (Gore-Tex, W. L. Gore and Associates, Inc., Naperville, IL).

Right ventricular outflow reconstruction using a tube graft can be performed with or without cardiopulmonary bypass.[25] Generally, the size of the conduit is limited to that which can be conveniently anastomosed to the hypoplastic central pulmonary artery. (The most frequently used graft diameters range from 10 to 14 mm.)

NONVALVED CONDUITS FOR CORRECTIVE OPERATION

A competent valve in a PV–PA reconstruction is advantageous at the time of complete correction because ventricular failure early postoperatively can result from periods of intraoperative global ischemia, ventricular incisions, and postoperative pulmonary arterial hypertension due to peripheral pulmonary artery stenoses, reactive pulmonary hypertension, pulmonary vascular obstructive disease, or combinations thereof. Valveless conduits, however, have been used with success in situations where appropriate-sized valved grafts are not available or in patients in whom the postoperative hemodynamic results are both highly predictable and favorable.

Neonates with truncus arteriosus have undergone successful correction utilizing nonvalved conduits. Spicer et al[26] reported five survivors among seven infants undergoing repair of truncus arteriosus using polytetrafluoroethylene (Gore-Tex) grafts, which ranged in size from 8 to 10 mm. These authors selected the nonvalved conduits because of difficulties related to insertion of the smallest available porcine-valved conduit (12 mm), but it should be noted again that pulmonary vascular reactivity and hypertension may compromise right ventricular function if pulmonary insufficiency is present. In the series reported by Spicer et al., the ratio of pulmonary-to-systemic resistance was 0.3 or less for each of the five survivors and 0.63 in both of the patients who died postoperatively.[26]

We have used nonvalved conduits during initial repair of complex lesions in 27 patients. Each patient fulfilled strict selection criteria, which included: (*a*) normal pulmonary artery size and distribution, (*b*) normal pulmonary arteriolar resistance, (*c*) a competent right AV valve, and (*d*) near-normal function of the pulmonary ventricle. Early results of these highly selected patients have been good, but one patient with corrected transposition of the great arteries subsequently received a valve in the PV – PA connection at the time of reoperation for tricuspid (systemic atrioventricular) valve replacement.

In all recent operations in which nonvalved conduits have been used for PV – PA reconstruction for total correction, we have used Dacron tube grafts. We are evaluating collagen-impregnated Dacron grafts (Tascon Medical, Metronic Blood Systems, Inc., Minneapolis, MN) which have real and theoretical advantages. These grafts have a relatively loose weave, are easy to anastomose to thin-walled pulmonary arteries, and they conform easily to the contour of the heart. Bleeding through the conduit is minimal after systemic heparinization is reversed with protamine. Other groups have had early success with polytetrafluoroethylene Gore-Tex tube grafts, but additional care is needed during insertion to avoid kinking of the graft.[27]

NONVALVED CONDUITS FOR REPLACEMENT OF OBSTRUCTED PULMONARY VENTRICLE-PULMONARY ARTERY VALVED CONDUITS

As previously noted, many patients surviving intial repair with PV – PA conduits, especially those who have correction during infancy and those with composite conduits constructed of Dacron and integral glutaraldehyde-fixed porcine valves, will require late reoperation because of somatic growth, conduit obstruction, or both.[28] A review of the first 100 patients at the Mayo Clinic who underwent reoperation for conduit obstruction demonstrated that operative risk was low (7% overall and 0% for those with conduit obstruction and no associated defects), and transconduit gradients were effectively relieved (preoperatively 81 ± 26 mm Hg; postoperatively 7 ± 8 mm Hg).[29] Many patients requiring reoperation for obstructed PV–PA conduits will fulfill the previous criteria for nonvalved conduits. In these patients, a nonvalved conduit is employed if the anticipated after-repair peak systolic pressure in the pulmonary ventricle is 50 mm Hg or less, in the hope of decreasing the need for additional conduit changes in the future.

Downing et al. reported on the early experience from our institution with 26 patients who underwent replacement of obstructed PV–PA valved conduits with nonvalved grafts, and results are encouraging.[30] All patients had satisfactory relief or transconduit gradients, and mean pulmonary ventricular systolic pressure decreased from 91 ± 20 mm Hg to 23 ± 9 mm Hg after conduit replacement. Fifteen of the 22 patients had Dacron tube grafts used to re-establish PV–PA continuity. The other 11 patients had PV–PA continuity restored by autogenous reconstruction.[31] With this technique, the stenotic Dacron conduit is excised, and care is taken to preserve the surrounding fibrous bed that leads from the ventriculotomy to the pulmonary artery. The anterior roof of this new pathway is supplemented by a large patch of autogenous or glutaraldehyde-preserved bovine pericardium. Essential features of the procedure are illustrated in Figure 15.1.

The method of autogenous reconstruction has the potential to avoid reoperation due to obstruction, and large pathways can consistently be obtained. It is not known whether these conduits will enlarge with somatic growth of the patient, and it is possible that the walls of the pathway will calcify, especially if heterologous pericardium is used for the roof. This, however, would not be expected to interfere with hemodynamic function. If patients develop late dilatation of the pulmonary ventricle or insufficiency of the right AV valve, insertion of a valve in the PV–PA connection would be relatively simple.

Replacement of obstructed PV–PA conduits with nonvalved grafts might be expected to reduce the need for future operations due to heterograft valve calcification, and the method of autogenous reconstruction may avoid complications of peel formation within Dacron tubes. Applied in properly selected patients, these techniques should yield the same generally satisfactory survival and functional results that have been observed in patients with residual pulmonary insufficiency after repair of tetralogy of Fallot.[21]

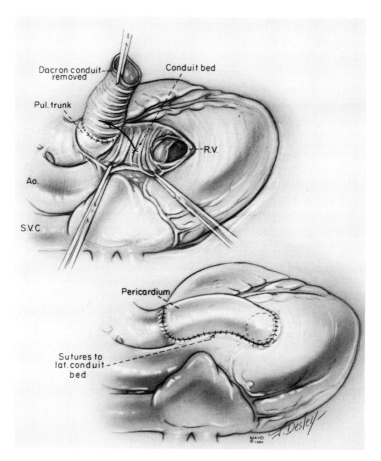

FIGURE 15.1 Illustration of steps in autogenous reconstruction of the pulmonary ventricle-to-pulmonary artery pathway. The obstructed PV–PA conduit is excised, and care is taken to leave the surrounding fibrous bed intact. Pericardium is then sutured to the edge of the pathway as a roof in order to make a wide communication from the ventricle to the pulmonary artery. Abbreviations: Ao = aorta; SVC = superior vena cava; RV = right ventricle.

SUMMARY

Extracardiac conduits have been used to correct pulmonary ventricle-to-pulmonary artery (PV–PA) discontinuity in a variety of complex congenital cardiac malformations. A competent valve in the PV–PA conduit provides the most physiologic repair, but prosthetic valves, especially heterografts, can cause late conduit obstruction. Long-term results following repair of tetralogy of Fallot demonstrate that absence of a functioning pulmonary valve is compatible with good late survival and functional status. Therefore, carefully selected patients may be candidates for nonvalved conduits during (*a*) staged correction of pulmonary atresia with ventricular septal defect and hypoplastic pulmonary arteries; (*b*) total correction of complex lesions with highly favorable and predictable postrepair hemodynamics; and (*c*) replacement of obstructed PV–PA conduits. This chapter reviews our experience with nonvalved extracardiac PV–PA conduits and presents a new method for autogenous reconstruction of the PV–PA connection at the time of conduit explantation.

REFERENCES

1. Klinner W, Zenker R. Experience with correction of Fallot's tetralogy in 178 cases. Surgery 1965;57:353–357.
2. Rastelli GC, Ongley PA, Davis GD, et al. Surgical repair for pulmonary valve atresia with coronary-pulmonary artery fistula: report of a case. Mayo Clin Proc 1965;40:521–527.
3. Ross DN, Somerville J. Correction of pulmonary atresia with a homograft aortic valve. Lancet 1966;2:1446–1447.
4. Rastelli GC, McGoon DC, Wallace RB. Anatomic correction of transposition of the great arteries with ventricular septal defect and subpulmonary stenosis. J Thorac Cardiovasc Surg 1969;58:545–552.
5. McGoon DC, Rastelli GC, Ongley PA. An operation for the correction of truncus arteriosus. JAMA 1968;205:59–63.
6. McGoon DC, Rastelli GC, Wallace RB. Discontinuity between right ventricle and pulmonary artery: surgical treatment. Ann Surg 1970;172:680–689.
7. Feldt RH, Mair DD, Danielson GK, et al. Current status of the septation procedure for univentricular heart. J Thorac Cardiovasc Surg 1981;82:93–97.
8. McGoon DC, Danielson GK, Puga FJ, et al. Late results after extracardiac conduit repair for congenital cardiac defects. Am J Cardiol 1982;49:1741–1749.
9. Moodie DS, Mair DD, Fulton RE, et al. Aortic homograft obstruction. J Thorac Cardiovasc Surg 1976;72:553–561.
10. Saravalli OA, Somerville J, Jefferson KE. Calcification of aortic homografts used for reconstruction of the right ventricular outflow tract. J Thorac Cardiovasc Surg 1980;80:909–920.
11. Fontan F, Choussat A, Deville C, et al. Aortic valve homografts in the surgical treatment of complex cardiac malformations. J Thorac Cardiovasc Surg 1984;87:649–657.
12. di Carlo D, de Leval MR, Stark J. "Fresh" antibiotic sterilized aortic homografts in extracardiac valved conduits. Long-term results. Thorac Cardiovasc Surgeon 1984;32:10–14.
13. Kay PH, Ross DN. Fifteen years' experience with the aortic homograft: the conduit of choice for right ventricular outflow tract reconstruction. Ann Thorac Surg 1985;40:360–364.
14. Kirklin JW, Barratt-Boyes BG. Aortic valve disease, Chapter 12, Method of homograft valve preparation, Appendix 12C. In: Cardiac Surgery. John Wiley & Sons, New York, 1986; pp 421–422.
15. Edwards WD, Agarwal KC, Feldt RH, et al. Surgical pathology of obstructed, right-sided, porcine-valved extracardiac conduits. Arch Pathol Lab Med 1983;107:400–405.

16. Agarwal KC, Edwards WD, Feldt RH, et al. Pathogenesis of nonobstructive fibrous peels in right-sided porcine-valved extracardiac conduits. J Thorac Cardiovasc Surg 1982;83:584–589.

17. Agarwal KC, Edwards WD, Feldt RH, et al. Clinicopathological correlates of obstructed right-sided porcine-valved extracardiac conduits. J Thorac Cardiovasc Surg 1981;81:591–601.

18. Vergesslich KA, Gersony WM, Steeg CN, et al. Postoperative assessment of porcine-valved right ventricular-pulmonary artery conduits. Am J Cardiol 1984;53:202–205.

19. Stewart S, Manning J, Alexson C, et al. The Hancock external valved conduit. A dichotomy between late clinical results and late cardiac catheterization findings. J Thorac Cardiovasc Surg 1983;86:562–569.

20. Schaff HV, Danielson GK, Puga FJ. Truncus arteriosus. In, Arcienegas E (ed): Pediatric Cardiac Surgery. Year Book Medical Publishers, Chicago, 1985, pp 247–256.

21. Fuster V, McGoon DC, Kennedy MA, et al. Long-term evaluation (12 to 22 years) of open-heart surgery for tetralogy of Fallot. Am J Cardiol 1980;46:635–642.

22. Fiore AC, Peigh PS, Robison RJ, et al. Valved and nonvalved right ventricular-pulmonary arterial extracardiac conduits. J Thorac Cardiovasc Surg 1983;86:490–497.

23. Piehler JM, Danielson GK, McGoon DC, et al. Management of pulmonary atresia with ventricular septal defect and hypoplastic pulmonary arteries by right ventricular outflow construction. J Thorac Cardiovasc Surg 1980;80:552–567.

24. Gill CC, Moodie DS, McGoon DC. Staged surgical management of pulmonary atresia with diminutive pulmonary arteries. J Thorac Cardiovasc Surg 1977;73:436–442.

25. Puga FJ, Uretzky G: Establishment of right ventricle-hypoplastic pulmonary artery continuity without the use of extracorporeal circulation. J Thorac Cardiovasc Surg 1982;83:74–80.

26. Spicer RL, Behrendt D, Crowley DC, et al. Repair of truncus arteriosus in neonates with the use of a valveless conduit. Circulation 1984;70(suppl 1):26–29.

27. Molina JE. Use of polytetrafluoroethylene (Gore-Tex) grafts for the construction of right ventricle-pulmonary artery conduits. Ann Thorac Surg 1985;40:405–407.

28. Ebert PA, Turley K, Stanger P, et al. Surgical treatment of truncus arteriosus in the first 6 months of life. Ann Surg 1984;200:451–456.

29. Schaff HV, DiDonato RM, Danielson GK, et al. Reoperation for obstructed pulmonary ventricle-pulmonary artery conduits. J Thorac Cardiovasc Surg 1984;88:334–343.

30. Downing TP, Danielson GK, Schaff HV, et al. Replacement of obstructed right ventricular-pulmonary arterial valved conduits with nonvalved conduits in children. Circulation 1985;72(Suppl 2):84–87.

31. Danielson GK, Downing TP, Schaff HV, et al. Replacement of valved right ventricle-to-pulmonary artery conduits with a xenograft or homograft patch (in preparation).

Section III
THE MITRAL VALVE

CHAPTER 16

The Morphology of the Mitral Valve with Regard to Congenital Malformations

Siew Yen Ho, PhD, and
Robert H. Anderson, MD, FRC Path

SUMMARY

The mitral valve complex consists of the annulus, two leaflets, chords, and two groups of papillary muscles. Due to the close arrangement of the papillary muscles, the interchordal spaces serve as important pathways for the dispersion of flow from the mitral orifice to the left ventricle. Congenital malformations of the mitral valve can be considered in anatomical terms by focusing either on the entire valve or on each valve component separately. Alternatively, the whole valve can be considered in functional terms. The functional approach considers each leaflet in terms of normal, prolapsed, or restricted motion. Anatomically, dysplasia and miniaturization are lesions that affect the entire valve. Lesions at the level of the annulus are absent of the left atrioventricular connection, an imperforate valve, Ebstein's malformation, dual orifice mitral valve, and overriding valve. An absent connection is distinguished from an imperforate valve, although the two entities are similar functionally. Lesions affecting the leaflets include prolapse and clefts. The latter, when affecting the aortic leaflet of a mitral valve, is distinguished from a cleft of the left valve (which is basically a trifoliate valve) in hearts with atrioventricular septal defect. The mitral arcade, parachute mitral valve, and the straddling valve are considered as lesions that affect the chords and papillary muscles.

INTRODUCTION

The mitral valve is characterized anatomically by its two-leaflet arrangement. Although the term "bicuspid valve" has been used on occasion, the adjective "mitral" is still preferred for description, the analogy being with the bishop's mitre. Four major anatomic components make up the mitral valve complex: annulus, leaflets, chords, and papillary muscles. The precise mechanism and timing of closure of this valve remain enigmatic.[1] It is well recognized, however, that its normal function is dependent upon a delicate coordination of all its components together with the adjacent atrial and ventricular walls.[2] In the open state (ventricular diastole), the valve is like a funnel extending from the annulus to the free margins of the leaflets. Chords anchor the leaflets to the papillary muscles. The apparently wide gap between the papillary muscles as displayed in some texts is artefactual (Fig. 16.1a). In reality the papillary muscles and chords are in close apposition, as shown when the valve is revealed by removal of the parietal walls of the ventricle (Fig. 16.1b). By virtue of this arrangement, the interchordal spaces serve as important pathways for the dispersion of flow from the mitral orifice to the left ventricle.

In the West, mitral valve disease in children is primarily due to congeni-

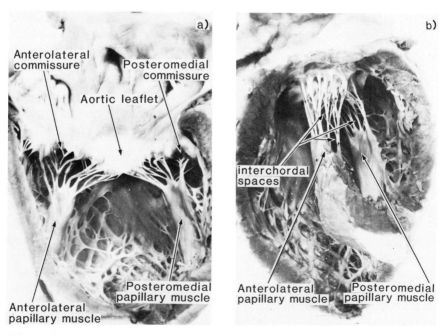

FIGURE 16.1 The mitral valve is dissected to show the artefactual separation of its papillary muscles in **(a)** and the usual arrangement in **(b)**.

tal malformations of the individual valve components or the entire apparatus, although acquired disease, particularly of rheumatic aetiology, must not be ignored. From an anatomic standpoint, the defects can be considered in terms of each unit of the valve complex. This approach may be criticized as oversimplistic because clinically it is often difficult to determine whether mitral valve disease takes the form of stenosis or insufficiency. In some instances the valve may present with abnormal anatomy; for example it may have a dual orifice, yet function normally. In contrast, functional derangements are not always accompanied by gross pathology of the valve apparatus. Moreover, lesions affecting different valvar components, for instance annular hypoplasia, parachute valve and arcade lesion, can have the same functional stenotic effect. In this review we shall first consider mitral valve disease in anatomic terms that permit an insight into the function of each element[3] and then give an account of the functional approach. We will also discuss separately the left atrioventricular valve in atrioventricular septal defects ("endocardial cushion defects"). Contrary to popular opinion, this valve is a three-leaflet structure with scant resemblance to a morphologically mitral valve.

THE NORMAL MITRAL VALVE

As discussed, the picturesque term "mitral" owes its origin to the resemblance that the atrial aspect view of the valve has to a plan view of a bishop's mitre. Although the basic structure of the mitral valve is well known, descriptions differ with regard to its detailed anatomy. This is partly due to a wide variation in anatomy within the normal range and partly due to the various terminologies applied to its subunits. The major units of the valve are the annulus, leaflets, chords, and papillary muscles.

The mitral annulus comprises of a fibrous ring that anteriorly is in continuity with the aortic valve leaflets. The two expanded portions of this fibrous continuity are the left and right fibrous trigones. In a few hearts, the mitral valve is separated from the aortic valve by a muscular fold, but this is considered within the normal spectrum.[4] The valve characteristically has two discrete leaflets. Accessory leaflets are rare and their presence has been disputed.[5,6] It is important in this respect to distinguish an accessory leaflet from the normal "scallops" of the mural leaflet (see below). The aortic (anterior, septal, or superior) and the mural (posterior, ventricular, or inferior) leaflets are separated by the posteromedial and anterolateral commissures (Fig. 16.2a). It is difficult to choose an entirely appropriate term to describe the different leaflets, particularly the "anterior" one. In the normal heart, the term aortic leaflet is most accurate because the leaflet is neither directly anterior, superior, or septal. But in malformed hearts, particularly

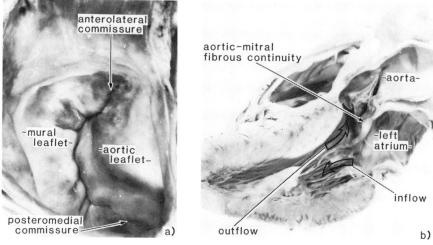

FIGURE 16.2 The atrial view of the mitral valve in **(a)** shows the arrangement of its two leaflets. A simulated parasternal long-axis view of the heart in **(b)** shows the aortic leaflet suspended between the left ventricular inflow and outflow tracts.

with abnormal venticuloarterial connections, this leaflet may be pulmonary, truncal, or it may not be in fibrous continuity with any arterial valve. Despite these caveats, we will use the term aortic leaflet in this work as the most accurate option. The aortic leaflet is semicircular or triangular and is attached to considerably less than one-half the circumference of the annulus. Hinged on its annulus, this leaflet hangs like a curtain between the inflow and outflow tracts of the left ventricle (Fig. 16.2b). In closed position, it forms the greater part of the atrial floor. The mural leaflet, in contrast, has less height but has a more expansive attachment at the mitral annulus. In this respect, the term mural is entirely appropriate because the leaflet is attached to the parietal ventricular wall. It has a scalloped contour, usually displaying three scallops, although five or more scallops may be normal variants. At their free margins, both leaflets have an opaque rough zone that is the region of leaflet coaption during ventricular systole. From the rough zone to the annular insertion is the translucent clear zone of the leaflets.

The chords supporting the mitral valve are mainly inserted into the rough zone on the ventricular aspect of the leaflets. Various classifications have been used for their description.[7,8] In simple terms, they may be divided into commissural (interleaflet) chords and leaflet chords. The anterolateral and posteromedial commissural chords arise as a short stem from the tips of their corresponding papillary muscles and branch almost immediately like the struts of a fan to insert into the free margin of the commissures (Fig.

16.1a). The posteromedial commissural chord fans out more extensively than its anterolateral counterpart.

Leaflet chords may be further classified into rough zone chords and strut chords of the aortic leaflet, and into rough zone chords, cleft chords, and basal chords of the mural leaflet. The strut chords are thicker tendinous structures (Fig. 16.3a) inserting into specific anterior leaflet positions,[8] which have been described as "critical."[9] The cleft chords support the breaches between the scallops of the mural leaflet. They are miniature fan-shaped structures that may be indistinguishable from commissural chords, hence some of the problems in distinguishing the posteromedial and anterolateral scallops from accessory leaflets. The basal part of the scallops may be further supported by chords that arise directly from the mural ventricular myocardium (the basal chords) (Fig. 16.3b). The rough zone chords provide the maximal support for both leaflets, each leaflet being supported by chords arising from both sets of papillary muscle groups. Rough zone chords divide soon after their origin from the papillary muscle to insert into the free margin, the ventricular aspect of the closure line and the intermediate region. The chords show considerable variation in structure, number, and distribution. Some show persistence of a muscular core up to the leaflet margin. This appearance should not be mistaken for rheumatic changes.

Two papillary muscle groups support the mitral valve leaflets. They are situated in close proximity and in anterolateral and posteromedial positions

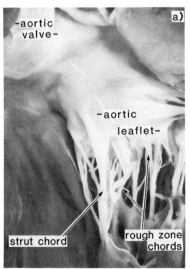
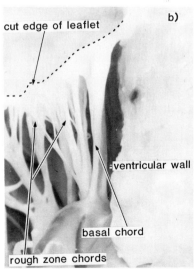

FIGURE 16.3 A left ventricular outflow view **(a)** shows the thicker strut chord and the more slender rough zone chords. The basal part of the mural leaflet is dissected in **(b)** to show the chordal arrangement.

respectively (Figs. 16.1b, and 16.4). A single pillarlike muscle usually occupies the anterolateral position whereas there is more variation in posteromedial position. The different morphology of the papillary muscle affects the chordal distribution. The bases of the papillary muscles are attached to the junction of the middle and lower thirds of the left ventricle.

THE ABNORMAL VALVE

Congenital disease of the mitral valve can affect one or more components of the mitral valve. Although each anatomic unit can be considered separately, more usually the lesion is a generalized deformity.

Lesions Affecting the Whole Valve
The Dysplastic Mitral Valve

This is an abnormal development of the entire valve, and it is the most common cause of isolated congenital mitral valve stenosis.[10] This covers a

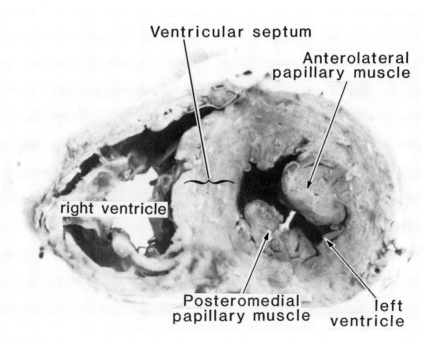

FIGURE 16.4 A short axis section through the ventricular mass shows the arrangement of the two papillary muscle groups supporting the mitral valve.

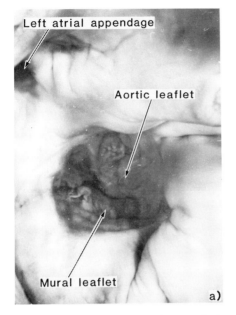
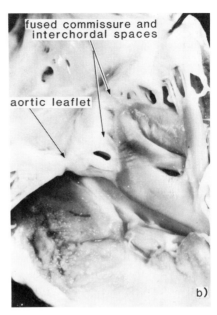

FIGURE 16.5 Left atrial view of a stenotic dysplastic valve is shown in **(a)**. Another dysplastic valve in ventricular view **(b)** shows a partial arcade formation with commissural fusion, obliteration of the interchordal spaces and leaflet thickening.

wide range of abnormalities in which the leaflets and chords are usually thickened, the commissures fused, and interchordal spaces obliterated[11,12] (Fig. 16.5). To this group can be added the funnel-shaped valve in which there is marked thickening and retraction of leaflet tissue in the presence of fused chords with normal papillary muscle arrangement[13]; the valve with reduced interpapillary muscle space[10]; and those valves with abnormally large and high origin of the papillary muscles together with thickened leaflets.[3,7] All of these lesions can cause mitral stenosis.

The Miniaturized Valve

All the components are present in this malformation and do not appear diseased. It is usually found in hearts with hypoplasia of the left ventricle where the entire valve apparatus is diminished in size (Fig. 16.6). The miniaturized valve may be functionally competent but stenotic purely in terms of its size.

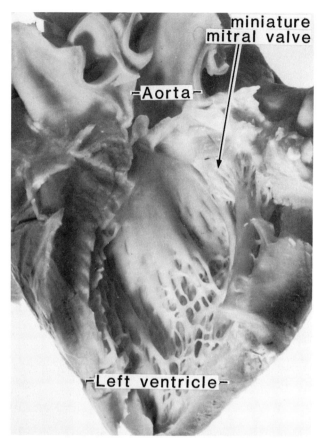

FIGURE 16.6 The mitral valve is miniatuarized although all its components are normally formed.

Lesions Affecting the Annulus

Malformations of the annulus can affect the effective mitral orifice. Included in this group are hearts with absent left atrioventricular connection; an imperforate valve; Ebstein's malformation; dual orifice mitral valve; and those with an overriding valve.

Absent Atrioventricular Connection

This is the most common variety of so-called mitral atresia. In this form the entire valve is absent. The left atrium has a muscular floor that is separated from the ventricular mass by the fibro-fatty tissue of the atrioventricular groove ("sulcus tissue"; Fig. 16.7a). In these hearts it is more appropriate to

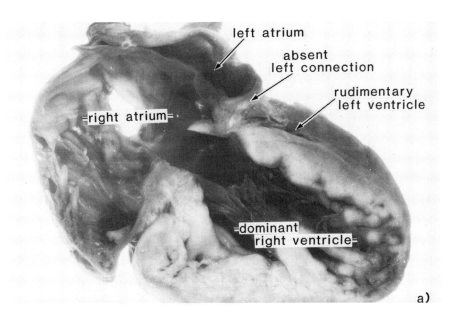

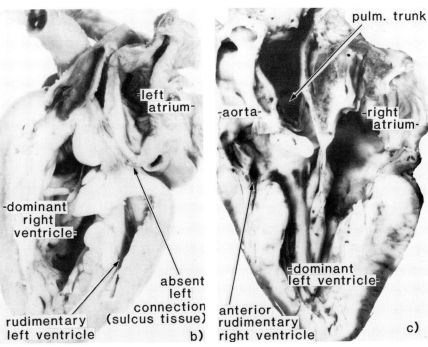

FIGURE 16.7 A four-chamber section in **(a)** shows the blind floor of the left atrium, which is separated from the ventricular mass by sulcus tissue. The right atrium opens into a dominant right ventricle. A similar heart in simulated parasternal long axis section **(b)** shows the posteroinferior position of the rudimentary left ventricle. Another heart **(c)** with dominance of the left ventricle in the presence of absent left atrioventricular connection is sectioned in similar fashion to show the anterior position of the rudimentary right ventricle.

speak of absent left atrioventricular connection rather than to imagine the morphology of a nonexistent valve. Be that as it may, pulmonary venous return leaves the left atrium usually by way of an associated atrial septal defect to the right atrium. The right atrium, although usually connected to a dominant morphologically right ventricle (Fig. 16.7b) can also be connected to a dominant morphologically left ventricle (Fig. 16.7c), or even, very rarely, to a solitary and indeterminate ventricle. It is this variety that underscores the advisability of using the term "left" rather than mitral to describe the arrangement. The left atrial anatomy is identical in each, as is the hemodynamic result and clinical presentation of the absent connection. Yet, when the right ventricle is dominant, it can be presumed that the absent connection was destined to become a mitral valve. In contrast, when the left ventricle is dominant, the valve may have become mitral or tricuspid depending on the position of the rudimentary right ventricle.[14] It is so much simpler and accurate to describe the arrangement as absent left atrioventricular connection.

Imperforate Mitral Valve

Behaving functionally like hearts with absent left atrioventricular connections are those with an imperforate mitral valve membrane.[15] The imperforate variant is a rare cause of mitral atresia. A membrane, instead of a muscular floor, interposes between the left atrium and a hypoplastic left ventricle (Fig. 16.8). The atrioventricular connection is therefore formed and obstructed rather than being absent. The valve membrane, supported by hypoplastic papillary muscles, tends to bulge into the ventricle. Although a concordant atrioventricular connection is usual, similar imperforate valves may be seen in double inlet ventricles, or on the right side in hearts with discordant atrioventricular connection and usually arranged atrial chambers.

Ebstein's Malformation

Usually a malformation of the tricuspid valve, the anatomic lesion termed Ebstein's malformation (see Chapter 23) occasionally affects the morphologically mitral valve. It is important to note that it truly is the morphologically mitral valve that is involved and not, as frequently described,[3] the tricuspid valve in mitral position in hearts with discordant atrioventricular connections. When afflicting the mitral valve, as first described by Ruschaupt et al,[16] Ebstein's malformation results in displacement of the annular insertion of the mural leaflet apically relative to the atrioventricular junction leaving a proximal atrialized ventricular portion (Fig. 16.9). Both leaflets also tend to be dysplastic.

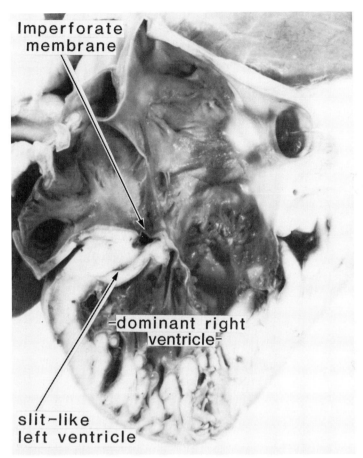

FIGURE 16.8 A section of a heart viewed from the back shows an imperforate membrane between the left-sided atrium and the tiny left ventricle.

Dual Orifice Mitral Valve

Dual orifice can be the consequence of two distinct malformations (Fig. 16.10). In one, the valve orifice is divided simply by fusion of leaflet tissue. In the other, the whole mitral apparatus is duplicated. The former deformity is sometimes seen in isolation,[17] but more often it occurs in the left component of the basically common atrioventricular valve in hearts with atrioventricular septal defect[18] (see below). In duplication of the true mitral valve, each orifice is surrounded by its own leaflets, which in turn are supported by their own sets of chords and papillary muscles. Hearts with this malformation have sometimes been described as having "double outlet left atrium."[19]

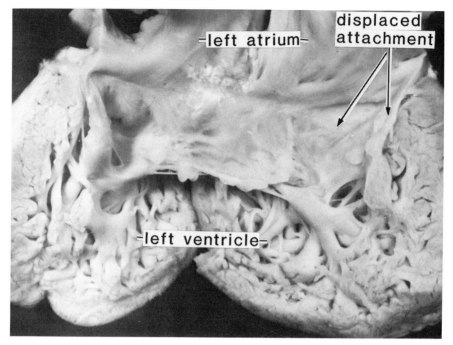

FIGURE 16.9 An Ebstein's malformation of the mitral valve. (Heart photographed courtesy of Dr. J. R. Zuberbuhler.)

Overriding Mitral Valve

The essence of this malformation is that the annulus of the mitral valve is so connected that the orifice opens to more than one ventricle. The overriding valve usually, but not always, exists with straddling of its tensor apparatus across the ventricular septum (Fig. 16.11). When override is such that most of the left atrium opens to the right instead of to the left ventricle, then the heart is categorized as having a double-inlet atrioventricular connection.[20]

Lesions Affecting the Leaflets

Cleft Mitral Valve

The cleft mitral valve is an anomaly that occurs rarely in isolation.[3] It is to be distinguished from the so-called cleft mitral valve seen in association with most forms of atrioventricular septal defect. (This will be considered in detail below.) In hearts with intact atrioventricular septal structures, the true cleft is seen in the aortic leaflet of the mitral valve with its apex pointing to the aortic root (Fig. 16.12). Chordal attachments anchoring one segment of the cleft

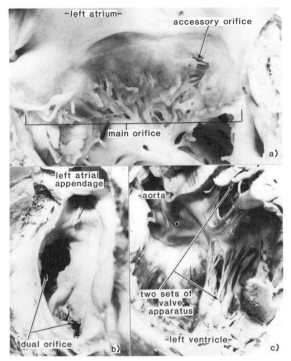

FIGURE 16.10 Two forms of dual orifice mitral valve. An accessory orifice in association with a main orifice is shown in **(a)**. Left atrial view of another heart shows two valve orifices in **(b)** and the left ventricular view **(c)** shows two sets of well formed tension apparatus.

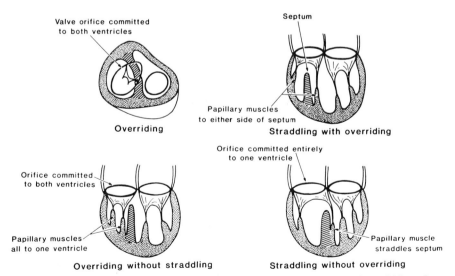

FIGURE 16.11 A diagram showing the distinction between straddling and overidding of an atrioventricular valve.

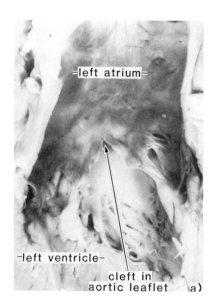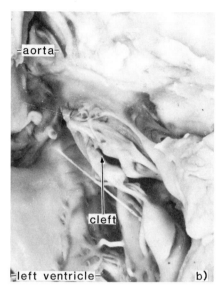

FIGURE 16.12 The aortic leaflet displayed in **(a)** shows a breach in leaflet tissue. The outflow tract view **(b)** shows the cleft pointing to the aorta.

leaflet to the septum can narrow the left ventricular outflow tract.[21] Clefts giving rise to congenital mitral insufficiency can also occur in the mural leaflet.[22] These are exaggerations of the usual breaches between the scallops of this leaflet. A cleft of the mitral valve with intact atrioventricular septal structures is occasionally seen in association with complete transposition or with double outlet right ventricle with subpulmonary defect (Taussig-Bing anomaly). It has been noted that a straddling mitral valve in the latter lesion often has a cleft of its straddling leaflet.[23]

Mitral Prolapse

Domelike extrusions of the valve leaflet into the left atrium during ventricular systole occur either because the leaflet or the chords (or both) are too long or redundant. It has been suggested that minor variations in chordal anatomy leading to unequal leaflet support may render a valve vulnerable to prolapse.[24] The prolapsing leaflet is usually thickened and has a floppy appearance due to mucoid changes in the central tissue core. Generally a feature of the aging heart, cases of mitral valve prolapse have been reported in children with Marfan's syndrome where the valve deformity is considered to be congenital.[7]

Lesions Affecting Chords and Papillary Muscles

Mitral Arcade

An arcade lesion is produced by direct union of the aortic leaflet with the papillary muscles and fusion of the papillary muscles beneath the free margin of the leaflet (Fig. 16.13). The chords are short and thickly muscularised resulting in limited leaflet movement. The arcade lesion (originally described by Layman and Edwards[25]) is included as one of the variants of the hammock valve.[13] The hammock valve describes the atrial view as seen by the surgeon with its numerous intermingled chords attached to a complex of hypertrophied papillary muscles sometimes arranged in an arcade.

The Parachute Mitral Valve

Different definitions have been given for the parachute mitral valve, but they all describe a funnellike malformation. Swan et al[26] first reported a case with a unique mitral valve: the chords were shortened and inserted into the apex of a double-bellied papillary muscle such that, when viewed from the atrial aspect, the mitral valve resembled the inverted top of a salt-shaker (Fig. 16.14a). The term "parachute valve" was not coined until 1961 and was used

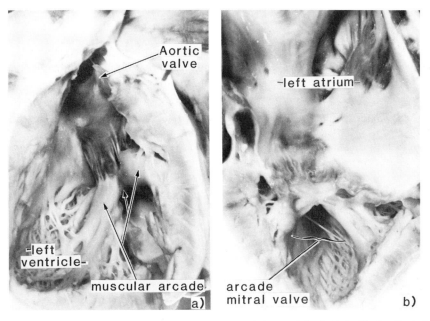

FIGURE 16.13 Fusion of the papillary muscles beneath the aortic leaflet **(a)** with direct insertion of the leaflet to the papillary muscles **(b)** forms an arcade lesion.

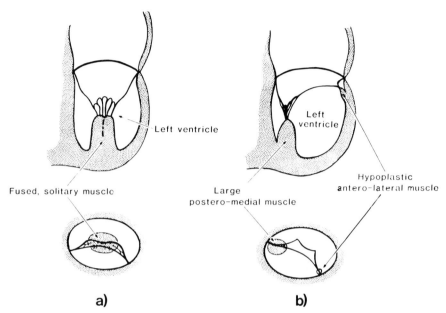

FIGURE 16.14 The parachute valve as originally described by Swan et al **(a)** is contrasted with a form described by Ruckman and Van Praagh **(b)**.

to describe the valve in a heart with congenitally corrected transposition.[27] Two leaflets and commissures are usually discernible[28] in the parachute valve, but the chords converge to insert into one major or sole papillary muscle. The presence of a solitary muscle is the classical form,[3] but Ruckman and Van Praagh[10] included cases with hypoplasia of the anterolateral papillary muscle (Fig. 16.14b). If two discernible papillary muscles are present, but one is hypoplastic, then this could be better described as partial muscle hypoplasia (Fig. 16.15) rather than parachute deformity.[19] Although Ruckman and Van Praagh[10] excluded cases with chordal attachment to each of two fused papillary muscles, others[28] have included them as partial parachute valves. These definitions and criteria seem over-rigid when free egress of flow in all types is dependent on the available interchordal spaces. The parachute mitral valve is frequently associated with left heart obstructive lesions such as supravalvar ring of the left atrium, subaortic stenosis, and aortic coarctation[28,30] and occasionally with right-sided lesions.[31]

Straddling Mitral Valve

A straddling valve is defined as one in which the tension apparatus is attached to both sides of the ventricular septum (Fig. 16.11). When present in hearts with concordant atrioventricular connections, the mitral valve straddles through an anterior septal defect (Fig. 16.16). This is usually seen with either the Taussig-Bing variant of double outlet right ventricle[32] or else with complete transposition. A straddling valve can exist without overriding of its valve orifice.

THE LEFT ATRIOVENTRICULAR VALVE IN ATRIOVENTRICULAR SEPTAL DEFECT

The description of the left valve in so-called endocardial cushion defects, repair of which is crucial in successful surgery, is bedevilled by accounts of a

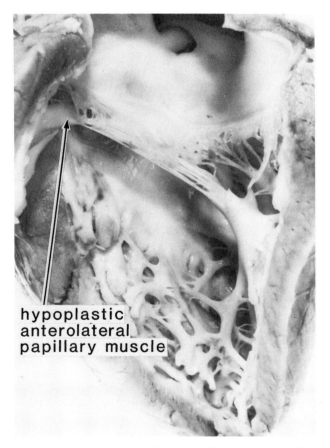

hypoplastic
anterolateral
papillary muscle

FIGURE 16.15 Hypoplasia of the anterolateral papillary muscle produces a tunnellike deformity.

"cleft mitral valve." We have described and illustrated above the morphology of a cloven aortic leaflet of the mitral valve in hearts with intact atrioventricular septal structures. The lesion points into the left ventricular outflow tract (Fig. 16.12). Suture of the two halves of the cloven leaflet restores the morphology of the normal mitral valve. The so-called cleft in atrioventricular septal defects bears no resemblance to this lesion. Indeed, the left atrioventricular valve in hearts with deficient atrioventricular septation bears scant resemblance to a mitral or bifoliate valve. This fact was first noted by Peacock,[33] who described the valve succinctly and accurately as a "tricuspid structure." Rastelli et al[34] then pointed to the inadvisability of describing a "cleft" in the mitral valve. Carpentier[35] subsequently emphasized the essential three-leaflet nature of the left valve. His observations have been amply confirmed by subsequent echocardiographic investigations,[36,37] along with the measurements of Penkoske et al.[38] Taken together, these works show that the left atrioventricular valve in atrioventricular septal defect differs from the normal mitral valve in terms of annular attachment, its leaflet arrangement, and the morphology of its papillary muscles within the left ventricle. Indeed, its only resemblance with the mitral valve is that it guards the inlet of the morphologically left ventricle. Some, however, seem reticent to accept these differences, arguing that there is little reason for not calling the structure a mitral valve, so long as it is recognized to be a deformed mitral valve. In support of this, they cite the case of the aortic valve, which continues to be called the aortic valve irrespective of whether it has one, two, or more leaflets. Here they miss the principle of the naming of anatomic structures. The aortic valve is called the aortic valve because it guards the aortic orifice, irrespective of the ventricle to which the aorta is connected. The mitral valve is called mitral because it has two leaflets, not in virtue of its position within the heart. There is no reason, therefore, to continue to describe a left atrioventricular valve as mitral when it unequivocally possesses three leaflets as in an atrioventricular septal defect.

It is important to note that this three-leaflet arrangement of the left valve (Fig. 16.17) is seen irrespective of whether an atrioventricular septal defect has a common orifice (complete defect) or separate right and left atrioventricular valve orifices (partial defect). The so-called cleft in all these lesions is the space between the left ventricular components of two bridging leaflets (the two leaflets that span the septum and are attached within both the right and left ventricles). Whether the space should be considered a commissure is moot.[39] It certainly is not a cleft in the aortic leaflet of the normal mitral valve. This is readily evident from the fact that the cleft points to the septum, not the outflow tract, and that the two components of the bridging leaflets take up more than two-thirds of the annular circumference (Fig. 16.17) This discussion has no bearing on whether the space between the left ventricular

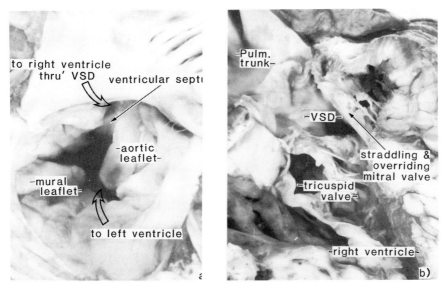

FIGURE 16.16 A left atrial view **(a)** shows overriding of the mitral valve across the ventricular septum. The right ventricular view **(b)** shows straddling of tension apparatus across an anterior ventricular septal defect.

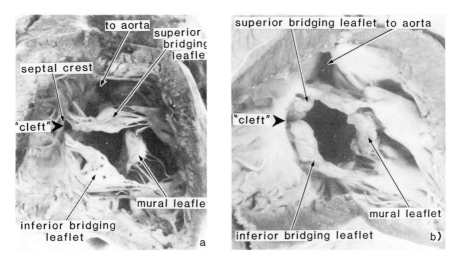

FIGURE 16.17 In hearts with atrioventricular septal defect the left component of the atrioventricular valve is trileaflet whether the septal crest is exposed **(a)** or covered by bridging leaflet tissue **(b)**. In each type the cleft points away from the aorta.

components of the bridging leaflets should be closed during surgery. That point remains unresolved and cannot be influenced by purely anatomic studies. Nonetheless, the functional studies that will be required to resolve this problem will be greatly aided if it is recognized that (as Peacock[33] indicated) the left valve in atrioventricular septal defect is basically a three-leaflet structure.

THE FUNCTIONAL APPROACH

It is well known that normal function of the mitral valve depends upon the integrity and condition of its individual components and their interaction with the contracting myocardium.[2] Although dysfunction is not always accompanied by gross pathology of the valve apparatus,[29] more than one defect can affect the same valve. Furthermore, anatomically heterogenous lesions can give rise to the same type of valvar dysfunction, thereby producing similar clinical states. The functional approach[40] is useful in surgical planning where the aim is to restore function rather than reconstruct the anatomy. It considers lesions that cause mitral insufficiency and mitral stenosis.[40] As the valve leaflets play the major role in guarding the atrioventricular orifice, their mobility is the key to valvar function. The functional approach (Table 16.1) considers motion of the aortic and mural leaflets separately in terms of normal, prolapse, or restricted motion.

TABLE 16.1 The Functional Approach[a]

Leaflet Motion	Congenital Malformations
Normal	Annulus dilatation
	Leaflet defect
	Cleft leaflet
Prolapsed	Chord agenesis
	Chord elongation
	Papillary muscle degeneration
Restricted	With normal papillary muscles
	Commissural fusion
	Short chords
	Ebstein's malformation
	With abnormal papillary muscles
	Parachute valve
	Hammock valve
	Absent papillary muscle(s)

[a]Adapted from Carpentier.[40]

REFERENCES

1. Little RC. The closure of the mitral valve: a continuing controversy. Circulation 1979;59:615–618.
2. Perloff JK, Roberts WC. The mitral apparatus. Functional anatomy of mitral regurgitation. Circulation 1972;46:227–239.
3. Davachi F, Moller JH, Edwards JE. Diseases of the mitral valve in infancy. An anatomic analysis of 55 cases. Circulation 1971;43:565–579.
4. Rosenquist GC, Clark EB, Sweeney LJ, et al. The normal spectrum of mitral and aortic valve discontinuity. Circulation 1976;54:298–301.
5. Rusted IE, Schiefley CH, Edwards JE. Studies of the mitral valve. I. Anatomic features of the normal mitral valve and associated structures. Circulation 1952;6:825.
6. Ranganatham N, Lam JHC, Wigle ED, et al. Morphology of the human mitral valve. II. The valve leaflets. Circulation 1970;41:459–467.
7. Roberts WC, Perloff JK. Mitral valvular disease. Ann Int Med 1972;77:939–975.
8. Lam JHC, Ranganathan N, Wigle ED, et al. Morphology of the human mitral valve. I. Chordae Tendineae: A new classification. Circulation 1970;41:449–458.
9. Brock RC. The surgical and pathological anatomy of the normal mitral valve. Br Heart J 1952;14:489–513.
10. Ruckman RN, Van Praagh R. Anatomic types of congenital mitral stenosis: report of 49 cases with consideration of diagnosis and surgical implications. Am J Cardiol 1978;42:592–601.
11. Ferencz C, Johnson AL, Wiglesworth FW. Congenital mitral stenosis. Circulation 1954;9:61–179.
12. Daoud G, Kaplan S, Perrin EV, et al. Congenital mitral stenosis. Circulation 1963;27:185–196.
13. Carpentier A, Branchini B, Cour JC, et al. Congenital malformations of the mitral valve in children. Pathology and surgical treatment. J Thorac Cardiovasc Surg 1976;72:854–866.
14. Restivo A, Ho SY, Anderson RH, et al. Absent left atrioventricular connection with right atrium connected to morphologically left ventricular chamber, rudimentary right ventricular chamber, and ventriculoarterial discordance. Problem of mitral versus tricuspid atresia. Br Heart J 1982;48:240–248.
15. Rigby ML Gibson DG, Joseph MC, et al. Recognition of imperforate atrioventricular valves by two dimensional echocardiography. Br Heart J 1982;47:329–336.
16. Ruschhaupt DG, Bharati S, Lev M. Mitral valve malformation of Ebstein type in absence of corrected transposition. Am J Cardiol 1976;38:109–112.
17. Edwards JE, Burchell HB. Pathologic anatomy of mitral insufficiency. Mayo Clin Proc 1958;33:497.
18. Ugarte M, de Salamanca FE, Quero M. Endocardial cushion defects. An anatomical study of 54 specimens. Br Heart J 1976;38:674–682.
19. Bini RM, Pellegrino PA, Mazzucco A, et al. Tricuspid atresia with double-outlet left atrium. Chest 1980;78:109–111.
20. Keeton BR, Macartney FJ, Hunter S, et al. Univentricular heart of right ventricular type with double or common inlet. Circulation 1979;59:403–411.
21. Sellers RD, Lillehei CW, Edwards JE. Subaortic stenosis caused by anomalies of the atrioventricular valves. J Thorac Cardiovasc Surg 1964;48:289–302.
22. Creech O, Ledbetter MK, Reemtsma K. Congenital mitral insufficiency with cleft posterior leaflet. Circulation 1962;25:390–394.
23. Soto B, Ceballos R, Nath PH, et al. Overriding atrioventricular valves. An angiographic-anatomical correlate. Int J Cardiol 1985 (in press).

24. Becker AE, Dewit APM. Mitral valve apparatus. Br Heart J 1979;42:680–689.
25. Layman TE, Edwards JE. Anomalous mitral arcade: A type of congenital mitral insufficiency. Circulation 1967;35:389–395.
26. Swan H, Trapnell JM, Denst J. Congenital mitral stenosis and systemic right ventricle with associated pulmonary vascular changes frustrating surgical repair of patent ductus arteriosus and coarctation of the aorta. Am Heart J 1949;38:914–923.
27. Schiebler GL, Edwards JE, Burchell HB, et al. Congenital corrected transposition of the great vessels: a study of 33 cases. Pediatrics 1961;2:s849.
28. Shone JD, Sellers RD, Anderson RC, et al. The developmental complex of "parachute mitral valve," supravalvular ring of left atrium, subaortic stenosis, and coarctation of the aorta. Am J Cardiol 1963;11:714–725.
29. Becker AE. Valve pathology in the paediatric age group. Pediatr Cardiol 1983;5:345–360.
30. Rosenquist GC. Congenital mitral valve disease associated with coarctation of the aorta. A spectrum that includes parachute deformity of the mitral valve. Circulation 1974;49:985–993.
31. Glancy DL, Chang MY, Dorney ER, et al. Parachute mitral valve. Further observations and associated lesions. Am J Cardiol 1971;27:309–313.
32. Kitamura N, Takao A, Ando M, et al. Taussig-Bing heart with mitral valve straddling: case reports and post-mortem study. Circulation 1974;49:761–767.
33. Peacock TB. Malformation of the heart consisting in an imperfection of the auricular and ventricular septa. Trans Pathol Soc (London) 1846;1:61–62.
34. Rastelli GC, Kirklin JW, Titus JL. Anatomic observations on complete form of persistent common atrioventricular canal with special reference to atrioventricular valves. Mayo Clin Proc 1966;41:296–308.
35. Carpentier A. Surgical anatomy and management of the mitral component of atrioventricular canal defects. In, Anderson RH and Shinebourne EA (eds): Paediatric Cardiology 1977. Churchill Livingstone, Edinburgh, 1978, pp 477–486.
36. Chin AJ, Bierman F, Sanders SP, et al. Subxyphoid 2-dimensional echocardiographic identification of left ventricular papillary muscle anomalies in complete common atrioventricular canal. Am J Cardiol 1983;51:1695–1700.
37. Ebels TJ, Meijboom EJ, Anderson RH, et al. Anatomic and functional "obstruction" of the outflow tract in atrioventricular septal defects with separate valve orifices ("ostium primum atrial septal defect"): an echocardiographic study. Am J Cardiol 1984;54:843–847.
38. Penkoske PA, Neches WH, Anderson RH, et al. Further observations on the morphology of atrioventricular septal defects. J Thor Card Surg 1985;90:611–622.
39. Anderson RH, Zuberbuhler JR, Penkoske PA, et al. Of clefts, commissures, and things. J Thor Card Surg 1985;605–610.
40. Carpentier A. Mitral valve reconstruction in children. In Anderson RH, Macartney FJ, Shinebourne EA, Tynan M (eds): Paediatric Cardiology 5. Churchill Livingston, Edinburgh, 1983, pp 361–368.

CHAPTER 17

A Consideration of the Morphology and Diagnostic Features of Certain Congenital Abnormalities of the Mitral Valve

Robert M. Freedom, MD, FRCP(C), FACC,
and Jeffrey F. Smallhorn, MD, FRACP, FRCP(C)

There is now an extensive literature devoted both to the anatomy and function of the normal mitral valve as well as to those heterogeneous congenital anomalies of the left ventricular inlet.[1-9] Ho and Anderson, in the preceding chapter, have elegantly displayed in word and picture the anatomy of the normal mitral valve and its support mechanism, and as well they have focused attention on the morphology on some of the more common congenital anomalies of the mitral valve. In this chapter, we will extend those morphological observations on certain congenital anomalies of the mitral valve, showing the value of angiography and cross-sectional echocardiography in their diagnosis.

THE MITRAL VALVE ANNULUS

The preoperative quantification or measurement of the mitral valve annulus may be very important in the management of the patient with obstruction at the left ventricular inlet.[10-13] It has become increasingly evident that cross-sectional echocardiographic examination of the mitral valve using both the left parasternal long axis and the subcostal four-chamber echocardiographic projections provides reasonable information about the mitral annulus.

185

CONGENITAL MITRAL STENOSIS

Ruckman and Van Praagh have defined four anatomic types of congenital mitral stenosis[4]: (a) typical congenital mitral stenosis with short chordae tendineae, attenuation of interchordal spaces and reduction of the distance between papillary muscles (Fig. 17.1); (b) so-called hypoplastic congenital mitral stenosis (this variety is usually associated with the hypoplastic left heart syndrome); (c) so-called parachute deformity of the mitral valve; and (d) supravalvular stenosing mitral ring. Among those patients considered to have typical mitral stenosis, some patients may exhibit abnormal chordal attachments to the left ventricular septal surface or free wall, or the thickened mitral valve attached directly onto the papillary muscles. Other patients exhibit rather impressive reduction in the interpapillary muscle distance, the papillary muscles of the left ventricle being abnormally close together or even fused, reminiscent of the parachute deformity. Ruckman and Van Praagh characterize so-called hypoplastic mitral stenosis as that form of congenital left ventricular inflow obstruction in which all components of the mitral valve were in miniature.[4] The mitral annulus and mitral valve orifice are both small. These authors describe the chordae tendineae as shortened, but not thickened, and the papillary muscles as small, often incorporated into the endocardial sclerosis.

THE PARACHUTE DEFORMITY OF THE MITRAL VALVE

The parachute deformity is a condition in which the chordae tendineae of the mitral valve converge to insert either onto a single papillary muscle or

---

FIGURE 17.1 Congenital mitral stenosis (typical type according to Ruckman and Van Praagh). **(a)** Internal view of severely enlarged left atrium *(LA)* and mitral valve. Two papillary muscles *(X)* are present. The free valve margin is thickened; the chordal tendineae are short and thick, and the interchordal spaces are attenuated. **(b)** Hypoplastic form of mitral valve stenosis in a neonate with aortic atresia, small left ventricle *(white asterisk),* and markedly hypertrophied myocardium. **(c)** Systolic frame of a left ventricular angiogram *(LV)* in a patient with severe mitral stenosis and markedly thickened mitral valve and support mechanism *(black asterisk).* **(d)** Appearance of a stenotic mitral valve *(black asterisk)* in a neonate with critical aortic stenosis and persistence of so-called spongy myocardium. **(e)** Praecordial long axis cut in mitral stenosis due to annular hypoplasia. This patient also had an associated ventricular septal defect. Note the normal sized left ventricle. Also observe the dilated coronary sinus. Abbreviations: Ao = aorta; CS = coronary sinus; LA = left atrium; LV = left ventricle; MV = mitral valve; MA = mitral annulus; RV = right ventricle. **(f)** Subcostal four-chamber cut in congenital mitral stenosis. Note that this patient has two papillary muscles. It is difficult to differentiate between the mitral leaflets, the chordae, and the papillary muscles due to the significant stenosis. Also observe the enlarged left atrium. Abbreviations: AN = annulus; LA = left atrium; PM = papillary muscle; RA = right atrium; RV = right ventricle.

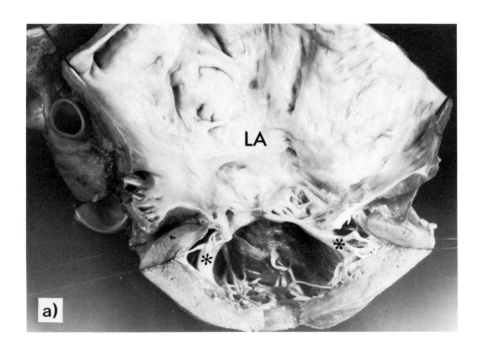

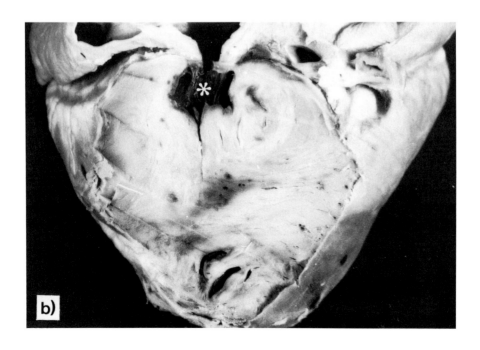

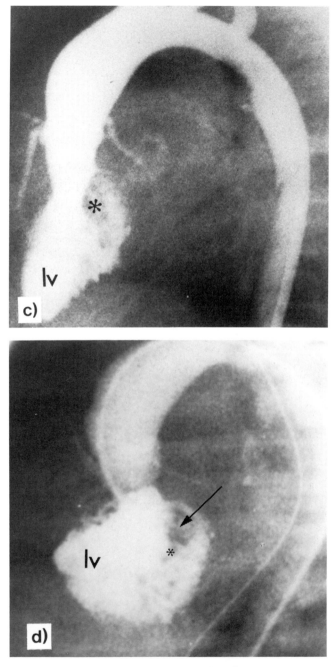

FIGURE 17.1 *(continued)*

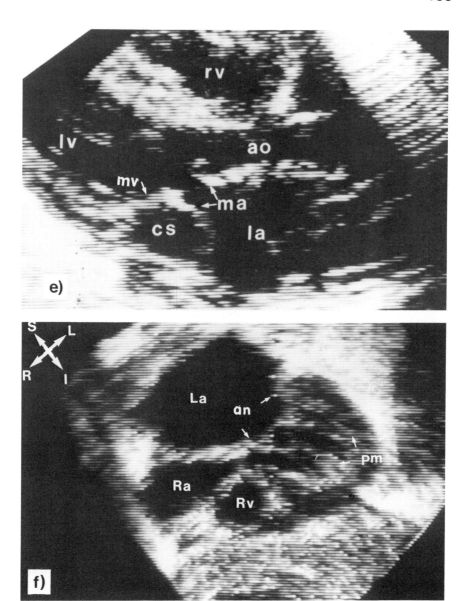

FIGURE 17.1 *(continued)*

onto a cluster of malpositioned contiguous papillary muscles[2,4,14-21] (Fig. 17.2). Such a deformity can occur in relative isolation, but its best known association is with the Shone complex: supravalvular stenosing mitral ring, subaortic stenosis, and coarctation of the aorta. A number of other reports have extended the association of the parachute mitral valve with any form of left ventricular outflow tract obstruction, coarctation of the aorta, transposition of the great arteries, atrioventricular septal defect, and univentricular atrioventricular connection.[22,23]

The parachute deformity of the mitral valve in its classical form has a solitary posteromedial papillary muscle onto which the mitral tensor or support apparatus converge. Usually this deformity is associated with some thickening of the free valve margin, shortening of the chordae tendineae, and attenuation of the interchordal spaces. All these factors tend to restrict flow through the mitral valve. Although such restriction and the appearance of a solitary papillary muscle can be recognized angiographically, the angiocardiographic findings may not always be convincing. Macartney et al have called attention to the so-called "egg-timer" or "hour-glass" deformity as visualized on left ventriculography as helpful to the diagnosis of the parachute deformity.[2,19,24] We, too, have found the appearance useful to the diagnosis of this entity (Fig. 17.2).

Today, however, we would consider cross-sectional echocardiography probably superior to angiography in the recognition of the parachute deformity. The left ventricle can be imaged in several cuts, and one can usually be convinced of a significant distortion in papillary muscle number or structure.

SUPRAVALVULAR STENOSING MITRAL RING

The supravalvular stenosing mitral ring is an unusual cause of left ventricular inflow obstruction, and this must be differentiated from the classical left atrial membrane of cor triatriatum. The membrane of cor triatriatum is positioned superiorly to the ostium of the left atrial appendage, while the supravalvular stenosing mitral ring is inferior to the left atrial appendage ostium, and is usually within a few millimeters of the mitral valve ring.[2,4,14,15,24-27]

The supravalvular stenosing mitral ring can occur in isolation, but this is most uncommon; more frequently this rare case of left ventricular inflow tract obstruction is in association with the Shone's complex: parachute deformity of the mitral valve, subaortic stenosis, and coarctation of the aorta.[14,15] The supravalvular stenosing mitral ring is usually circumferential, or nearly so, and is composed of fibroelastic tissue. The mitral valve may be normal or abnormal in configuration (Fig. 17.3).

The diagnosis of a supravalvular stenosing mitral ring should be considered in any patient with left ventricular inlet and outlet obstruction. The diagnosis can be made by left atrial angiography or by left ventricular angiography (in the presence of mitral regurgitation). Probably the right anterior oblique or hepatoclavicular projections should profile the circumferential radiolucency that partitions the left atrium inferior to the ostium of the left atrial appendage.[24] Although cardiac angiography can make the diagnosis of a supravalvular stenosing mitral ring, our experience indicates that cross-sectional echocardiographic interrogation is more reliable in establishing this diagnosis. One can readily visualize, without overlapping structures, the mitral valve, its annulus, and the points of opening of the mitral valve. A supravalvular stenosing mitral ring is readily seen within the context of these landmarks. (Fig. 17.3)

"ANOMALOUS MITRAL ARCADE"

Nearly 20 years ago, Layman and Edward[28] called attention to the anomalous mitral arcade as a specific type of congenital mitral insufficiency. The "arcade" is formed by the papillary muscles, the lower edge of the anterior mitral leaflet, and the intervening chordae. Chordae tendineae between the anterolateral papillary muscle and the aortic leaflet of the mitral valve are markedly attenuated, and, in essence, there is direct union of this papillary muscle and the aortic leaflet of the mitral valve. The arcade deformity is uncommon, or at least it is uncommonly recognized as such. Castaneda et al[29] reported an unusual case of congenital mitral stenosis in which functional obstruction at the left ventricular inlet resulted both from the anomalous arcade and obstructing papillary muscles. Frech et al[30] called attention again to the association of the anomalous mitral arcade with enlarged papillary muscles. In one of their two patients, the huge papillary muscles formed a narrow channel under the mitral valve, and this presumably was the basis for the mitral stenosis (Fig. 17.2a).

From the available clinical reports and from our own limited patient material, the mitral arcade can be found in patients with congenital mitral regurgitation, or stenosis, or both. We are not convinced that there are specific angiographic features of the anomalous mitral arcade, but this is contentious. Nor do we not have enough clinical experience with echocardiographic examination to formulate diagnostic criteria.[31]

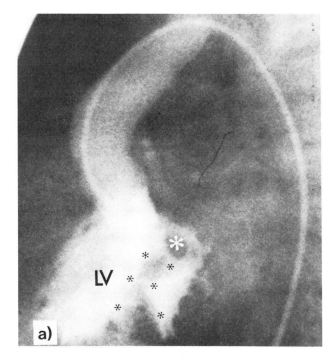

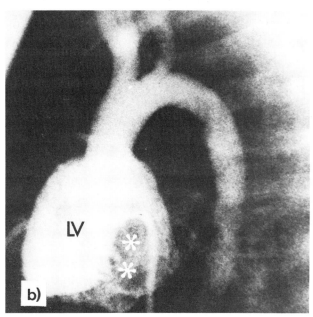

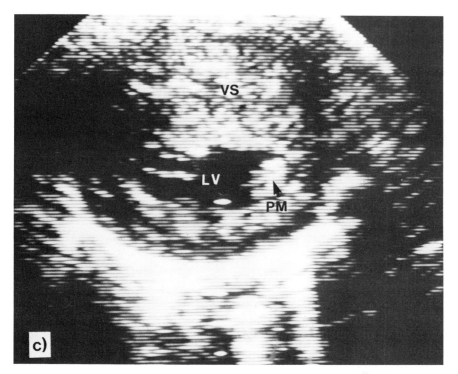

FIGURE 17.2 Parachute deformity of mitral valve. **(a)** This left ventricular *(LV)* angiogram in the left anterior oblique projection demonstrates the so-called "egg timer" deformity. The restrictive mitral orifice *(white asterisk)* and the abnormal contour of the mitral apparatus converging *(black asterisk)* onto a solitary left ventricular papillary muscle are clearly evident. **(b)** A patient with congenital mitral stenosis and enlarged papillary muscles in a parachute configuration. **(c)** Praecordial short-axis cut in mitral stenosis and a single papillary muscle. Abbreviations: LV = left ventricle; PM = papillary muscle; VS = ventricular septum.

ISOLATED ANTERIOR MITRAL CLEFT

The isolated cleft of the anterior or aortic leaflet of the mitral valve results in congenital mitral regurgitation (Fig. 17.4).[32,33] This type of cleft must be differentiated from the so-called cleft associated with the atrioventricular septal defect.[32] The isolated cleft is a constant defect in the aortic leaflet of the mitral valve and cross-sectional echocardiographic interrogation shows that this cleft in this situation points towards the left ventricular outflow tract. Conversely, the so-called cleft of the atrioventricular septal defect is situated between the anterior and posterior bridging leaflets and the cleft points towards the interventricular septum rather than the left ventricular outflow tract.[32]

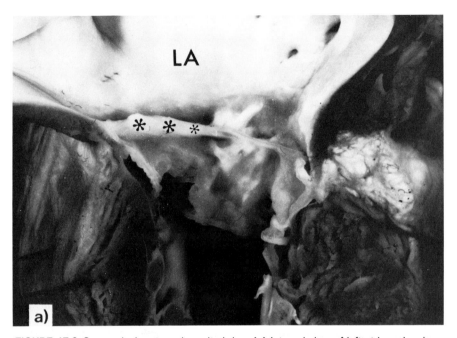

FIGURE 17.3 Supravalvular stenosing mitral ring. **(a)** Internal view of left atrium showing a circumferential supravalvular stenosing mitral ring *(black asterisk)*. The mitral valve in this patient was also abnormal. **(b)** This left atriogram *(LA)* filmed in the right anterior oblique projection shows a supravalvular stenosing mitral ring *(arrows)* inferior to the dilated left atrial appendage. The mitral valve *(black asterisk)* is stenotic in this patient. **(c)** Praecordial long-axis cut in mitral stenosis due to a supramitral mitral ring. Note the large left atrium and the supramitral membrane attached to the mitral leaflets. Abbreviations: AO = aorta; LA = left atrium; LV = left ventricle; MV = mitral valve; SMM = supramitral membrane; RV = right ventricle.

The anterior mitral cleft can occur in isolation, but it has now been associated with a wide range of congenitally malformed hearts including those with a straddling mitral valve. There is little angiographic information in patients with isolated cleft in the aortic leaflet of the mitral valve. We are persuaded, however, by the accumulation of clinical evidence that cross-sectional echocardiographic examination along with Doppler interrogation is the method of choice in establishing this diagnosis (Fig. 17.4).

THE EBSTEIN-LIKE MALFORMATION OF THE MITRAL VALVE

While displacement and dysplasia of the morphologically tricuspid valve has been well described in patients with atrioventricular concordance or discor-

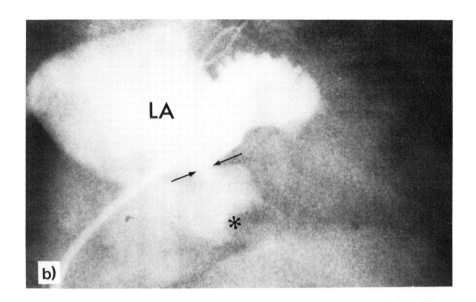

b)

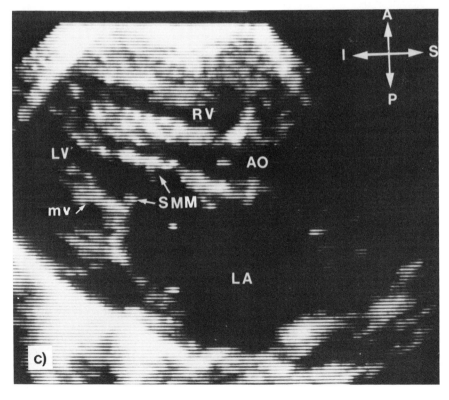

c)

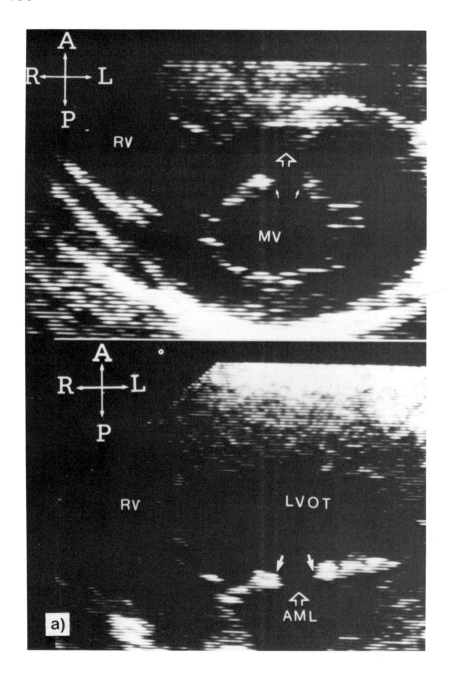

a)

FIGURE 17.4 Isolated anterior mitral cleft. **(a)** Praecordial short-axis views from a patient with isolated anterior mitral cleft. Note that the cleft in the anterior mitral leaflet points towards the left ventricular outflow tract and not towards the right ventricle as seen in patients with an atrioventricular septal defect. **(b)** The upper picture is a praecordial long-axis cut of a patient with a cleft anterior mitral leaflet and chordae from the leaflet inserting to the left ventricular outflow tract. This frame is taken during systole. The lower picture is from the same picture taken during diastole demonstrating the persistent chordae inserting into the outflow tract. Abbreviations: AML = anterior mitral leaflet; LVOT = left ventricular outflow tract; MV = mitral valve, RV = right ventricle; Ao = aorta; CH = chordae; LA = left atrium; LV = left ventricle; MV = mitral valve.

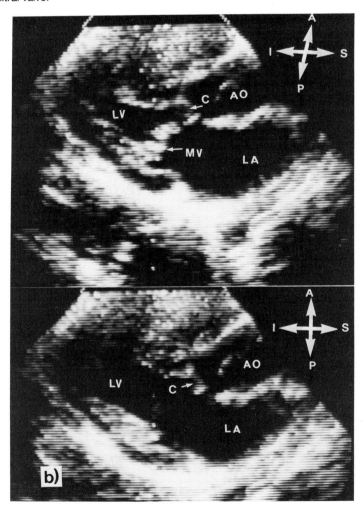

dance, there are now a few well documented examples of displacement of the mural leaflet of the mitral valve from the left atrioventricular groove.[34,35] Such displacement results in mitral regurgitation.[34,35] We have not had the opportunity to study such a patient, but cross-sectional echocardiography with Doppler interrogation is likely to be the most efficacious way of recognizing this anomaly.

DOUBLE-OUTLET LEFT ATRIUM

The diagnosis of double-outlet left atrium (Fig. 17.5) was first made in the context of a complex form of atrioventricular septal defect in which striking malalignment between atrial and ventricular septa was evident.[36,37] Among patients with atrioventricular septal defect, we and others have recognized patients with double-outlet right atrium as well as double-outlet left atrium. But the term "double-outlet atrium" embraces not only those hearts with malalignment between atrial and ventricular septa, but other hearts with straddling or overriding of one or both atrioventricular valves, or those with an accessory atrioventricular orifice.[38-53]

Numerous papers have addressed the morphological features of a straddling mitral valve, and the types of congenital heart disease in which a straddling mitral valve had been recognized.[41-44,46-49] Suffice it to say, a straddling mitral valve cannot occur in isolation. The mere presence of a straddling mitral valve necessitates an anteriorly positioned ventricular septal defect. It is the aortic or anterior leaflet of the mitral valve that usually straddles, not the mural leaflet. Morphologically, straddling can be relatively mild or very severe. When severe straddling and overriding is present, there may be difficulty in differentiation from a univentricular atrioventricular connection. But even a minor degree of straddling implies important surgical management implications. While the straddling mitral valve can be identified in patients with relatively "simple" lesions such as isolated ventricular septal defect or tetralogy of Fallot, its most common association is with double-outlet right ventricle of the Taussig-Bing type; transposition of the great arteries; right atrioventricular valve atresia; or superoinferior ventricles with crossed atrioventricular connections. A straddling mitral valve has been recognized in patients with atrioventricular discordance, but this is distinctly uncommon.

Selective left atriography or ventriculography can be used to diagnose the straddling mitral valve (Fig. 17.5), but anomalies of the atrioventricular junction are best addressed by cross sectional echocardiographic interrogation.

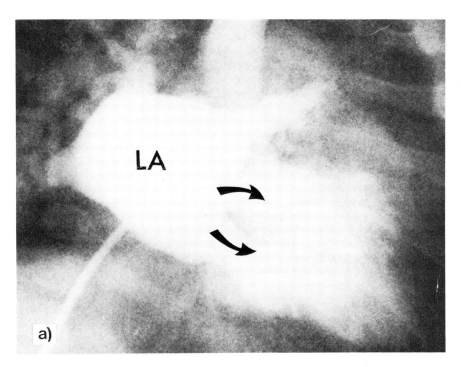

FIGURE 17.5 Various forms of double-outlet left atrium. **(a)** Left atriogram *(LA)* clearly showing a double orifice *(arrows)* mitral valve. **(b,c)** Absent right atrioventricular connection and double-outlet left atrium. **(b)** Internal view of morphologically right atrium *(RA)* showing no connection with the ventricular mass. **(c)** The basis for the double-outlet left atrium is the straddling anterior leaflet *(asterisk)* of the mitral valve. **(d)** Straddling mitral valve as the aetiology of double-outlet left atrium *(LA)* in a patient with transposition and severe left ventricular outlet obstruction. Note the anterior leaflet *(asterisks)* of the mitral valve crosses the ventricular septal defect, inserting into the right ventricle *(white asterisk)*. **(e)** Virtual double-inlet univentricular connection of right ventricular type. This internal view of the left atrium shows that the mitral valve *(black asterisks)* is committed in its entirety to the right ventricle *(white asterisk)*, and the morphologically left ventricle *(LV)* is globally underdeveloped. **(f)** Left atriogram *(LA)* of a different patient followed in hepatoclavicular projection clearly showing a straddling mitral valve (necropsy-confirmed). **(g)** Praecordial long-axis cut from a patient with double orifice mitral valve. Note the two orifices indicated by the *arrows* each with its own tension apparatus. **(h)** A praecordial long-axis cut from a patient with double-outlet right ventricle and straddling mitral valve. Note the chordae from the anterior mitral leaflet cross the ventricular septal defect and insert into the right ventricle. The lower picture is a similar cut from a different patient demonstrating anatomical features. **(i)** Praecordial four-chamber cut in a patient with double-outlet right atrium and atrioventricular septal defect. Note that the right atrium is committed to both the right ventricle and the left ventricle. This patient had an associated restricted ostium primum atrial septal defect. Abbreviations: Ao = aorta; LA = left atrium; LV = left ventricle; OR1 = orifice 1; OR2 = orifice 2; CH = chordae; MV = mitral valve; RA = right atrium; RV = right ventricle; VS = ventricular septum. (Figure 17.5e provided by Dr. C. Belcourt, Halifax, Nova Scotia.)

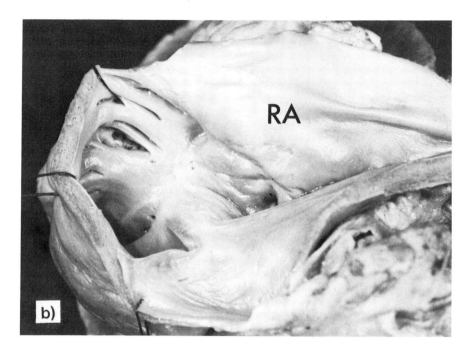

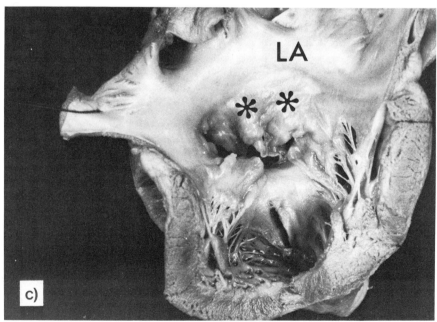

FIGURE 17.5 *(continued)*

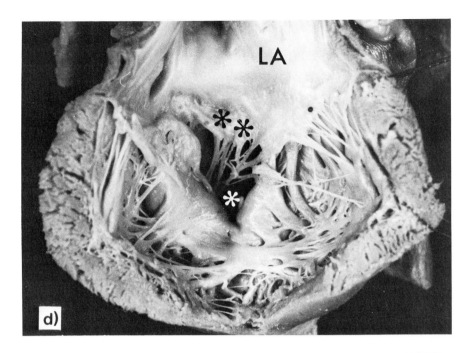

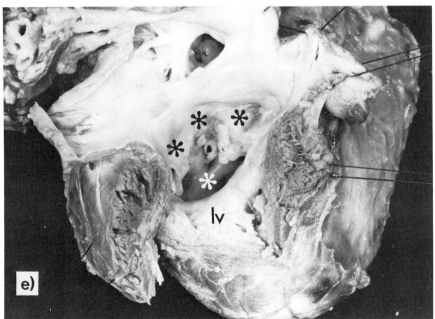

FIGURE 17.5 *(continued)*

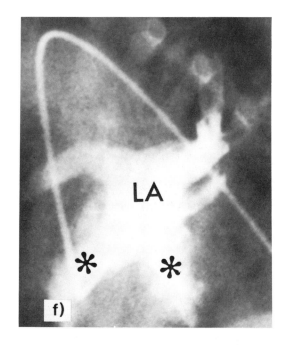

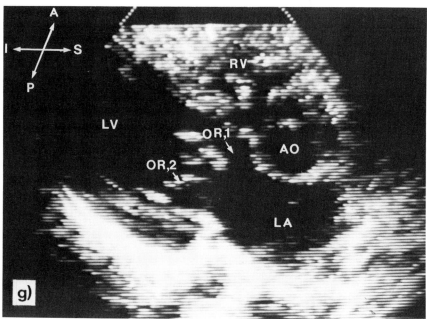

FIGURE 17.5 *(continued)*

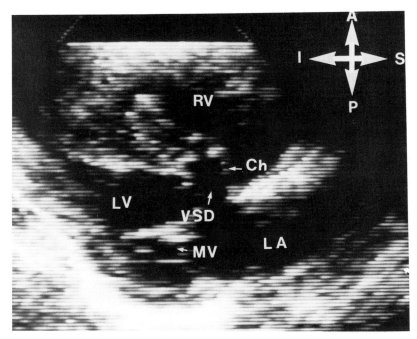

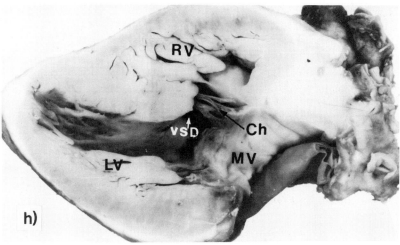

FIGURE 17.5 *(continued)*

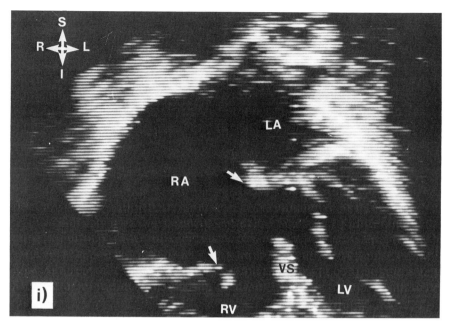

FIGURE 17.5 *(continued)*

LEFT VENTRICULAR OUTFLOW TRACT OBSTRUCTION AND CONGENITAL ANOMALIES OF THE MITRAL VALVE

That congenital obstruction to left ventricular inlet may coexist with congenital anomalies of left ventricular outflow tract obstruction is amply documented, but both can occur in isolation. Thus, congenital mitral stenosis is common in neonates with severe aortic stenosis or atresia, and supravalvular mitral stenosis occurs with subaortic stenosis and coarctation of the aorta in the constellation of Shone's complex.

Yet, congenital anomalies of the mitral valve — or, more frequently, its support apparatus — can participate in and be morphologically responsible for subaortic stenosis (Fig. 17.6). We have previously summarized our experience with these congenital malformations.[54] The so-called Björk deformity of the mitral valve is characterized by malattachment of the chordae tendineae from the aortic leaflet of the mitral valve to the ventricular septal surface.[55] When these chordal attachments are sufficiently dense, they may obstruct the left ventricular outlet.[56,57] A straddling mitral valve, especially when there are abnormal chordal attachments, may obstruct the left ventricular outlet. Thus, when the ventriculoarterial connections are concordant, a straddling mitral valve may participate in subaortic stenosis. Subpulmonary

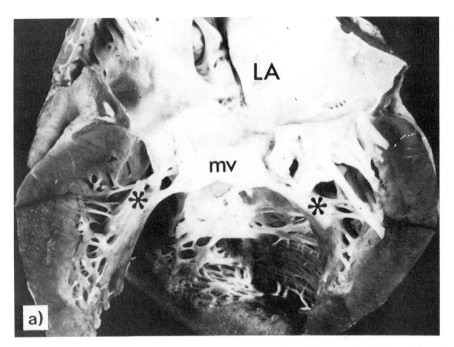

FIGURE 17.6 Left ventricular inlet and outlet obstruction. **(a – e)** Same patient internal view of left atrium *(LA)* showing a grossly abnormal and stenotic mitral valve *(MV)*, with two papillary muscles *(asterisks)*. **(b)** Internal view of left ventricle and aortic *(AO)* outflow tract. Note the diffuse endocardial sclerosis *(large black asterisk)* beneath the aortic valve. Thick chordal attachments *(x)* from the anterior mitral valve *(mv)* participate in the severe left ventricular outflow tract obstruction. **(c,d)** Left ventricular *(LV)* angiogams showing the severe subaortic obstruction *(black asterisk)*. **(e)** Praecordial long-axis cut in mitral stenosis and associated left ventricular outflow tract obstruction. Note the thickend mitral valve and the chordal attachment from the anterior mitral leaflet inserting into the left ventricular outflow tract. **(f,g)** A different patient with Shone's constellation. **(f)** The aortogram *(AO)* shows a bizarre aortic valve and a mild coarctation *(asterisk)*. **(g)** This left ventriculogram *(LV)* shows a tunnel form *(asterisk)* of subaortic stenosis, with considerable separation between aortic valve and mitral valve *(white arrows)*. This patient also has mitral stenosis. Abbreviations: Ao = aorta; CH = chordae; LA = left atrium; LV = left ventricle.

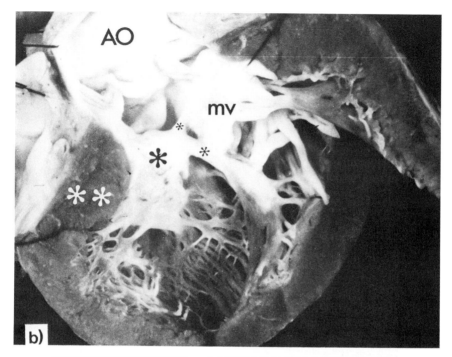

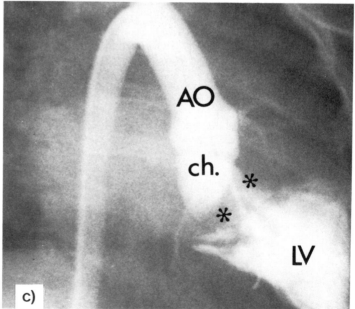

FIGURE 17.6 *(continued)*

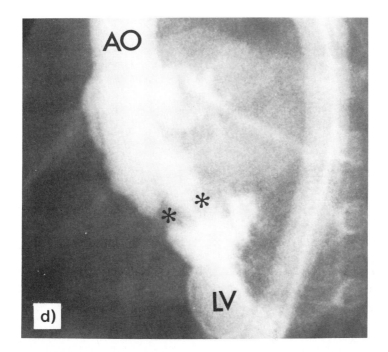

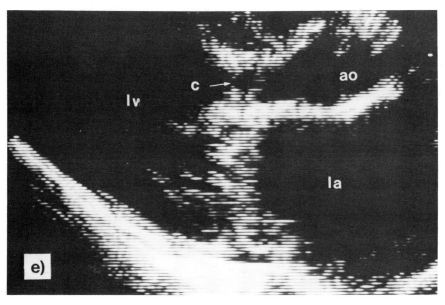

FIGURE 17.6 *(continued)*

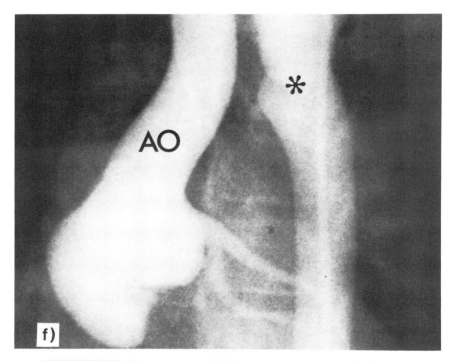

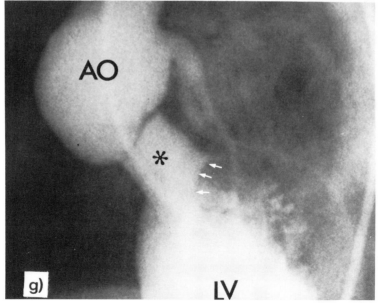

FIGURE 17.6 *(continued)*

obstruction may have its morphologic basis in a straddling mitral valve when the ventriculoarterial connections are discordant, or double-outlet right ventricle. Other diverse mechanisms intimately associated with the mitral valve that have been implicated in the genesis of subaortic stenosis include supernumerary mitral valve, parachute accessory anterior mitral valve leaflet, or accessory or dysplastic tissue tags originating from the mitral valve.[58-62] Both left ventricular angiography and cross-sectional echocardiography provide valuable diagnostic information (Fig. 17.6).

THE ANATOMY OF "MITRAL ATRESIA"

It is evident that the morphologic bases for so-called mitral atresia are either an (*a*) absent atrioventricular connection; or (*b*) an imperforate atrioventricular connection.[63-66] Angiocardiography will only rarely differentiate between an absent connection (in which the floor of the left atrium is separated from the left ventricular cavity by atrioventricular sulcus tissue) and a truly imperforate mitral valve. Yet, while angiography (using either selective left atrial or left ventricular angiography) is unlikely to provide anatomic information about the morphologic basis for mitral atresia, cross-sectional echocardiography is able to make this differentiation.[67]

The ability to differentiate between an absent atrioventricular connection and an imperforate one is rarely of clinical importance (that is, in the surgical management of the patient), but we agree in the intrinsic differences between these two forms of mitral atresia.

REFERENCES

1. Davachi F, Moller JH, Edwards JE. Diseases of the mitral valve in infancy. An Anatomic Analysis of 55 cases. Circulation 1971;43:565–579.
2. Macartney FJ, Bain HH, Ionescu MI, Deverall PB, Scott O. Angiocardiographic pathologic correlations in congenital mitral valve anomalies. Europ J Cardiol 1976;4:191–211.
3. Rosenquist GC. Congenital mitral valve disease associated with coarctation of the aorta. A spectrum that includes parachute deformity of the mitral valve. Circulation 1974;49:985–993.
4. Ruckman RN, Van Praagh R. Anatomic types of congenital mitral stenosis: report of 49 autopsy cases with consideration of diagnosis and surgical implications. Am J Cardiol 1978;42:598–601.
5. Carpentier A, Branchini B, Cour JC, Asfaou E, Villani M, Deloche E, Relland J, D'Allaines CI, Blindeau PB, Piwnica A, Parenzan L, and Brom G. Congenital malformations of the mitral valve in children. Pathology and Surgical Treatment. J Thorac Cardiovasc Surg 1976;72:854–866.
6. Collins-Nakai RL, Rosenthal A, Castaneda AR, Bernhard WF, Nadas AS. Congenital mitral stenosis. A review of 20 years of experience. Circulation 1977;56:1039–1047.

7. Snider AR, Roge CL, Schiller NB, Silverman NH. Congenital left ventricular inflow obstruction evaluated by two-dimensional echocardiography. Circulation 1980;61:848–855.
8. Roberts WC. Morphologic features of the normal and abnormal mitral valve. Am J Cardiol 1983;51:1005–1028.
9. Smallhorn JF, Tommasini G, Deanfield J, Douglas J, Gibson D, Macartney FJ. Congenital mitral stenosis. Anatomical and functional assessment by echocardiography. Br Heart J 1981;45:527–534.
10. Riggs TW, Lapin GD, Paul MH, Muster AJ, Berry TE. Measurement of mitral valve orifice in infants and children by two-dimensional echocardiography. J Am Coll Cardiol 1983;1:873–878.
11. Gutgesell HP, Cheatham J, Latson LA, Nihill MR, Mullins CE. Atrioventricular valve abnormalities in infancy: Two-dimensional echocardiographic and angiocardiographic comparison. J Am Coll Cardiol 1983;2:531–537.
12. Grenadier E, Sahn DJ, Valdes-Crus LM, Allen HD, Oliveira Lima C, Goldberg SJ. Two-dimensional echo Doppler study of congenital disorders of the mitral valve. Am Heart J 1984;107:319–325.
13. Gutgesell HP, Bricker JT, Colvin EV, Latson LA, Hawkins EP. Atrioventricular valve anular diameter: two-dimensional echocardiographic autopsy correlation. Am J Cardiol 1984;53:1652–1655.
14. Shone JD, Sellers RD, Anderson RC, Adams P Jr, Lillehei CW, Edwards JE. The developmental complex of "parachute mitral valve" supravalvular ring of left atrium, subaortic stenosis, and coarctation of aorta. Am J Cardiol 1963;11:714–725.
15. Carey LS, Sellers RD, Shone JD. Radiologic findings in the developmental complex of parachute mitral valve, supravalvular ring of left atrium, subaortic stenosis and coarctation of aorta. Radiology 1964;82:1–10.
16. Simon AL, Friedman WF, Roberts WC. The angiographic features of a case of parachute mitral valve. Am Heart J 1969;77:809–813.
17. Glancy DL, Chang MY, Dorney ER, Roberts WC. Parachute mitral valve. Further observations and associated lesions. Am J Cardiol 1971;27:309–313.
18. Schachner A, Varsano I, Levy MJ. The parachute mitral valve complex. Case report and review of the literature. J Thorac Cardiovasc Surg 1975;70:451–457.
19. Macartney FJ, Scott O, Ionescu MI, Deverall PB. Diagnosis and management of parachute mitral valve and supravalvular mitral ring. Br Heart J 1974;36:641–652.
20. Deutsch V, Yahini JH, Shem-Tov A, Neufeld HN. The parachute mitral valve complex: Angiographic observations. Chest 1974;65:262–268.
21. Shrivastava S, Moller JH, Tadavarthy M, Fukuda T, Edwards JE. Clinical pathologic conference. Am Heart J 1976;91:513–519.
22. David I, Castaneda AR, Van Praagh R. Potentially parachute mitral valve in common atrioventricular canal. Pathologic anatomy and surgical importance. J Thorac Cardiovasc Surg 1982;84:178.
23. Ilbawi MN, Idriss FS, Deleon SY, Riggs TW, Muster AJ, Berry TE, Paul MH. Unusual mitral valve abnormalities complicating surgical repair of endocardial cushion defects. J Thorac Cardiovasc Surg 1983;85:697.
24. Freedom RM, Culham JAG, Moes CAF. Angiocardiography of Congenital Heart Disease. McMillan, New York, 1984, p 320–325.
25. Manubens R, Krovetz LJ, Adams PJr. Supravalvular stenosing ring of the left atrium. Am Heart J 1960;60:286–295.
26. Srinivasan V, Lewin AN, Peironi D, Levinsky L, Gomez Alicea JR, Subramanian S. Supravalvular stenosing ring of the left atrium: case report and review of the literature. Cardiovasc Dis Bull Texas Heart Inst 1980;7:149–158.
27. Isner JM, Salem DN, Seaver PR, Payne DD, Cleveland RJ. Supravalvular stenosing ring of

the left atrium associated with bilateral atrioventricular valvular regurgitation. Am Heart J 1983;106:1150–1153.

28. Layman TE, Edwards JE. Anomalous mitral arcade. A type of congenital mitral insufficiency. Circulation 1967;35:389–395.

29. Castaneda AR, Anderson RC, Edwards JE. Congenital mitral stenosis resulting from anomalous arcade and obstructing papillary muscles. Report of correction by use of ball valve prosthesis. Am J Cardiol 1969;24:237–240.

30. Frech RS, White RI Jr, Bessinger FB, Amplatz K. Anomalous mitral arcade with enlarged papillary muscles. Angiographic study of two cases. Radiology 1972;103:633–636.

31. Parr GVS, Fripp RR, Whitman V, Bharati S, Lev M. Anomalous mitral arcade. Echocardiographic and angiographic recognition. Pediatr Cardiol 1983;4:163–165.

32. Smallhorn JF, de Leval M, Stark J, Somerville J, Taylor JFN, Anderson RH, Macartney FJ. Isolated anterior mitral cleft. Two dimensional echocardiographic assessment and differentiation from "clefts" associated with atrioventricular septal defect. Br Heart J 1982;48:109–116.

33. Di Segni E, Edwards JE. Cleft anterior leaflet of the mitral valve with intact septa. A study of 20 cases. Am J Cardiol 1983;51:919–926.

34. Actis-Dato A, Milocco I. Anomalous attachment of the mitral valve to the ventricular wall. Am J Cardiol 1966;17:278–281.

35. Ruschhaupt DG, Bharati S, Lev M. Mitral valve malformation of Ebstein type in absence of corrected transposition. Am J Cardiol 1976;38:109–112.

36. Horiuchi T, Saji K, Osuka Y, Sato K, Okada Y. Successful correction of double outlet left atrium associated with complete atrioventricular canal and l-loop double outlet right ventricle with stenosis of the pulmonary artery. J Cardiovasc Surg 1976;17:157–161.

37. Van Mierop LHS. Pathology and pathogenesis of endocardial cushion defects: Surgical implications. In, Davila JC (ed): Second Henry Ford Hospital International Symposium on Cardiac Surgery. Appleton-Century-Crofts, New York, 1977, pp 201–207.

38. Rosenberg J, Roberts WC. Double orifice mitral valve. Arch Pathol 1968;86:77–80.

39. Mercer JL, Tubbs OS. Successful surgical management of double mitral valve with subaortic stenosis. J Thorac Cardiovasc Surg 1974;67:440–442.

40. Ancalmo N, Ochsner JL, Mills NL, King TD. Double mitral valve. Angiology 1977;28:95–100.

41. Freedom RM, Bini R, Dische R, Rowe RD. The straddling mitral valve: morphological observations and clinical implications. Eur J Cardiol 1978;8:27–50.

42. Aziz, KU, Paul MH, Muster AJ, Idriss FS. Positional abnormalities of atrioventricular valves in transposition of the great arteries including double outlet right ventricle, atrioventricular valve straddling, and malattachment. Am J Cardiol 1979;44:1135–1145.

43. Milo S, Yen Ho S, Macartney FJ, Wilkinson JL, Becker AE, Wenink ACG, Gittenberger de Groot A, Anderson RH. Straddling and overriding atrioventricular valves: morphology and classification. Am J Cardiol 1979;44:1122–1134.

44. Freedom RM, Duncan WJ, Rowe RD. The straddling and overriding atrioventricular valve: morphological and diagnostic features. In, Galucci V, Bini RM, Thiene G, (eds): Selected Topics in Cardiac Surgery. Patron Editors, Bologna, 1980;297–328.

45. Bini RM, Pellegrino PA, Mazzucco A, Gallucci V, Milanesi O, Maddalema F, Thiene G. Tricuspid atresia with double-outlet left atrium. Chest 1980;78:109–111.

46. Otero Coto E, Calabro R, Marsico F, Lopez Arranz JS. Right atrial outlet atresia with straddling left atrioventricular valve. A form of double outlet atrium. Br Heart J 1981;45:317–324.

47. Smallhorn JF, Tommasini G, Macartney FJ. Detection and assessment of straddling and overriding atrioventricular valves by two dimensional echocardiography. Br Heart J 1981;46:262–284.

48. Wenink ACG, Gittenberger de Groot AC. Straddling mitral and tricuspid valves. Morphologic differences and developmental backgrounds. Am J Cardiol 1982;49:1957–1970.

49. Yen Ho S, Milo S, Anderson RH, Macartney FJ, Goodwin A, Becker AE, Wenink ACG, Gerlis LM, Wilkinson JC. Straddling atrioventricular valve with absent atrioventricular connection. Report of 10 cases. Br Heart J 1982;47:344–352.

50. Edwards BS, Edwards WD, Bambara JF, Van Der Bel-Kahn J, Edwards JE. Anomalies of the left atrium and mitral valve. Cords, flaps and duplication of valve. Arch Pathol Lab Med 1983;107:29–33.

51. Wilkinson JC. Accessory atrioventricular orifices and "double outlet atrium." Int J Cardiol 1984;6:163–165.

52. Gerlis LM, Anderson RH, Dickinson DF. Duplication of the left atrioventricular valve in double inlet left ventricle: a triple inlet ventricle? Int J Cardiol 1984;6:157–161.

53. Otero Coto E, Quero Jiminez M, Deverall PB. Rare anomalies of atrioventricular connection: hidden or supernumerary valves with imperforate right atrioventricular connection. Int J Cardiol 1984;6:149–156.

54. Freedom RM, Dische MR, Rowe RD. Pathologic anatomy of subaortic stenosis and atresia in the first year of life. Am J Cardiol 1977;39:1035–1044.

55. Bjork VO, Hultquist G, Lodin H. Subaortic stenosis produced by an abnormally placed anterior mitral leaflet. J Thorac Cardiovasc Surg 1961;41:659–669.

56. Sellers RD, Lillehei CW, Edwards JE. Subaortic stenosis caused by anomalies of the atrioventricular valves. J Thorac Cardiovasc Surg 1964;48:289–302.

57. Van Praagh R, Corwin RD, Dahlquist EHJr, Freedom RM, Mattiolo L, Nebesar RA. Tetralogy of Fallot with severe left ventricular outflow tract obstruction due to anomalous attachment of the mitral valve to the ventricular septum. Am J Cardiol 1970;26:93–101.

58. Mathewson JW, Riemenschneider TA, McGough EC, Condon VR. Left ventricular outflow tract obstruction. Produced by redundant mitral valve tissue in a neonate. Clinical, angiographic and operative findings. Circulation 1976;53:196–199.

59. Cooperberg P, Hazell S, Ashmore PG. Parachute accessory anterior mitral valve leaflet causing left ventricular outflow tract obstruction. Report of a case with emphasis of the echocardiographic findings. Circulation 1976;53:908–911.

60. Hatem J, Sade RM, Taylor A, Usher BW, Upshur JK. Supernumerary mitral valve producing subaortic stenosis. Chest 1981;79:483–486.

61. Wright PW, Whittner RS. Obstruction of the left ventricular outflow tract by the mitral valve due to a muscle band. J Thorac Cardiovasc Surg 1983;85:938–940.

62. Nanton MA, Belcourt CL, Gills DA, Krause VW, Roy DL. Left ventricular outflow tract obstruction owing to accessory endocardial cushion tissue. J Thorac Cardiovasc Surg 1979;78:537.

63. Ando M, Satomi G,f Takao A. Atresia of tricuspid or mitral orifice: Anatomic spectrum and morphogenetic hypothesis. In, Van Praagh R, Takao A (eds): Etiology and Morphogenesis of Congenital Heart Disease. Futura Press, Mt. Kisco, New York, 1980, p 421.

64. Thiene G, Daliento L, Frescura C, De Tommasi M, Macartney FJ, Anderson RH. Atresia of the left atrioventricular orifice: anatomical investigation in 62 cases. Br Heart J 1981;45:393–401.

65. Shore D, Jones O, Rigby ML, Anderson RH, Lincoln C. Atresia of left atrioventricular connection. Surgical considerations. Br Heart J 1982;47:35–40.

66. Gittenberger de Groot AC, Wenink ACG. Mitral atresia. Morphological details. Br Heart J 1984;51:252–258.

67. Rigby ML, Gibson DG, Joseph MC, Lincoln JCR, Shinebourne EA, Shore DF, Anderson RH. Recognition of imperforae atrioventricular valves by two dimensional echocardiography. Br Heart J 1982;47:329–336.

CHAPTER 18

Mitral Valve Reconstruction in Children

Sylvain Chauvaud, MD, and
Alain Carpentier, MD, PhD

Mitral valve disease in children deals with two major problems. Bioprosthesis have a high rate of calcifications and mechanical valve replacement is limited by anticoagulation therapy and thromboembolism. In such a situation mitral valve repair is specially indicated in children.

CONGENITAL MALFORMATIONS OF THE MITRAL VALVE

Congenital malformations of the mitral valve have several peculiar features: *(a)* The lesions are complex and multivarious and therefore difficult to recognize prior to and during the operation; *(b)* They are frequently associated with other congenital lesions which may hide or be hidden by the mitral malformation.

CLASSIFICATION

The mitral malformation is classified as to whether the valve is incompetent or stenotic, whether the motion of the leaflets is normal, prolapsed or restricted, and whether the papillary muscles are normal or not (Table 18.1).

This classification is based on angiocardiography, echocardiography, and examination of the mitral valve during the operation as seen from the left atrium. The lesions must be analyzed in a sequential manner: *(a)* the atrium: sometimes jet lesions on the atrial wall and adjacent leaflet indicate prolapse of the opposite leaflet; *(b)* valve function is assessed by determining

213

TABLE 18.1 Pathophysiologic Classification

Mitral Valve Incompetence	Mitral Valve Stenosis
Type I: Normal leaflet motion	Type A: Normal papillary muscles
Type II: Leaflet prolapse	Type B: Abnormal papillary muscles
Type III: Restricted leaflet motion	
A. With normal papillary muscles	
B. With abnormal papillary muscles	

whether the valve is stenotic or incompetent, evaluating the motion of anterior and posterior leaflet (normal, prolapsed or restricted); and *(c)* one must determine whether or not the annulus is dilated, deformed, or both, by comparing available leaflet tissue and orifice area and recognize defects of leaflets tissue.

When more than one anomaly is present the primary lesion serves to classify the malformation. Mitral valve diseases of atrioventricular defect, corrected transposition, univentricular heart, and left ventricular hypoplasia are excluded from the classification.

The pathophysiological classification has proved to be an important guideline in the application of the techniques of valve reconstructions. The major aim of surgical repair is to restore normal function than to restore a normal anatomy.

CONGENITAL MITRAL VALVE STENOSIS
Mitral Valve Stenosis with Normal Papillary Muscles
Papillary Muscle Commissure Fusion

The tip of the two papillary muscles is directly implanted on the commissure without any chordae tendinae (Fig. 18.1). The commissural areas are fused and thickened. The motion of the leaflet is restricted. The orifice of the mitral valve, situated between the two papillary muscles, is severely narrowed. A "form fruste" may exist with short chordae. The anomaly is treated by commissurotomy, papillary muscle fenestration and removal of secondary chordae.

Excess Valvar Tissue

The interchordal spaces are obstructed by abnormal valvar tissue. The mitral valve apparatus is otherwise normal (Fig. 18.2). Interchordal space obliteration must be corrected by chordae fenestration in order to remove the excess tissue.

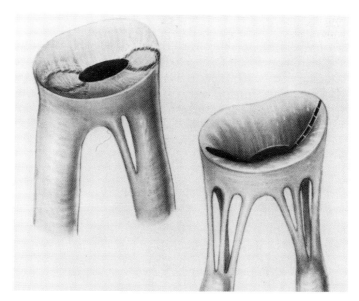

FIGURE 18.1 Papillary muscle commissure fusion. The two papillary muscles are implanted on the commissure without any intermediate chordae tendinae. This condition is treated by commissurotomy and papillary muscle fenestration.

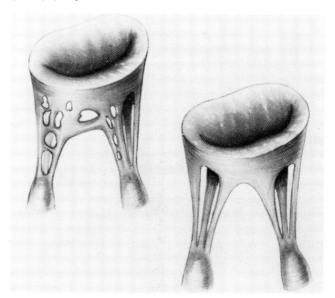

FIGURE 18.2 Excess valvar tissue. The spaces between the chordae tendinae are obstructed by abnormal valvar tissue. In some cases a bridge of valvar tissue joins the anterior and posterior leaflets. Interchordal space obliteration is corrected by fenestration and removal of excess tissue which obliterates the interchordal spaces.

Supravalvular Ring

A circumferential ridge of connecting tissue is attached to the anterior leaflet below its insertion on the annulus or to the atrium slightly above the attachment of the mural leaflet (Fig. 18.3). Depending on the diameter of the ring, various degrees of obstruction may exist. The supravalvular ring is sometimes isolated, but it could be associated with any kind of mitral valve. In the latter conditions the ring may only play a part of the functional obstruction. Surgical correction consists of resection of the fibrous tissue, taking care not to injure the anterior leaflet.

Mitral Valve Stenosis with Abnormal Papillary Muscles

Parachute Mitral Valve

This type of malformation is one of the most frequent lesions causing mitral valve stenosis. All chordae are attached to a single papillary muscle. The single papillary muscle is formed either from fusion of two papillary muscles or from the development of one papillary muscle. The second one is either hypoplastic or adherent to the muscular ventricular wall without any chordal connection (Fig. 18.4). The stenosis results from obliteration of the

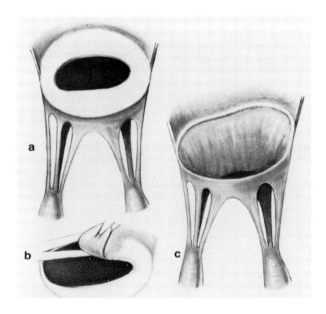

FIGURE 18.3 Supra-valvular ring. The ridge of abnormal tissue is attached on the anterior leaflet or on the atrial wall **(a)**. The fibrous tissue has to be resected **(b** and **c)** taking care not to injure the anterior leaflet.

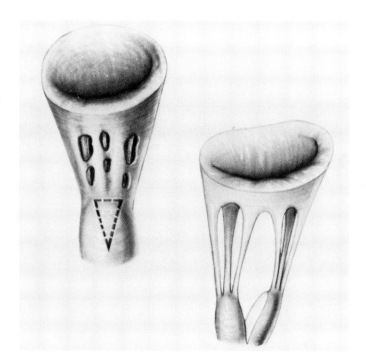

FIGURE 18.4 Parachute mitral valve. In this condition, all the chordae tendinae are attached to a single papillary muscle. The stenosis results from obliteration of the interchordal spaces by excess valvular tissue. Correction is obtained by splitting the papillary muscle and fenestration of the interchordal spaces.

interchordal spaces by excess valvular tissue. In some cases a commissural cleft is the only orifice connecting left atrium and ventricle.

The parachute mitral valve can be corrected by splitting the papillary muscle and fenestrating the interchordal space. A characteristic association of a parachute mitral valve, a supravalvular ring, a subvalvular aortic stenosis and a coarctation of the aorta has been described by Shone.

Hammock Valve

The two papillary muscles are replaced by numerous papillary muscles, and muscular and fibrous bands implanted high on the posterior wall of the left ventricle, just underneath the mural leaflet. The mitral valve orifice is obstructed by intermixed chordae and abnormal papillary muscle (Fig. 18.5). There is not one central orifice but several. This condition is difficult to correct by reconstructive techniques. The goal is to separate the anterior from the posterior leaflet and to remove all the chordae and papillary muscles not attached to the free edge of the leaflets.

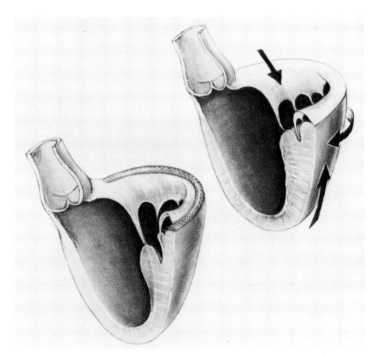

FIGURE 18.5 Hammock valve. The chordae tendinae are implanted on fibrous and muscular bands which are situated on the upper part of the posterior wall of the left ventricle. There is a lateral and upward displacement of the subvalvular apparatus. The obstruction is due to intermixed chordae and abnormal muscle tissue. The goal of the surgical procedure is to separate the anterior from the posterior leaflet and to remove all the chordae and papillary muscles which are not attached on the free edges of the leaflets.

CONGENITAL MITRAL VALVE INCOMPETENCE
Normal Leaflet Motion

Annulus Dilatation and Deformation

We have encountered this malformation in five cases of mitral valve incompetence (diagnosed within the first few weeks of life) without coarctation or subvalvular aortic stenosis. The anteroposterior axis of the mitral orifice is greater than the transverse axis. The dilatation mainly affects the mural leaflet; the aortic leaflet is normal. (Fig. 18.6). In some cases, minor abnormalities of mitral valve tissue such as excess tissue or imperforated interchordal spaces may be present and further support the diagnosis of congenital origin.

This condition can always be treated with reconstructive surgery; a prosthetic ring or an annuloplasty is possible in most of the cases. The selection of the ring is based on the measurement of the base of aortic leaflet not affected by the dilatation. This measured annuloplasty treats the dilatation and the deformation of the annulus without impairing leaflet motion or reducing the orifice area. If the operation is necessary before age 10 years, it is better to avoid the use of a prosthetic ring which may create stenosis at a later age. In this situation, mitral valve incompetence may be corrected by rectangular resection of the mural leaflet, annulus plication, and suture of the leaflet edges. The resection should be electively performed in the sites of indentations of the mural leaflet.

Cleft Leaflet

In this condition the cleft is situated in the anterior leaflet and separates the leaflet into two hemileaflets. Chordae tendinae are often attached to the free edges of the cleft. The orifice of the mitral valve may be dilated, but the papillary muscles are normally situated (Fig. 18.7).

Closure of the cleft after resection of the abnormal chordae can be performed in most of the cases. It may be necessary to use a pericardial patch to close the gap between the edges of the leaflet if the edges are rolled, fibrotic, or retracted.

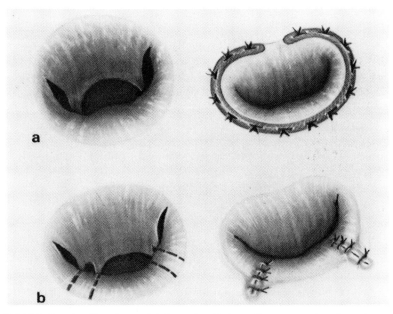

FIGURE 18.6 Annulus dilatation and deformation. Deformation occurs when the anteroposterior axis of the mitral orifice is greater than the transverse axis. The dilatation affects the mural leaflet (posterior); the aortic leaflet (anterior) is normal. A prosthetic ring (annuloplasty) is used for larger hearts **(a)**. In young patients (before the age of 10 years) we prefer to avoid the use of a prosthetic ring, the dilatation of the annulus is treated by rectangular resection of the mural leaflet and annulus plication **(b)**.

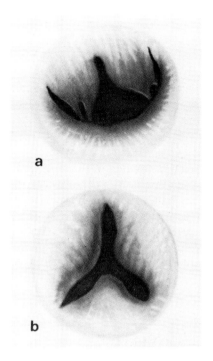

FIGURE 18.7 Cleft leaflet. The cleft separates the anterior leaflet in two hemi leaflets **(a)**. The two papillary muscles are normal. Closure of the cleft is obtained by suturing the edges of the hemi valves **(b)**.

Leaflet Defect

Localized agenesis of leaflet tissue may be encountered, particularly in the mural leaflet (Fig. 18.8). This lesion is treated by rectangular resection of the corresponding part of the leaflet and suture of the free edges.

Prolapsed Leaflet

In this condition, the free edge of one or two leaflets overrides the plane of the orifice during systole. It is a functional definition that excludes the billowing mitral valve with excess valvular tissue, which is ballooning during the systole.

Absent Chordae

Absence of one or several marginal chordae tendinae attached to the free edge of the leaflets leads to prolapse of the corresponding portion of the leaflet (Fig. 18.9). The prolapsed part of the leaflet may be completely free of chordae. This condition is corrected by rectangular leaflet resection and suture.

Elongated Chordae Tendinae

Chordal elongation usually involves all the chordae tendinae arising from one of the papillary muscles. The corresponding portion of the leaflet tissue is prolapsed within the atrium during systole (Fig. 18.10). Elongated chordae had been encountered in Barlow's syndrome with excess valvular tissue and in Marfan's syndrome.

Chordal elongation is treated by shortening the chordae. A groove is made in the papillary muscle, and a suture is passed through each side of the groove and around the elongated chordae. Tying the suture buries the excessive length of the chordae in the groove, which is subsequently closed. If present, associated dilatation of the annulus is corrected by annulus remodeling by using a prosthetic ring.

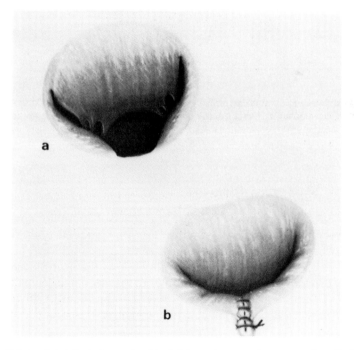

FIGURE 18.8 Leaflet defect. Agenesis of leaflet tissue is more often encountered in the mural leaflet. The free edge of the defect is either free of chordae or attached to thin chordae tendinae. The defect of the mural leaflet is treated by rectangular resection of the corresponding part of the leaflet **(a)**. A defect of the anterior leaflet is treated by a pericardial patch or a direct suture depending on the size of the defect **(b)**.

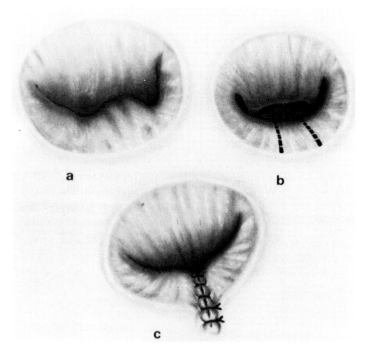

FIGURE 18.9 Absent chordae. Absence of marginal chordae of the free edge of the mural leaflet leads to prolapse **(a)**. The correction of this condition is obtained by rectangular resection of the prolapsed leaflet **(b)** and suture **(c)**.

Elongated Papillary Muscle

Papillary muscle elongation may exist in absence of anomalous origin of the left coronary artery. The papillary muscle is thin, flattened, and elongated to such an extent that it can prolapse through the mitral orifice. The papillary muscle is either white and fibrotic or, yellowish with a necrotic appearance. Histology usually shows scar tissue similar to that seen in a healed infarction (Fig. 18.11). Infarcted areas may also be seen in the adjacent subendocardic layer of the left ventricule, demonstrating associated abnormal vascularization.

Papillary muscle elongation can be corrected by the technique of papillary muscle shortening. A groove is created within the muscular wall of the left ventricle just above the implantation of the papillary muscle. The inferior portion of the papillary muscle is buried in the trench, which is subsequently closed.

RESTRICTED LEAFLET MOTION

This group is further subdivided into two subgroups according to whether or not there are abnormal papillary muscles.

Restricted Leaflet Motion with Normal Papillary Muscles

Commissure Fusion

The lesions are similar to that described in rheumatic valve disease. In congenital lesions, however, the interchordal tissue is thin, delicate, and multiperforated; in rheumatic disease the tissue is thickened and yellowish. Chordae tendinae are often short. Mitral valve incompetence is due to retraction of the anterior or posterior leaflet, or annulus dilatation, or both (Fig. 18.12).

This condition is treated by commissurotomy and annulus remodeling. Commissurotomy may prove to be difficult because an incision in the abnormal commissural tissue may create commissural incompetence.

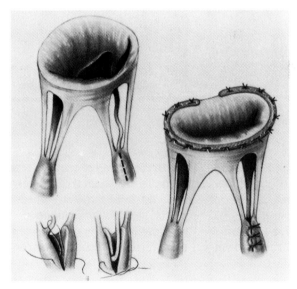

FIGURE 18.10 Elongated chordae tendinae. Chordae elongation usually involves all the chordae arising from one or two papillary muscles. Prolapse of the corresponding leaflet is treated by shortening of the chordae. The tip of the papillary muscle is split and suture is passed around the elongated chordae and through each side of the groove. The excessive length of chordae is buried in the papillary muscle by tying the suture, then the groove is closed. Elongation of two or three chordae of the mural leaflet can be treated either by chordae shortening or by resection and suture of the prolapsed portion of the leaflet.

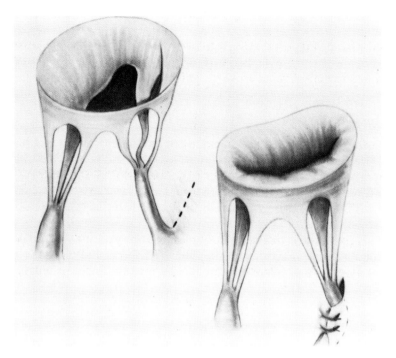

FIGURE 18.11 Elongated papillary muscle. The papillary muscle is white or yellowish, thin, flattened, and elongated. Correction of the prolapse is obtained with creating a groove in the muscular wall of the left ventricle. The inferior portion of the papillary muscle is buried in the trench.

Short Chordae

Short chordae tendinae may limit the mobility of the leaflet, creating mitral valve incompetence. Papillary muscles are normal or hypertrophied. Chordae are well delineated, only slightly thickened and not fused. The interchordal spaces are tremendously reduced and create an associated stenosis (Fig. 18.13). Surgical correction of this malformation consists of fenestration of the papillary muscle to enlarge the interchordal spaces and restore the mobility of the leaflets.

Restricted Leaflet Motion with Abnormal Papillary Muscles

Parachute Mitral Valve

In this condition all the chordae tendinae are attached to a single papillary muscle. The interchordal spaces are obliterated this leading to stenosis (Fig. 18.14). Valvular incompetence may result from various associated lesions: cleft leaflet, short chordae or annulus dilatation.

The correction of this anomaly is treated by the following reconstructive techniques: the single papillary muscle is split, or more accurately fenestrated by removing a triangular piece of muscular tissue so as to separate it in two parts, anterior and posterior. The interchordal spaces are fenestrated so as to relieve the subvalvular stenosis. The incompetence is treated by leaflet suture, or annulus remodeling depending on its mechanism.

Hammock Valve

The valvar orifice is obstructed by intermixed chordae and papillary muscles implanted high on the posterior wall of the left ventricule just underneath the mural leaflet. The leaflet tissue may be totally normal. It may also be abnormal, however, with no delineation between the anterior and posterior leaflet. Chordae from the anterior leaflet cross the orifice, this giving the appearance of the hammock. A hammock valve is usually a stenotic lesion; however, it may be purely incompetent or both stenotic and incompetent. Valvar incompetence may be due to cleft leaflet, anterior leaflet hypoplasia, short chordae, or annulus dilatation.

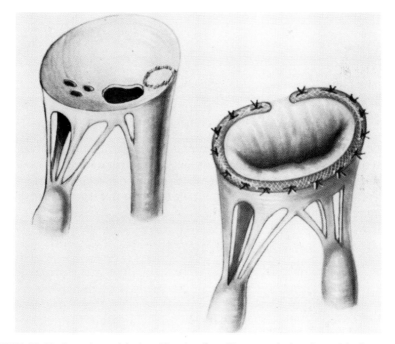

FIGURE 18.12 Commissural fusion. The tip of papillary muscle is adherent to the commissures. Chordae tendinae are short. Commissurotomy leads to mobilization of the leaflet tissue but can create commissural incompetence. The use of a prosthetic ring, concentrating the plication at the commissure usually corrects the mitral valve incompetence.

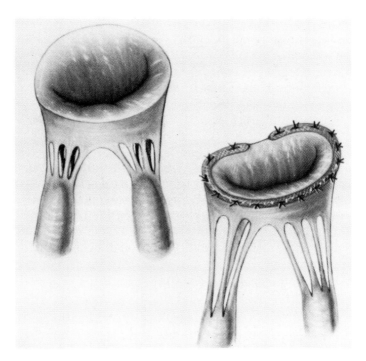

FIGURE 18.13 Short chordae. The leaflet mobility is impaired by the shortness of the chordae tendinae. The annulus fibrosus is often enlarged and dilated, probably secondary to mitral valve incompetence. Correction is obtained by fenestration of the papillary muscle which restores the mobility of the leaflets.

The hammock valve is the congenital mitral valve malformation most difficult to correct by reconstructive surgery. The operation consists of excision of excess papillary muscle underneath the mural leaflet, fenestration of the interchordal spaces, and correction of the incompetence by suture of a cleft and remodeling of the annulus.

Papillary Muscle Hypoplasia or Agenesis

Poor development or absence of one or both papillary muscles may lead to mitral valve incompetence. Chordae are attached to a single papillary muscle and/or various points of the ventricule wall (Fig. 18.15). Valve incompetence is due to either abnormal tension on these chordae or to underdevelopment of the leaflet tissue. The most frequent anomaly is anterior papillary muscle hypoplasia, with an underdeveloped corresponding half anterior valve. When one papillary muscle is hypoplastic or absent, the distinction with a parachute mitral valve may be difficult. The surgical correction may be performed using a modified prosthetic ring. The curvature of the anterior commissure is modified so as to conform to the lack of tissue of the anterior commissure.

CONTROL OF REPAIR

The repair is controlled by injecting saline through the mitral valve into the left ventricle. The result is judged to be satisfactory when *(a)* the closure line of the two leaflets is parallel to the annulus supporting the mural leaflet; and *(b)* there is a good surface of coaptation between the two leaflets. An asymmetric line of closure would indicate a residual prolapse or a residual restricted motion of one leaflet.

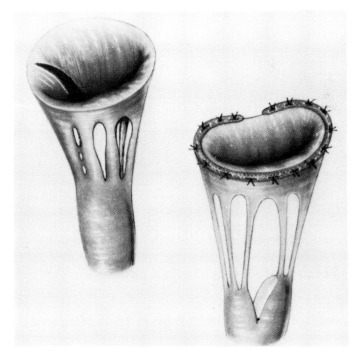

FIGURE 18.14 Parachute mitral valve. Chordae tendinae are attached to a single papillary muscle. Valvular incompetence may result from several mechanisms: cleft leaflet is treated by leaflet suture, annulus dilatation is corrected by annulus remodeling. The single papillary muscle is split or fenestrated to allow a normal motion of the valvular tissue.

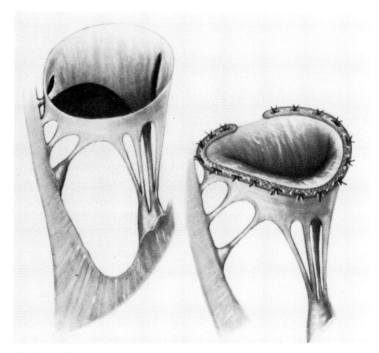

FIGURE 18.15 Papillary muscle hypoplasia or agenesis. The most frequent lesion is anterior papillary muscle hypoplasia. The corresponding half of the anterior leaflet is underdeveloped as is the anterior commissure creating a so-called cleft commissure responsible for the mitral valve incompetence. The surgical correction is performed using a modified prosthetic ring to conform the lack of tissue of the anterior commissure.

CLINICAL RESULTS

Between 1970 and 1984, 72 children have been operated on in Broussais Hospital. Valve repair was performed in 52 patients and valve replacement in 20 patients. Associated congenital lesions were present for 60% of the patients. The average age was 3 years in a group of 24 patients operated upon for mitral valve stenosis (Table 18.2). Eight patients died after the operation due to low cardiac output, six of whom had severe preoperative pulmonary vascular obstructive disease.

For mitral valve incompetence (Table 18.3), 48 children were operated on (mean age, 6 years; range, 9 months to 12 years). Six patients died after the operation, three of whom underwent valvular replacement. The mean clinical follow-up period was 6.6 years (range, 1 – 14 years) for 40 patients. Five children died during the long-term follow up, two after reoperation, two of unknown causes, and one of fibroelastosis of the left ventricule. Reoperation

TABLE 18.2 Mitral Valve Stenosis

	Patients
Type A: Normal papillary muscles	
Papillary muscle commissure fusion	8
Excess valvular tissue	2
Supravalvular ring	3
Type B: Abnormal papillary muscles	
Parachute valve	4
Hammock valve	5

was performed for eight patients, in six of whom a second valve repair was performed.

ACQUIRED MITRAL VALVE INCOMPETENCE

In patients less than 12 years of age, acquired mitral valve incompetence is characterized by rheumatic disease, which is the main cause of valvular dysfunction.

TABLE 18.3 Mitral Valve Incompetence

	Patients
Type I: Normal leaflet motion	
Annulus dilatation	5
Cleft leaflet	8
Leaflet defect	2
Type II: Prolapsed leaflet	
Absent chordae	2
Elongated chordae	15
Elongated papillary muscle	5
Type III: Restricted leaflet motion	
Normal papillary	
Commissure fusion	3
Short chordae	1
Abnormal papillary muscle	
Parachute valve	3
Hammock valve	3
Papillary muscle agenesis	1

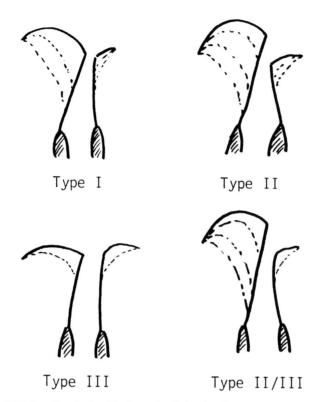

Type I   Type II

Type III   Type II/III

FIGURE 18.16 Functional classification of mitral valve incompetence according to leaflet motion.

Classification

The mitral valve incompetence is classified to whether the motion of the leaflet is normal, prolapsed, or restricted (Fig. 18.16). This classification is based on angiocardiography, echocardiography, and clinical examination of the mitral valve during the operation. In *type I*, the motion of the leaflet is normal; valvar incompetence is due to annulus enlargement. In *type II*, prolapsed leaflet is present with elongated or ruptured chordae tendinae. In *type III*, the motion of the leaflet is restricted by retraction and fibrosis of chordae associated with fusion of the commissures. Lesions are often associated on the same patient; for example, a prolapsed anterior leaflet type II may be associated with a restricted motion of the posterior leaflet.

Surgical Techniques

There are five basic techniques used, either separately or in combination.

Annulus Remodeling

Annulus remodeling by means of a prosthetic ring restores the normal shape and, therefore, the normal function of the valve. Ring selection is based on measurement of the base of the aortic leaflet that is not affected by the dilatation (Fig. 18.17). Sutures are placed through the annulus around the whole periphery of the mitral ring (Fig. 18.18).

Chordae Tendinae Shortening

Chordae elongation is responsible of prolapsed leaflet (type II), mainly on the anterior leaflet. If all of the chordae arising from a papillary muscle are elongated, a shortening plasty of the chordae should be performed. The tip of the papillary muscle is incised longitudinally. A stay suture is passed through

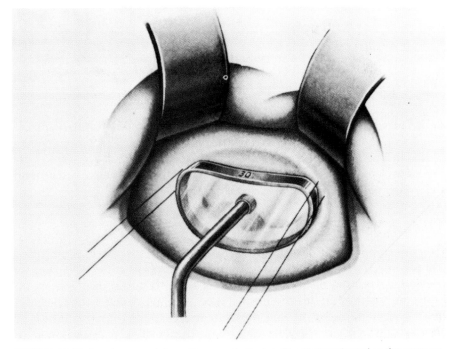

FIGURE 18.17 Annulus remodeling with a prosthetic ring. The ring is selected on the measurement of the anterior leaflet between anterior and posterior commissures.

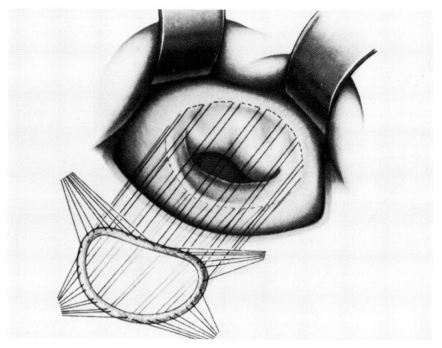

FIGURE 18.18 The suture of the prosthetic ring are placed through the annulus.

or tied around the chordae at a distance from the tip of the papillary muscle equal to one-half of the excess length of the chordae. This suture is then passed through the papillary muscle at the base of the trench in order to bury the excess length of the chordae. The papillary muscle is then closed around the buried portion of the chordae (Fig. 18.19).

Transposition of Chordae Tendinae

Rupture of main chordae of the anterior valve is responsible of prolapsed leaflet (type II). In the past, we recommended replacing the valve because triangular resection of the anterior leaflet leads to mitral insufficiency on both commissures. In this condition it is possible to perform a transposition of chordae tendinae from the posterior leaflet to the anterior leaflet. A chordae of the posterior leaflet with a small piece of valvular tissue is individualized in front of the ruptured chordae of the anterior leaflet. The chordae are detached and sutured on the free edge of the anterior leaflet.

Resection of the Mural Leaflet

Prolapse of the mural leaflet due to elongated or ruptured chordae is treated by quadrangular resection of the mural leaflet (Fig. 18.20). Two guide sutures are placed around the normal chordae at the limits of the prolapsed part of the leaflet *(AA)*. The distance between these two chordae is projected down to the annulus *(BB)*, so that a rectangle is formed, which corresponds to the prolapsed portion of the leaflet. This tissue is removed. A "U" suture is placed into the annulus in order to approximate the free edges of the leaflet, which are then sutured using interrupted 5/0 sutures. A prosthetic ring is placed to reinforce the repair and to remodel the annulus.

Mobilization of the Leaflet

In type III, leaflet motion is impaired by shortening and retraction of the chordae, commissure fusion, chordae, and/or leaflet thickening. The mobi-

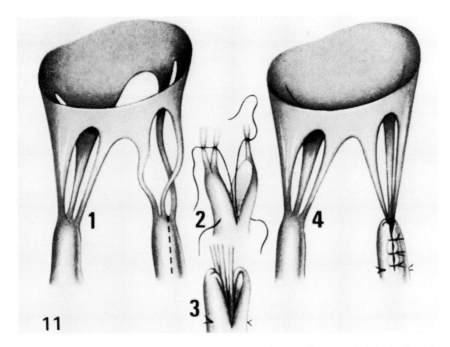

FIGURE 18.19 Chordae tendinae shortening. The tip of the papillary muscle is incised and the elongated chordae are buried in the trench.

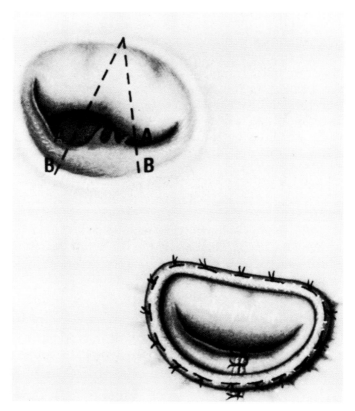

FIGURE 18.20 Resection of the mural leaflet. Prolapse of the mural leaflet is treated by rectangular resection (B). A prosthetic ring is placed to remodel the annulus.

lization of the leaflet may be achieved by a commissurotomy, a resection of the secondary chordae, and a fenestration of fused chordae by resection of a triangular portion of the fibrous tissue (Fig. 18.21).

CLINICAL RESULTS

From 1969 to 1984, 89 children under 12 years of age have been operated on for an acquired mitral valve insufficiency by using Carpentier's techniques. Mortality is 2.2%. The mean follow-up is 5.8 years (1–15 years) for 77

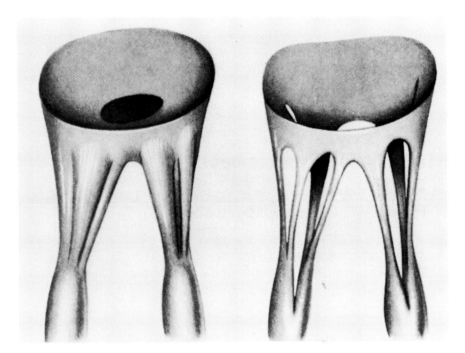

FIGURE 18.21 Mobilization of the leaflet. Commissural fusion is treated by commissurotomy, fused chordae are fenestrated and interchordal fibrous tissue is resected.

patients (88% of surviving patients). Of these, 86% of the patients are in functional class (NYHA) I or II, 12% in class III and 2% in class IV. Actuarial survival rate is 90% ± 8.7% at 9 years. Thirteen children have been reoperated on (17%) with one hospital death.

CHAPTER 19

Mitral Valve Replacement in Children
A Twenty-One-Year Experience

John W. Brown, MD, Jerald L. Cooper,
William R. Deschner, MD, and
Harold King, MD

Thirty-nine mitral valve replacements in 27 children, utilizing mechanical and tissues prostheses, during a 21-year period (December 1963 to December 1984) are reviewed. There were 16 boys and 11 girls, who ranged in age from 11 months to 19.5 years (mean, 12 years 2 months). Etiology of the initial valve disease was congenital in 15/27 (55%) and acquired in 12/33 (45%). Ten tissue and 29 mechanical prostheses were used. Hospital records and postoperative interviews were reviewed to determine early and late mortality and major valve-related complications, which included thromboemboli, endocarditis, primary valve failure, and major bleeding 2° to anticoagulation. Two early and five late deaths occurred in children receiving mechanical mitral valves (all prior to 12/75), and one early (prior to 1975) and one late death (1978 & 1980) occurred in patients receiving tissue mitral valves. No early deaths and only one late death occurred since 1978. The follow-up period for the 10 patients with tissue mitral valve replacements is 39 months, and for the 29 patients with mechanical mitral valve replacements, it is 63 months. During these periods, five major valve-related complications occurred in the patients who received tissue mitral valves, and four of the five complications were related to calcific degeneration and primary tissue failure. Eight complications occurred in the patients with mechanical mitral valves and 6/8 were in patients with currently obsolete mechanical prostheses. When the actuarial incidence of major valve-related complications for current model mechanical and tissue valves are compared, patients with mechanical prostheses have fewer postoperative problems and superior prosthetic durability than patients with tissue valves.

Our results with valve replacement in children are compared with other recently reported series, and we concur that mitral valve replacement can be accomplished with low mortality and low risk of thromboemboli, bleeding, or valve outgrowth. The high incidence of early (<5 years) primary tissue failure in biologic valves make them a low priority choice except in very limited clinical situations.

Mitral valve replacement in adult patients was first successfully carried out by Starr in 1961.[1] Relatively few institutions published their experience with valve replacement in children until the mid- to late 1970s, and at that time the operative risks and postoperative complications rate were high[2-6]; mechanical prostheses were used exclusively in the 1960s and early 1970s. Bioprosthetic valves were introduced in the early to mid-1970s and were initially felt to be better suited for children because they had a lower profile than the then-popular caged-ball prostheses. They did not require long term anticoagulation therapy, and they demonstrated a very low incidence of thromboemboli. The advantage of a central flow orifice of the heterograft valve was offset by their relatively poor orifice-to-annular ratio in the small sizes. Reports of lower operative mortality for valve replacement utilizing tissue valves in children were soon followed by reports of an alarmingly high incidence of accelerated primary tissue failure in children as compared with adults receiving tissue valves.[7-23]

The recent preference for mechanical over tissue valves for mitral valve replacement in children has been increased by the introduction of mechanical prostheses with improved hemodynamic design and lower thromboembolic risks than previously available valves. Careful clinical trials of mechanical valves in children without anticoagulation therapy are currently in progress.[24,25] The addition of "anticalcification chemicals" to tissue fixatives and low pressure fixation of tissue valves may improve their durability in children, but these claims are currently unproven.

This retrospective review of 39 mitral valves in 27 children over a 21-year period will elucidate the problems encountered with the early years of mechanical valve replacement in children, demonstrate our enthusiasm for the tissue valves in the mid- to late 1970s, and demonstrate their early failure. The review will further demonstrate our current preference for mechanical mitral prostheses for children in most clinical situations.

We have not included in this review our patients with right ventricular valves or valved conduits for the right or left ventricles.

PATIENTS AND METHODS

Thirty-nine mitral prosthetic valves were inserted in 27 children ranging in age from 11 months to 19.5 years. The preoperative clinical characteristics of groups are shown in Table 19.1. Fifteen children had congenital abnormalities and 12 had rheumatic causes for their valve dysfunction. Four valve replacements were done for endocarditis. Three had miscellaneous causes. Several patients had combined congenital and acquired valvular disease. The pathologic process affecting valves is shown in Table 19.2. There were 16 males and 11 females in the group. In all, 10 tissue valves (all heterografts) were inserted in the mitral position and 29 mechanical valves were inserted. These groups include three patients who had double valve replacement. Table 19.3 shows the types of valves used in this series: 13 of the 16 Starr-Edwards ball valve prostheses and two Beall valves were used in the period 1963–1976, five of the Starr-Edwards ball valves were the currently obsolete type with a metal ball and cloth covered cage. All patients with this model Starr-Edwards prosthesis have undergone elective replacement or have died. Three Starr-Edwards Silastic ball mitral valves have been used since 1981.

The six Björk-Shiley mitral valves were used from 1975 to 1983. We began using St. Jude Medical valves in 1982 and have inserted five in the

TABLE 19.1 Preoperative Clinical Characteristics of Patients Receiving Mitral Prostheses

	Mitral Valve Replacement Group
Total number of patients	27[a]
Age	
Range	11 mo–19 yr 6 mo
Mean	10 yr 9 mo
Sex	
Male	16 (63.6%)
Female	11 (36.4%)
Valve type	
Tissue	10 (27.3%)
Mechanical	29 (72.7%)
Etiology	
Congenital	15 (45.5%)
Acquired	12 (54.5%)
Follow-up	
Range	2 mo–12 yr 11 mo
Mean	4 yr 8 mo
Previous valve replacement	12 (44%)

[a]Three of the 27 had both AVR and MVR.
Abbreviations: AVR = aortic valve replacement; MVR = mitral valve replacement.

TABLE 19.2 Pathologic Valvular Lesion Requiring Valve Replacement

Pathology	Tissue	Mechanical
Congenital		
Pure MR	1	3
Pure MS	—	4
MS + MR	—	1
MR + TR	1	—
MR + AR	1	1
AS + AR + MR	—	1
Total	3	10
Acquired rheumatic		
Pure MR	2	6
MR + MS	—	4
MR + AS	—	1
AR + MR	5	1
Total	7	12
Endocarditis		
Pure MR	2	2
AR + AS	1	1
Total	3	3
Other		
Cardiomyopathy/MR	1	1
Liposarcoma/MRMS	1	—
Total	2	1

Abbreviations: MR = mitral regurgitation; MS = mitral stenosis; AR = aortic regurgitation; AS = aortic stenosis.

TABLE 19.3 Distribution of 39 Mechanical and Tissue Valves Used for MVR as Initial on Subsequent Operations in 27 Children

Valves Used	MVR	AVR + MVR
Mechanical		
Starr-Edwards	15	1
St. Jude	5	—
Björk-Shiley	4	2
Beall	2	—
Total	26	3
Tissue		
Hancock porcine	4	1
Carpentier-Edwards	4	—
Ionescu-Shiley	1	—
Total	9	1

Abbreviations: MVR = mitral valve replacement; AVR = aortic valve replacement.

mitral position since that time. Eight of the 10 tissue heterograft valves were implanted between 1975 and 1981. A 19-mm Ionescu-Shiley valve was inserted in a 2-year-old in 1983, and a low-pressure fixed Hancock porcine valve was used in 1984 in a child who was not felt capable of enduring anticoagulation therapy.

RESULTS
Mortality

Nine deaths have occurred in the 27 patients over 21 years (33%): three were operative deaths (11.1%) and six were late deaths (22.2%). One early death and two late deaths occurred in patients undergoing double valve replacement. The late deaths occurred at a mean of 2.1 years after operation (range, 3 months to 8.4 years) with five of the six late deaths occurring in the first year after operation. All three operative deaths occurred among 16 valve replacements in the period 1963 through 1975 (19%). Two of the three early deaths were in patients who received mechanical valves. All but one of the late deaths occurred in patients operated on before 1978. One of the late deaths was a patient with a tissue valve and death was sudden and unexplained. The one late death in a patient with a tissue valve was secondary to endocarditis. Five late deaths were in patients with mechanical valves, and two of these patients had undergone double valve replacement. Both double valve patient deaths were sudden and unexplained. One double valve patient late death had received two Starr-Edwards valves, one was a patient with two Starr-Edwards valves, and one was a patient with two Björk-Shiley valves. The other two mechanical valve late deaths were due to endocarditis and hepatitis.

Follow-Up of Survivors

Sixteen of the 18 patients currently alive were available for follow-up examination within 2 months of submission of this manuscript. Two patients have moved to other states, but were alive several years after valve replacement. Follow-up data was obtained from hospital charts, office charts, and telephone interviews with the patients and/or their families. The follow-up period has been from 1 month to 13.5 years on the 18 survivors, with a mean follow-up period of 5.12 years on mechanical valves (range, 0.1 – 13 years) and 5.1 years on patients with tissue valves (range, 0.9 – 12 years).

Postoperative Valve-Related Complications

Postoperative valve-related complications have occured with four tissue valves and eight mechanical valves in children surviving operation, these are shown in Table 19.4.

Prosthetic Thrombosis and Thromboemboli

One mechanical valve (Beall) thrombosed in a patient taking Coumadin and required replacement 3 months after implantation. Only one postoperative embolus occurred in our series and this occured in a 9-year-old boy who underwent emergency mitral replacement with a porcine heterograft. He was noted to have a hemiparesis in the early postoperative period. His neurological deficit cleared completely within 10 days and he is currently neurologically normal.

Bleeding Secondary to Anticoagulation Therapy

Only one significant bleeding episode has occurred and this was in a child receiving warfarin and aspirin for a St. Jude Medical prosthesis. This patient required a 2-unit transfusion for epistaxis. The aspirin therapy has subsequently been discontinued. All patients who have mechanical valves are receiving warfarin and several recent patients are receiving warfarin and dipyridimole. An attempt has been made to keep their prothrombin times between 1.6 and 2 times the control value.

TABLE 19.4 Major Valve-Related Complications in Survivors of Mitral Valve Replacement with Tissue or Mechanical Prosthesis at Initial or Subsequent Operations

Complications	Tissue Prosthesis	Mechanical Prosthesis
Valve thrombosis and thromboemboli	1 (MVR)	1 (MVR)
Bleeding from anticoagulation	—	1 (MVR)
Endocarditis	—	2 (MVR)
Deterioration	4 (MVR)	4 (MVR)
Total	5	8
	10 = 50%	29 = 27%

Abbreviations: MVR = mitral valve replacement.

Endocarditis

Two episodes of postoperative endocarditis have occurred in the 24 patients who survived operation. These two episodes occurred 2 years and 8.4 years after mitral valve replacement with Starr-Edwards ball-valve prostheses. One of these two patients survived a second valve replacement and is currently well 1 year later. The other died during his first episode of endocarditis, 8.4 years after valve replacement.

Prosthetic Valve Deterioration

Four mechanical valves and four tissue valves have undergone functional deterioration and all 8 have been replaced. An early Starr-Edwards mitral prosthesis (Model 6000) developed ball variance 8 years after operation and became obstructed. A Beall valve developed severe disc wear and became regurgitant 10 years after operation. A mitral cloth-covered Starr-Edwards ball valve and a mitral Björk-Shiley valve developed tissue ingrowth and became obstructive 9.4 years and 8 years after insertion, respectively.

Six of the original 10 tissue valves are currently in place and functioning well. Four porcine heterografts have developed calcific degeneration and have become obstructive (at a mean of 4.2 years after operation) and have been replaced. Early and late deaths are shown in Table 19.5.

The actuarial incidence of major valve-related problems calculated by the Kaplan-Meier method[25] for our entire series is shown in Figures 19.1 and 19.2

Prosthetic Replacement

Nine patients have undergone replacement of their initial prosthetic valve. One patient has undergone a second and another has undergone a third prosthetic valve replacement. One Starr-Edwards Model 6000 valve was replaced after 8 years for ball variance. Two size 2M Starr-Edwards valves were replaced because the patients outgrew the prosthesis 10 years after insertion. Two other Starr-Edwards valves were removed: one due to endocarditis after 2 years, and one due to tissue ingrowth on a currently obsolete model. Two of two Beall valves were removed: one due to thrombosis after 3 months, and one due to prosthetic dysfunction secondary to disk wear after 10 years. One Björk-Shiley mitral valve was replaced after 8 years because of subannular tissue ingrowth.

Four porcine heterograft mitral valves were removed at a mean of 4.2 years (range, 2–6.4 years) for tissue degeneration. The overall mortality for

TABLE 19.5 Deaths Associated with Initial or Subsequent Mitral
Valve Replacement

	Tissue Prosthesis	Mechanical Prosthesis
Early deaths[a]	1	2
Late deaths	1	5

[a]Less than 3 months after operation.

re-replacement of prosthetic valves in our nine patients is 33%, with one
early and two late deaths.

DISCUSSION

The management of cardiac valve disease in children should conserve the
natural valve whenever possible because there is currently no prosthesis that

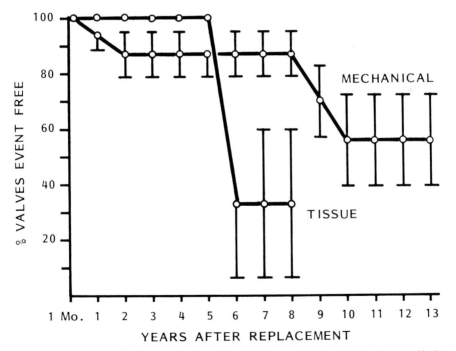

FIGURE 19.1 Actuarial incidence of major valve-related complications for all valves used in the
mitral position.

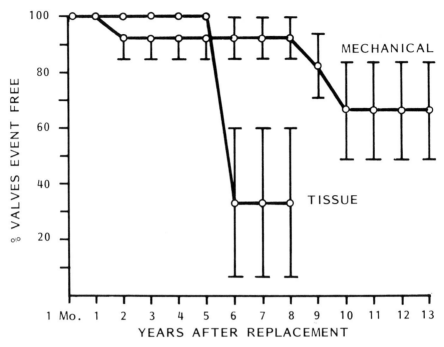

FIGURE 19.2 Actuarial incidence of major valve-related complications for current model valves used in the mitral position.

is totally free of thromboembolic and anticoagulation problems and that has an effective orifice that will not be outgrown by a small child. The durability of recently introduced mechanical valves seems superior to certain previously introduced designs, but many more years of follow-up studies will be required to substantiate this alleged superiority. The life-long need for prophylaxsis for bacterial endocarditis will remain a major concern throughout the child's life.

Major advancements in operative technique, perioperative care and prosthetic design, coupled with a more aggressive surgical approach to end-stage cardiac valvular disease in children, have greatly lowered the early and late mortality and morbidity rates. The first successful valve replacement in humans was reported in 1960–61.[1,27] Early series of valve replacement in children reported an overall mortality of 14%–42%, and many of these reports included children operated on through the mid-1970s.[2–6] Klint et al[4] reviewed the literature pertaining to 166 children undergoing valve replacement through 1972 and reported a 26% mortality, 5.4% thromboembolism rate and 4.8% bleeding rate, secondary to anticoagulation; the total complication rate due to thromboembolism or bleeding was 10.2%. In 1979, Sade et al[28] reviewed the literature on mechanical prostheses in children from the report by Klint et al in 1972 through 1978 and found reports on 314 additional mechanical valve replacements in children. Of these, 17.5% died early and 9.2% died late after valve replacement, for an overall mortality of 26.8%. Sade et al[27] also reported that 25/275 patients (9.1%) had thromboembolic episodes, 10 of 101 (9.9%) patients had bleeding episodes related to anticoagulation therapy, and 11 of 268 (4.1%)'developed prosthetic valve endocarditis. They went on to report on their series of 26 porcine prostheses in children and 24 more from the literature who had a 4% early and a 4% late mortality with only one-fourth the late complication rate seen with mechanical valves. They concluded that the safest prosthetic valve to use in children at that time was the porcine valve.

In preparation for this report, we reviewed the pediatric aortic and mitral valve replacement literature from 1979 to the present and found a total of 1446 children undergoing valve replacement reported from 21 pediatric centers (Tables 19.6 and 19.7). Many of these reports encompassed children operated on from the mid-1960s to the present. The primary author, city or institution, year published, years included, age of patients, and length of the follow-up period are included whenever available.

These reports are further broken down by the valve location (mitral and aortic) and by the type of prosthesis used (tissue, mechanical). Whenever possible, the mortality (early and late) and postoperative complications are broken down by valve type and valve location. The variation in reporting and statistical techniques and the number of years encompassed do not permit precise comparisons. However, certain conclusions can be drawn.

Reports that exclude their early experience (1963 – 1974) have mortalities for valve replacement ranging from 0% – 15%, which are quite similar to the mortality for valve replacement in adults during the same period. In our series of 27 patients, all early deaths occurred in the period prior to 1975. All but one of the late deaths occurred in patients operated on before 1978. Pass et al[24] reported no deaths in a series of 34 patients operated on from 1978 to 1983. Many factors are responsible for the decline in early and late mortality, including significantly better techniques of myocardial preservation, better prosthetic materials, and improved perioperative care. Without question, myocardial protection using cold potassium cardioplegia, used at our institution after 1975, has resulted in a marked reduction in operative mortality (0% since 1975).

Postoperative thromboemboli in children after valve replacement are much less frequent than previously reported. In 1970, Vidne and Levy[6] reported a 20% incidence of thromboemboli in children after valve replacement with mechanical prostheses. Klint et al,[4] in their review of 166 children, reported a 5.4% incidence of thromboemboli in children reviewed prior to 1972 and thromboemboli accounted for 30% of late deaths. There was also a 4.8% incidence of bleeding secondary to anticoagulation. Sade et

TABLE 19.6 Tissue Valve Series

First Author & Location	Years of Study	Date Pub.	No.	Mean Age (yr)	Postop. Follow-Up (months) (mean)	No. Valve	Mort E	Mort L	PVF	TE	SBE	BL
Sanders[19] Boston Childrens	74-78	1980	44	0.9-20 (12.2)	—	8 PH	0	0	1	0	0	0
Curcio[8a] Capetown South Africa	75-80	1981	54	<16	12-33 (22)	1 PH	0	1	1	—	—	—
Dunn[9] Multicentre	75-80	1981	227	<21.0	3-108 —	47 PH		3 (6%)	60%	—	—	—
Galioto[11] DC Childrens	76-79	1981	13	10-19	—	—	—	—	—	—	—	—
Gena[14] Yale	74-80	1982	31	20 (9.0)	— —	14 PH					0	1
Miller[17] Stanford	71-81	1982	41	20 —	(54)	9 PH	—	—	—	—	—	—
Williams[22] Mayo	73-80	1982	47	2-18 (10)	(35.3)	8 PH	—	—	1 (12%)	0	0	—
Mostefa-Kara[18] Marsalle FR	75-80	1984	43	5-18 —	24 —	—	—	—	—	—	—	—
Mechanical Valve Series												
Friedli[10] Geneva	69-79	1981	171	2-17 —	12-108 (43)	18 SE						
John[35] Veliore IN	67-81	1983	118	9-20 (15.4)	12-108 (61)	—	—	—	—	—	—	—
Henze[32] Stockholm	70-80	1984	17	4-12 (8)	2-10 (92)	2 BS						
Iyer[34] New Delhi	75-82	1984	136	6-20	3-96	50 BS	3 (6%) E	2 (4%) L	0	0	0	0
Pass[20] U. of South Carolina	79-82	1984	134	9-21 (12.8)	1-50 (24)	14 SJ	0	0	0	1	1	0

Abbreviations: A = aortic; AC = anticoagulation; A-P = aspirin/persantine; AVR = aortic valve replacement; B = Beall; Bio = biologic; BI = bleeding; BS = Björk-Shiley; C = Coumadin; DM = dura matter; E = early; KS = Kay Shiley; L = late; L-K = Lillehei-Kastor; M = mechanical; mPO = months postoperative; Mort = mortality; MVR = mitral valve replacement.

al[28] reported a 9% incidence of thromboemboli in 25/275 mechanical valves replaced during the period 1972–1978, and a 9.9% incidence of bleeding secondary to anticoagulation. This high incidence of thromboemboli with warfarin therapy is likely to be in part related to mechanical valve design or inadequate anticoagulation regimens during these early years; however, recent reports of mechanical valves show only a fraction of the thromboemboli and bleeding problems reported in these earlier series. John et al,[35] in a series of 97 children receiving Starr-Edwards ball mitral valves between 1967 and 1981 and reported in 1983, showed an overall incidence of thromboemboli of 2.8%, or 0.8% per 100 patients-years. Ninety percent of their patients were receiving warfarin. Freidli et al,[10] however, in a 1969–1979 series of 132 Starr-Edwards ball valves for both the aortic and mitral position, reported in 1981 an 11% incidence of the thromboemboli (3 per 100 patient-years), but only 22% of patients were receiving warfarin and 32% were receiving aspirin

TABLE 19.6 Tissue Value Series *(continued)*

	MVR												
	Mort		**Complications**					**Reoperations**					
No. Valve	E	L	PVF	TE	SBE	BL	AC	PVF	mPO	TE	SBE	OG	Other
28 PH	5 (18%)	2 (7%)	6	0	2	—		1A	7M	22–68	2	0	
7 PH		1 (14%)	7	—	—	—	all	1A	7M	12–33	0	0	
67 PH		5 (7%)	60%	—	—	—	—	5A	7M	—	1A	0	
13 PH &1 BP	(14%)	—	0	0	0	0	None	—	—	—	—	—	
8 PH		5 (16.1%)	7 (23%)	0	0	0	None	7	21–48	—	—	—	
15 PH	1 (2.4%) E	10 (25%) L	—	2 (1.3%)	3 (2%)	0	11%	4A	8M 1–94	—	—	—	
16 PH			2 (12.5%)	0	0	—	—	2A	3M 15–60	—	—	—	
47 PH	0	(14%)	2 (4.2%)	1	4	—	—	(5.5%)	—	—	—		
116 SE	5.9% E 8.7% L		0	3PPY 14 (11%)	43%	—	32% A-P 22% C	—	—	—	—	—	
97 SE	14 (11.8%)			1BS			91% C	No reop. in SE or BS valve					
11 BS	18 (17%) L		0	2SE	1	4							
13 BS	2 (12%) E 1 (6%) L		1	2	0	0	all	1	—	—	—	—	
61 BS	9 (15%) E 2 (3%) L		0	1	0	1	C + AP 100%	0	0			0	—
12 SJ	0	—	0	0	0	0	18%-AP 0%-C	0	0			0	—

OG = outgrown; PH = porcine heterograft; PO = postoperative; PPY = per patient year; PVF = primary valve failure; SBE = subacute bacterial endocarditis; SE = Starr-Edwards; SJ = St. Jude Medical; TE = thromboemboli; * = total; ( ) = percent; ( ) = combined AVR & MVR.

and/or dipyridamole. In 1984, Iyer et al[33] reported a series of 111 children receiving Björk-Shiley valves from 1975 to 1982 and reported only 1 child had thromboembolism, for incidence of 0.82% per patient-year; all of their patients were receiving Coumadin plus aspirin and/or dipyridamole. It is clear from their reports that anticoagulant therapy is important in preventing thromboemboli in children with most types of mechanical valves.

The recently introduced St. Jude Medical Valve has been shown to have a low incidence of thromboemboli. In 1984 Pass et al[24] reported a series of 34 children receiving 14 aortic and 12 mitral valves: none received Coumadin and only 18% received aspirin and/or dipryidamole; During a mean follow-up of 24 months, no patient had an embolus. Further follow-up studies in their small series, however, demonstrated that one child with a St. Jude pulmonary valve thrombosed the valve and one child with a St. Jude aortic valve had a coronary embolus. In spite of these two problems, Pass et al[24]

TABLE 19.7 Combined Mechanical and Tissue Valve Series

First Author & Institution	Years of Study	Date Publ	No. Pts	Mean Age (yr)	Follow-Up (months) (mean)	No. Valve	AVR Mort E	L	PVF	TE	SBE	BL
Sade[18] U. South Carolina	67–75 76–79	1979	24T 48–24M	2–18 (12½%) 2–18 (13%)		14 PH 7BS + B + KS						
Attie[30] Mexico City	64–80	1981	13PH 110 23DM 74M	(12.3) 6–15 (12.0) (13.2)	30–54 (40) 18–64 (23) 18–180 (75.6)	—						
Williams[23] Tor. Chldns	63–80	1981	92			35 PH 39* 11 M	0%		4 0	0 1	3 2	0 —
Human[33] Capetown, South Africa	72–79	1982	56	2–12 (9.4)		—	—			—		
Weinstein[25] U.C. at San Francisco	75–80	1982	7T 24 11M	2/3–19 (12.2)	1–59 (20.4)	3 PH 10* 7 BS	1	1	0	0	0	0
Gardner[13] Johns Hopkins	65–80	1982	64	1–17	1–180	6T 27* 21 M, SE BS, SJ	1	2	0 0	0 0	0 0	0 0
Armistead[29] Brmpt Hosp. London	66–79	1983	21	1/6–13 (9.1)	1–120 (14)	—	—			—		
Current Ind. University Series	63–84	1985	47	1–20 (12) 1–156	30A	9 Bio–7 PH 20* 56 M 11M–6BS, 4SJ	1 —	1 1	1 0	0 0	1 0	0 0

See Table 19.6 for explanation of abbreviations.

continue to contend that "the risk of thromboemboli in un-anticoagulated children with St. Jude Medical valve is no greater than that in anticoagulated adults," and that these results justify continuing the clinical investigation of the St. Jude Medical valve in children without postoperative anticoagulation. In our own series, all patients receiving mechanical valves, including St. Jude Medical valves, receive Coumadin and several are also receiving dipyridamole. The only child with thrombosis of a mechanical valve had a currently obsolete Beall valve. The only embolus in our entire series was in a child with a procine mitral valve.

The threat of bleeding from anticoagulation therapy in current series of valve replacement in children is much less than previously reported. The fear that children respond erratically to anticoagulation seems largely unfounded.

In the review of Klint et al,[4] 4.8% of children had bleeding secondary to

TABLE 19.7 Combined Mechanical and Tissue Valve Series *(continued)*

	MVR												
	Mort		**Complications**						**Reoperations**				
No. Valve	E	L	PVF	TE	SBE	BL	AC	PVF	mPO	TE	SBE	OG	Other
10 PH	1 (4%) E		1	0	(2)	0	0	—		5	3	—	
19BS + B + KS	1 (4%) L		0	(3)	(1)	(3)	c 100%						
	(6 (24%) E)												
	(2 (11%) L)												
13 PH	14%		16.3%	0	2.3%	—	0	—		—	—	—	
23 DM	2.3%		6.8%	23%	0	—	0						
74 M	1.3%		.85%	1.7%	.87%	—	(−100%)						
17 PH	32%	18%	3	1	1	—	A-P	—		—	—	(1)	
50*							(100%)						
33M-11BS			4	—	—	—	C + AP					(4)	
SE-8 B-4							(100%)						
33 PH	2% E		11	1	—	—	0	—		—	—		
24*M-17SE	2(4%)L												
5L-K, 2BS	1	E	—	2	1	—	C-100	—		—	—	1	
4 PH			0	0	0	0	AP-74%	—		—	—		
8*							74%						
3-BS, 1-B		1	0	0	0	0	C-21%	—		—	—	2	
11T			2	0	0	0	0	—		—	—		
24*	4	3					AP-32						
13M, SE													
BS, SJ			2	1	0	1	C-68%	—		—	—	1	
10 Bio			2	0	0	0	0	—		—	—	—	
8PH, 2H													
21*													
11M-10BS-			0	1	0	0	100%	—		—	—	—	
1SE													
9Bio-8PH	0	2	5	1	0	0	0	8	—	0	0	0	
33*													
24M-15SE	5	3	4	1	2	1	100%	2	—	0	1	2	
5SJ,2BS													

anticoagulation therapy. The review by Sade et al[28] showed a 9.9% incidence of bleeding. In our review of 1446 children, only 10 incidents of bleeding due to anticoagulation therapy could be documented since 1979 (an incidence of 0.7%). The cause for the reduction in bleeding in current series is not fully understood, but may be due to the fact that many surgeons and cardiologists are using lower dosages of warfarin-type anticoagulants. We found that a prothrombin time between 1.6 and 2.0 times the control valve gives the same protection from emboli and at a much lower risk of bleeding than more prolonged prothrombin times.

In our own series, only one patient had bleeding significant enough to warrant transfusion. This child had epistaxis while receiving Coumadin and aspirin. The substantially increased bleeding tendency with Coumadin plus aspirin is well recognized. After the above episode, our patient was switched from aspirin to Coumadin and dipyridamole, and no further bleeding has occurred.

The lower risk of anticoagulation and thromboembolic problems in children with mechanical prosthetic valves may be due to the childs faster heart rate and increased frequency of poppet or disk motion, which impedes thrombus formation. Some authors have suggested that the coagulation cascade is different in children, with the result that bleeding problems are less in children than adults on a regimen of Coumadin.[36,37] No evidence exists, however, of any difference in coagulation studies in children.[38]

Therapeutic levels of warfarin are felt to produce a significant risk during pregnancy to both mother and fetus.[36,38] Gandner et al[13] and others continue to feel that the older teenager who contemplates eventual pregnancy should have a tissue valve that does not require warfarin therapy. John et al,[35] however, in a recent report on mechanical valves in children, reported that 8/9 girls who became pregnant while receiving warfarin had normal children. Thus, the prospect of normal childbearing seems more favorable than previously thought in female patients receiving warfarin.

The risk of prosthetic valve endocarditis remains a life-long concern for any patient with a prosthetic cardiac valve. The frequency of prosthetic valve endocarditis ranges from 1% to 5%. In our series it was 7.4%, occurring in two patients with mechanical mitral valves. Most authors agree that the type of prosthesis does not alter the incidence of prosthetic endo-carditis.[1,4,7-14,18-20,22-24,29-35]

The potential need for reoperation in children with prosthetic heart valves depends largely on the durability of the prosthesis, the size orifice into which the prosthesis is inserted, and the effective orifice area of the prosthesis used. Children requiring valve replacement for congenital heart disease frequently have smaller hearts and their annular orifice is smaller than children of the same age affected by rheumatic valvular heart disease. Nine patients in our series underwent 12 repeat valve replacements, for an incidence of 33%; The one death during reoperation occurred after replacement of the third prosthetic valve. The two late deaths after repeat valve replacements occurred 6 months and 8 years, respectively, after the repeat procedure. The early and late mortality for re-replacement of a prosthetic valve in our series 1/9 was (11%) and 2/9 (22%), respectively. The six tissue valves that are currently functioning well will likely require replacement in the next few years.

Four porcine heterografts have undergone degeneration and required replacement. Outgrowth of the prosthesis has been an infrequent cause for reoperation, occurring in only two patients in our series.

The high operative mortality early in our experience with valve replacement in children, coupled with the fear of bleeding and thromboembolic problems, caused us (like many other institutions) to adopt tissue valves for children in the mid- to late 1970s. A total of ten tissue valves were used in our 27 patients. It is now clear that our reduction in operative mortality with tissue valve replacement was due primarily to better myocardial protection with potassium cardioplegia than to the tissue prosthesis. The disturbingly high incidence of tissue valve failure (40% in 5 years) and premature calcification seen in our series has also been born out by many other centers[6,7,8,11,13–18,22,23,28] (Tables 19.6 and 19.7). Tissue valves, with the possible exception of fresh aortic homografts, are less desirable than mechanical valves for the aortic and mitral position in children because of the more-than 50% incidence of primary tissue failure within 5 years of replacement.[9] The actuarial incidence of major valve related problems for currently available valves are shown in Figure 19.2 and show a less favorable prognosis for tissue valves. The modification of tissue valve fixation using low pressure instead of high pressure and the addition of anticalcification agents to tissue valves may improve their durability.

In summary, mitral valve replacement in children continues to be associated with significant risks. The low operative mortality for primary and repeat operations, coupled with the low incidence of thromboembolic and bleeding complications with currently available mechanical valves allows for considerably more optimism than previously held for valve replacement in children. Currently available tissue heterograft valves are prone to calcification and early tissue failure in the mitral position and cannot be recommended in children except under unusual circumstances. Tissue valves continue to be the valve of choice for the tricuspid and pulmonary position. On the basis of our current knowledge, we recommend mechanical mitral valves for children. We further recommend anticoagulant therapy for children with all types of mechanical valve prostheses, even though we are encouraged by the early reports of few thromboemboli with the St. Jude Medical prosthesis.

Surgical management of cardiac valve disease in children should be conservative, but this study and others confirm that valve replacement can be performed safely in children and the risks of postoperative problems continue to decline as prosthetic valves and perioperative care improves.

ACKNOWLEDGMENTS

The authors would like to gratefully acknowledge the secretarial assistance of Geri French, Carole Lorris, and Norma Hazelwood for the preparation of this manuscript.

REFERENCES

1. Starr A, Edwards ML. Mitral replacement: clinical experience with a ball valve prosthesis. Ann Surg 1961;154:726.
2. Berry BE, Ritter DG, Wallace RB, et al. Cardiac valve replacement in children. J Thorac Cardiovasc Surg 1974;68:705–710.

3. Bleiden LC, Castaneda AR, Nicoloff DM, et al. Prosthetic valve replacement in children. Results in 44 patients. Ann Thorac Surg 1972;14:545-552.
4. Klint R, Hernandez A, Weldon C, et al. Replacement of cardiac valve in children. J Pediatr 1972;80:980-987.
5. Matthews RA, Park SC, Neches WH, et al. Valve replacement in children and adolescents. J Thorac Cardiovasc Surg 1977;78:872-876.
6. Vidne B, Levy MJ. Heart valve replacement in children. Thorax 1970;25:57.
7. Bortolotti U, Milano A, Mazzacco A, et al. Alterazioni strutturali delle bioprotesi di hancock applicate in eta' pediatrica. G Ital Cardiol 1980;10:1520.
8. Brown JW, Girod DA, Hurwitz RA, et al. Apicoaortic valved conduits for complex left ventricular outflow obstruction-technical considerations and current status. Ann Thorac Surg 1984;38:162.
8a. Curcio CA, Commerford PJ, Rose AG, et al. Calcification of glutaraldehyde-preserved porcine xenografts in young patients. J Thorac Cardiovasc Surg 1981;81:621.
9. Dunn JM. Porcine valve durability in children. Ann Thorac Surg 1981;32:357.
10. Freidli B, Friendli GM, Ben Ismail M, et al. Remplacement valvulaire chez l'enfant: resultats et suites eloignees chez 171 opers. Schweiz Med Wschr 1981;111:1044.
11. Galioto FM Jr, Midgley FM, Kapur S, et al. Early failures of Ionescu-Shiley bioprosthesis after mitral valve replacement in children. J Thorac Cardiovasc Surg 1982;83:306.
12. Galioto FM Jr, Midgley FM, Shapiro SR, et al. Mitral valve replacement in infants and children. Pediatrics 1981;67:230.
13. Gardner TJ, Roland JA, Neill CA, et al. Valve replacement in children: a fifteen-year perspective. J Thorac Cardiovasc Surg 1982;83:178.
14. Geha AS, Hammond GL, Laks H, et al. Factors affecting performance and thromboembolism after porcine xenograft cardiac valve replacement. J Thorac Cardiovasc Surg 1982;83:277.
15. Geha AS, Laks HH, Stansel C Jr, et al. Late failure of porcine valve heterografts in children. J Thorac Surg 1979;78:351.
16. Kutsche LM, Oyer P, Shumway N, et al. An important complication of Hancock mitral valve replacement in children. Cardiovasc Surg 1979;60:I-98.
17. Miller DC, Stinson EB, Oyer PE, et al. The durability of porcine xenograft valves and conduits in children. Circulation 1982;66:I-172.
18. Mostefa-Kara M, Blin D, Langlet F, et al. Remplacement valvulaire mitral par bioprosthese chez l'enfant. Arch Mal Coeur 1984;77:161.
19. Sanders SP, Levy RJ, Freed MD, et al. Use of Hancock porcine xenografts in children and adolescents. Am J Cardiol 1980;46:429.
20. Silver MM, Pollock J, Silver MD. Calcification in porcine xenograft valves in children. Am J Cardiol 1980;45:687.
21. Thandroyen FT, Whitton IN, Pirie D, et al. Severe calcification of glutaraldehyde-preserved porcine xenografts in children. Am J Cardiol 1980;45:690.
22. Williams DB, Danielson GK, McGoon DC, et al. Porcine heterograft valve replacement in children. J Thorac Cardiovasc Surg 1982;84:446.
23. Williams WG, Pollock JC, Greiss DM, et al. Experience with aortic and mitral valve replacement in children. J Thorac Cardiovasc Surg 1981;81:326.
24. Pass HI, Sade RM, Crawford FA, et al. Cardiac valve prostheses in children without anticoagulation. J Thorac Cardiovasc Surg 1984;87:832.
25. Weinstein GS, Mavroudis C, Ebert PA. Preliminary experience with aspirin for anticoagulation in children with prosthetic cardiac valves. Ann Thorac Surg 1982;33:549.
26. Kaplan ES, Meier P. Nonparametric estimation from incomplete observations. J Am Stat Assoc 1955;53:457.

27. Harken DE, Soroff HS, Taylor WJ, et al. Partial and complete prosthesis in aortic insufficiency. J Thorac Cardiovasc Surg 1960;40:755.
28. Sade M, Ballenger JF, Hohn AR, et al. Cardiac valve replacement in children. J Thorac Cardiovasc Surg 1979;78:123.
29. Armistead SH, MacFarland R, Lange I, et al. Mitral valve surgery in infants and children. J Cardiovasc Surg 1983;24:144.
30. Attie F, Kuri J, Zanoniani C, et al. Mitral valve replacement in children with rheumatic heart disease. Circulation 1981;64:812.
31. Benmimoun EG, Friedli B, Rutishauser W, et al. Mitral valve replacement in children: comparative study of pre- and post-operative haemodynamics and left ventricular function. Br Heart J 1982;48.
32. Henze A, Lindblom D, Björk VO. Mechanical heart valves in children. Scand J Thorac Cardiovasc Surg 1984;18:155.
33. Human DG, Joffe HS, Fraser CB, et al. Mitral valve replacement in children. J Thorac Cardiovasc Surg 1982;83:873.
34. Iyer KS, Reddy KS, Rao IM, et al. Valve replacement in children under twenty years of age: experience with the Björk-Shiley prosthesis. J Thorac Cardiovasc Surg 1984;88:217.
35. John S, Bashi VV, Jairaj PS, et al. Mitral valve replacement in the young patient with rheumatic heart disease. J Thorac Cardiovasc Surg 1983;86:209.
36. Johnson M, Ramey E, Ramwell PW. Sex and age differences in human platelet aggregation. Nature 1975;253:355.
37. Russo R, Barlolotte U, Schevazappa L, Girolami A. Warfarin treatment during pregnancy: a clinical note. Haemastasis 1979;8:96.
38. Suschke J, Stehr K, Jacobi E, et al. Measurement of thrombocyte adhesion in children. Klein Paediatr 1973;185:287.
38a. ven der Horst RL, le Roux BT, Rogers NMA, Gotsman MS. Mitral valve replacement in childhood. A report of 51 patients. Am Heart J 1973;85:624–634.
39. Beadle EM, Suepher RV, Williams PP. Pregnancy in a patient with porcine xenografts. Am Heart J 1979;98:510.
40. Reading HW, Rosie R. Age and sex differences related to platelet aggregation. Biochem Soc Trans 1981;9:180.

CHAPTER 20

Repair of the Mitral Valve in Atrioventricular Defects

Alain Carpentier, MD, PhD, and
Sylvain Chauvaud, MD

Current techniques for the repair of atrioventricular defects must deal with two major problems: *(a)* leaflet dehiscence from the patch, which occurs in 5%–10% of those patients undergoing the procedure; and *(b)* residual or recurrent valvular incompetence, which occurs in 30%–60% of those patients suffering from valvular insufficiency before operation.[1,2]

ANATOMY

Anatomic studies in our laboratory show that the left atrioventricular valve in atrioventricular defect (AVD) is not a normal mitral valve with a cleft anterior leaflet. Instead, it is a three-leaflet valve with a large anterior leaflet, a less-developed posterior leaflet, and a triangular-shaped lateral leaflet. In this three-leaflet configuration, the lateral leaflet is attached to the left atrioventricular valve along one-fourth of its circumference, whereas the mural leaflet of a normal mitral valve is attached along approximately two-thirds of the circumference of the orifice. There are three commissures: one septal, one anterolateral, and one posterolateral; the so-called "cleft" is the septal commissure. In 50% of the patients presenting with left AVD, the septal commissure displays chordae arising from the septum and attaching to the free margin of both the anterior and posterior leaflets. This typical configuration can be seen whether the AVD is partial or complete. Papillary muscles are displaced laterally, and they are responsible for the displacement of the posterolateral and anterolateral commissures (Fig. 20.1).

The three-leaflet configuration is a common finding whatever the type

254

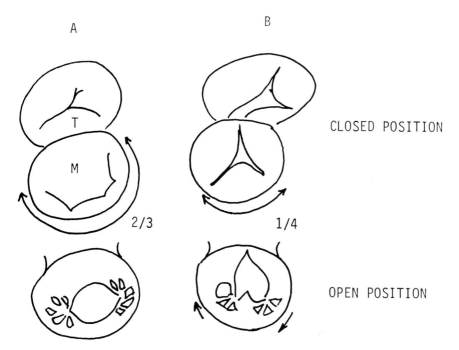

A   B

                                              CLOSED POSITION

T

M

2/3   1/4

                                              OPEN POSITION

FIGURE 20.1 Mitral valve in open and closed positions. **(A)** Normal valve. **(B)** Left atrioventricular valve in atrioventricular septal defect. *Arrows* indicate lateral displacement of papillary muscles.

of AVD. All the variations in the types of AVDs are located at the septal junction and depend on the extent of the involvement of the interventricular septum. The partial AVD is characterized by the absence of ventricular septal defect, and both left and right atrioventricular valves are attached on the crest of the muscular ventricular septum. In the complete AVD, the ventricular septal defect is below the atrioventricular valves. The intermediate AVD is characterized by a gap between the crest of the septum and the mitral–tricuspid junction; the gap is also obstructed by a fragile and sometimes perforated septum.

Variations in this three-leaflet configuration occur in 18.5% of the patients presenting with AVD (Fig. 20.2). Variations may result from a complete or partial fusion of one commissure, leading to either a two-leaflet valve or a double-orifice valve. A two-leaflet valve, however, is actually a three-leaflet valve with a fused commissure. Similarly, a double-orifice valve is actually a three-leaflet value with a bridge between the posterior and lateral leaflet. The only true variation is the parachute valve, which results from the presence of a single papillary muscle.

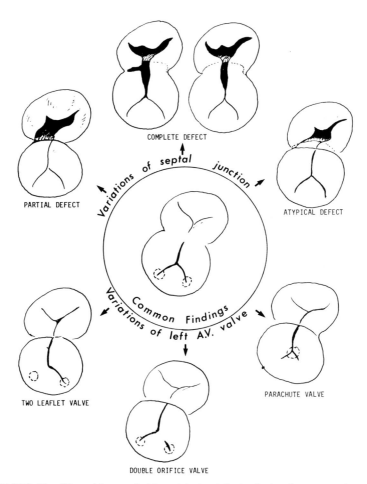

FIGURE 20.2 The different types of atrioventricular defects display the same atrioventricular valve configuration. The variations that distinguish them as three types are located only at the septal junction *(upper junction)*. The only true variation of the left atrioventricular valve *(lower portion)* is the parachute valve with its single papillary muscle *(dotted line)*. The two-leaflet and double-orifice valves result from partial or complete fusion of one commissure of the three-leaflet left atrioventricular valve.

MECHANISMS OF LEFT ATRIOVENTRICULAR VALVE INCOMPETENCE

The three-leaflet valve is functionally competent in 30% of the patients[3] presenting with AVD. It is important to note that valve incompetence does not necessarily result from a leak at the septal commissure. It may result from a leak at the anterolateral commissure, the posterolateral commissure, or at the center of the orifice. There may also be several associated sites of leakage.

TECHNIQUE IN COMPLETE ATRIOVENTRICULAR DEFECT

Analysis of the Lesions

The lesions should be analyzed while the heart is still beating and with the atrioventricular valve in the closed position. The aorta is cross-clamped at 25 °C. The right atrium is opened and saline is injected into the left ventricle to assess whether the regurgitant jets are coming from the septal commissure, the anterolateral commissure, the posterolateral commissure, and/or from the central portion of the valvular orifice. At this stage, two stay sutures are placed: the first one is to approximate the anterior and posterior leaflets at a level corresponding to the crest of the interventricular septum, and the second one is to approximate the three leaflets at the center of the orifice (Fig. 20.3). The valve is then analyzed in the open position to examine the subval-

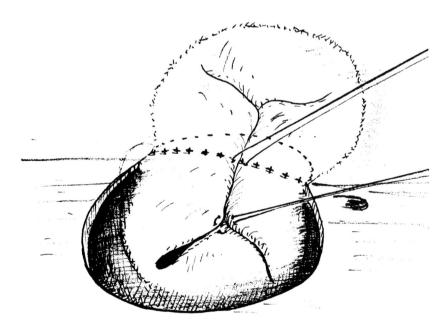

FIGURE 20.3 One stay suture placed at projected intercept of ventricular septum and valve leaflets approximates the anterior and posterior leaflets while another approximates the three leaflets in center.

vular apparatus; that is, the chordae and papillary muscles. The aorta is then unclamped for 2 minutes, after which cardioplegia is instituted.

Leaflet Mobilization

We prefer dividing the patch rather than the leaflets; the exception is the posterior component of the right atrioventricular valve, which is separated from the annulus. The fibrous tissue connecting the crest of the septum to the posterior component of the left atrioventricular valve is, however, carefully preserved (Fig. 20.4). Leaflet mobilization is completed by resecting occasional secondary chordae or fibrotic bands attaching the ventricular aspect of the leaflets to the septum. Marginal chordae attached to the free margin of the leaflets are preserved to avoid leaflet prolapse.

Suture of the Ventricular Patch

A large seminular ventricular patch is sutured to the right side of the septum using a continuous 3-0 prolene suture starting from the middle portion of the

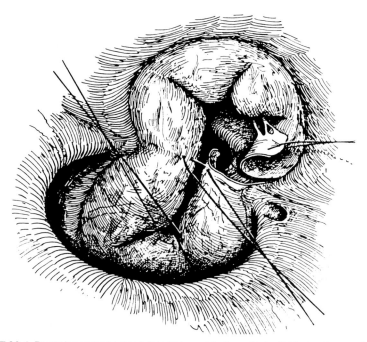

FIGURE 20.4 Posterior component of right atrioventricular valve is divided and separated from annulus to expose the area of the conduction bundle.

septum. The patch is extended posteriorly beyond the area of the bundle of His.

Valve Reconstruction

The free edge of the patch is tailored according to the amount of leaflet tissue available and a slight concave curve is fashioned to reproduce the downward displacement of the crest of the septum in AVD. At the level of the septal commissure, a 5-mm vertical incision is made within the free edge of the patch. The opposing surfaces of the anterior and posterior components are then introduced and sutured to facilitate their approximation (Fig. 20.5).

In AVDs associated with "hypoplastic anterior components" (Fig. 20.6), it may be necessary to divide the anterior component completely. The anterior and posterior components are sutured to the free edge of the ventricular patch together with the atrial patch by using mattress 4-0 monofilament sutures. The sutures are passed successively through the interventricular patch, the leaflet tissue, and the atrial patch. This technique of suturing preserves leaflet continuity and the two patches serve to pledget the suturing of leaflet tissue, thus preventing the sutures from tearing out and leaflet dehiscence (Fig. 20.7).

The competence of the left atrioventricular valve is assessed by injecting saline into the left ventricular cavity. Residual leaks at the anterolateral commissure can be corrected by an anulus plication of this commissure. Residual leak at the posterolateral commissure is treated by similar anulus plications. A significant central leak is treated by an anulus plication of the two commissures; no attempts should be made to correct a minimal central leak. The right atrioventricular valve is then reconstructed by suturing the posterior component to the atrial patch with a slight translation toward the anterior commissure to compensate for the lack of tissue in this area.

Suture of the Atrial Patch

The atrial patch is sutured so as to leave the coronary sinus on either the left or right side, according to its distance from the edge of the ostium primum (Fig. 20.8). When the coronary sinus ostium is far from the edge of the ostium primum, the suture is placed between these two structures and the coronary sinus is in the right atrium. When the distance between the coronary sinus and the ostium primum is very short, it is safer to place the suture around the coronary sinus ostium.

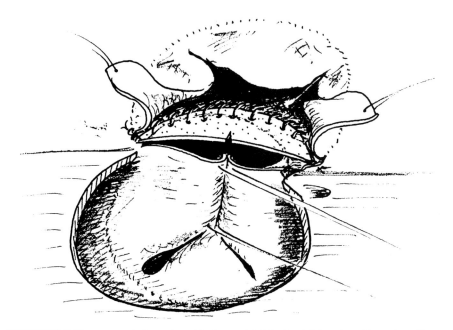

FIGURE 20.5 The crescent-shaped ventricular septal defect patch is sutured into place. Note the posterior extension beyond the area of the bundle of His. The superior edge is slightly concave, and a 5-mm vertical incision has been made at the level of the septal commissure. Opposing edges of anterior and posterior leaflets are introduced into incision in superior edge of ventricular septal defect patch and sutured into place. Undivided anterior leaflet is secured to rim of ventricular septal defect patch and atrial septal defect patch (in cross-section, *inset*).

TECHNIQUE IN PARTIAL ATRIOVENTRICULAR DEFECTS

The principles outlined above also guide the reconstruction of partial AVDs.

Leaflet Mobilization

Mobilization of the anterior and posterior components is critically important to the subsequent approximation of leaflets. The secondary chordae
(those chordae attached to the ventricular surface of the leaflets) are resected
whereas the marginal chordae (those attached to the free margin of the
leaflets or commissures) are carefully preserved (Fig. 20.9). Short chordae
arising from the papillary muscles also may restrict the motion of the leaflets,
but this can be corrected by splitting the papillary muscles.

Leaflet Approximation

A suture is placed at the center of the orifice to approximate the three leaflets (Fig. 20.10). The septal commissure is then reconstructed by plicating the attachment of this commissure to the septum. When necessary, the antero-lateral commissure and/or the posterolateral commissure are also plicated. Severe secondary lesions, such as thickening and retraction of the free edges of the leaflets, are frequent in older children and adults; these secondary lesions make it impossible to restore a good surface of apposition of the anterior and posterior components. In these instances it is necessary to close the septal commissure as in the current "classic" technique.

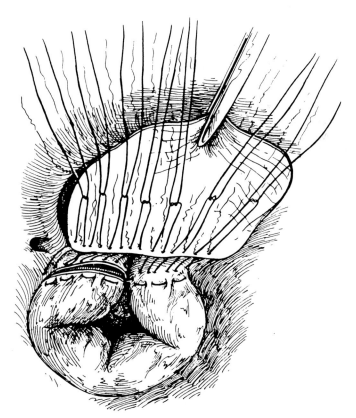

FIGURE 20.6 Divided anterior leaflets (Rastelli type A).

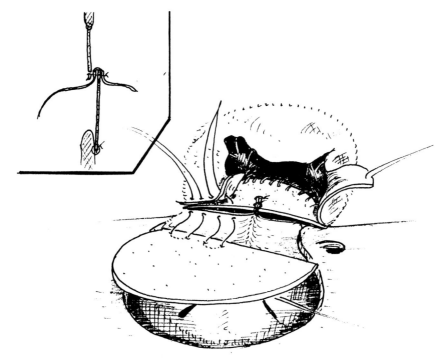

FIGURE 20.7 Divided leaflet is sutured to edges of ventricular and atrial patches in a manner preserving leaflet continuity *(inset)*.

Suture of Atrial Patch

The patch is sutured, leaving the coronary sinus on either the left or the right side according to the aformentioned criteria. The suture of the patch to the crest of the septum is performed with interrupted mattress sutures placed through the tricuspid annulus to avoid the bundle of His.

Intermediate Form

Although in some AVDs the mitral – tricuspid junction is as well delineated as in partial AVDs the junction does not adhere to the crest of the septum as it does in partial AVDs. There is a gap between the crest of the septum and the mitral – tricuspid junction, which is obstructed by a fragile and some-times perforated membranous septum. Correcting this form as if it were a partial AVD may lead to patch dehiscence from the mitral–tricuspid junction. We prefer to suture the patch to the right side of the septum after temporarily detaching the septal component of the right atrioventricular valve.

RESULTS

Since 1977, we have used this technique in 54 consecutive children, age 6 weeks to 15 years (mean age, 5 years 9 months). In this patient group, we encountered 21 complete, 23 partial, and 10 intermediate forms of AVDs; all but two patients with complete AVDs presented with moderate-to-severe mitral insufficiency. The characteristic three-leaflet left atrioventricular valve was present in 44 patients (81.5%), an atypical valve was present in eight patients (14.8%), and a double-orifice right atrioventricular valve was present in two patients (3.7%). Eight patients presented with associated

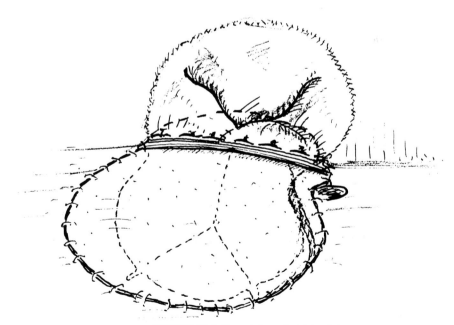

FIGURE 20.8 Completion of atrial patch.

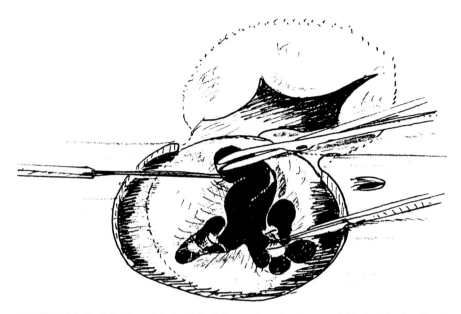

FIGURE 20.9 Partial atrioventricular defect. Secondary chordae are divided, while chordae at leaflet free margins are preserved. Short chordae can be lengthened by incising papillary muscles.

lesions. Four presented with a single atrium. Of these 54 children, three had previously undergone operation elsewhere for repair of a "mitral cleft."

There were nine hospital deaths 16.7%. This mortality reflects the peculiar selection of children who were referred to us on the basis of associated valvular incompetence and the fact that we do not reject patients with pulmonary hypertension. Ten patients with intermediate-type defects and 14 patients with complete-type defects were followed-up for a mean period of 5.2 years (0.5–8 years). There were three late deaths (12.5%): one due to atrioventricular block, one of unknown cause, and one noncardiac death. A second operation was necessary in two patients: one for iatrogenic aortic insufficiency, which could be repaired, and one for residual mitral insufficiency, which required a valve replacement. Incidence of atrioventricular block was 12%.

Clinical results as judged according to growth, functional class, and residual murmur, were grouped into three categories: *(a)* excellent: all variables were normal; *(b)* fair: functional class I, residual murmur, and without any cardiac insufficiency; and *(c)* poor: signs of residual mitral insufficiency and/or growth retardation, and poor function. Eighty-five percent of the children operated on had excellent results, 15% had fair results, and no patient had poor results.

Two-dimensional echocardiography and pulsed Doppler ultrasound studies were performed during follow-up examinations in 15 patients. They were then classified according to valvular and ventricular function: 12 patients (80%) had normal valve function and normal ventricular function; three patients (20%) had slightly abnormal valve function and normal ventricular function; none had abnormal valve function and abnormal ventricular function.

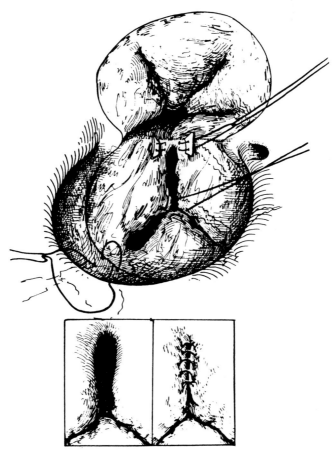

FIGURE 20.10 Three leaflets are approximated in center to align repair and septal commissure which are reconstructed by plicating the attachment of the commissure to the septum using pledgetted sutures.

CONCLUSIONS

Based on our clinical experience, we have made the following conclusions:

1. The three-leaflet left atrioventricular valve is a characteristic of AVDs, be they partial, intermediate, or complete.
2. Variations of the three-leaflet configuration are rare.
3. This valve is spontaneously competent in 30% of cases, and when it is not it should be repaired as a three-leaflet valve, not as a mitral valve.
4. Reestablishment of mitral–tricuspid leaflet continuity by the use of two separate septal patches minimizes leaflet dehiscence.
5. Suturing the atrial patch according to the technique described minimizes the risk of atrioventricular block.
6. Postoperative angiocardiography and catheterization are necessary to evaluate residual systolic murmurs.

REFERENCES

1. Castaneda AR, Nicoloff DM, Moller JH, et al. Surgical correction of complete atrio-ventricular canal utilizing ball-valve replacement of the mitral valve. J Thorac Cardiovasc Surg 1971;62:926.
2. McCabe JC, Engle MA, Gay WA, et al. Surgical treatment of endocardial cushion defects. Am J Cardiol 1977;39:72.
3. Somerville J. Clinical assessment of the function of the mitral valve in atrio-ventricular defects related to the anatomy. Am Heart J 1965;71:701.

CHAPTER 21

The Tricuspid Valve in Transposition of the Great Arteries

Peter J. Robinson, MB, FRACP, and
James F. N. Taylor, MD, FRCP, FACC

Rearrangement of atrial flow in transposition of the great arteries corrects the physiologic disturbance of blood flow pattern, but it leaves the anatomic relationship between the great arteries and ventricles unaltered. This raises concerns about the long-term functioning of the right ventricle as the systemic arterial ventricle and about the ability of the tricuspid valve to act as the systemic atrioventricular valve; the latter, because it would always be subject to systemic pressure. Fear that tricuspid valve failure would be a dominant feature in the period after surgical correction was enhanced by the frequency with which systemic atrioventricular valve (or left AV valve) regurgitation occurs in ventricular arterial discordance accompanied by atrioventricular discordance (corrected transposition). One should also consider the competance of the tricuspid valve in other anatomic situations, however, where for many years the right ventricle must sustain systemic pressure before surgical intervention. Tricuspid regurgitation is not a common feature in the tetralogy of Fallot, double-outlet right ventricle, or large ventricular septal defect associated with severe pulmonary vascular disease (at least until terminal myocardial failure ensues).

The tricuspid valve is the biological low-profile valve with large central orifice providing little obstruction to forward flow. It is supported on the ventricular side by a system of chordae and papillary muscles, which are more substantial structures in the hypertrophied right ventricle than in normal hearts; they are, however, less massive than their left ventricular counterparts. The basic structure of the tricuspid valve in transposition of the great arteries does not differ from that in the normal heart, although an autopsy series by Huhta et al[1] described a wide range of tricuspid valve abnormalities that can be seen in transposition associated with ventricular septal defects.

Our concern is with the survival of children after successful operations for transposition, and the nature of the problems that account for the falling population of survivors as shown by actuarial curves.[2] The experience with tricuspid valve function after intraatrial repair for transposition of the great arteries, occurring either as an isolated lesion (save for an associated atrial defect created by balloon septostomy) or with a ventricular septal defect or ductus arteriosus, is summarized in Table 21.1. Since 1964 our unit has undertaken a total of 725 Mustard and Senning operations and 80 Rastelli operations. The follow-up period has extended for a maximum of 21 years. In the early part of the series, many of the patients were in early childhood at the time of operation, whereas the procedure has been undertaken almost exclusively in infants during the last 10 years.

If subsequent tricuspid valve failure was significant occurrence, one would expect a steadily increasing number of children to return with this problem. This has not been the case in our experience. During this 21-year period (January 1964 – December 1984), there have been only ten occasions in which patients experienced tricuspid valve function impaired to such a degree that operative intervention was necessary to correct regurgitation. The majority of our patients are followed-up in our own clinics on an annual basis, and the Hospital receives reports on children residing outside England on a regular basis; thus we would be aware of further cases of clinically significant tricuspid valve regurgitation. We therefore believe that regurgitation is not a progressively significant feature in the follow-up of the patients as an isolated problem, and that it is uncommon as an associated feature. This is a different viewpoint from that expressed by Huhta et al[1] where there is a 14% incidence of surgically significant tricuspid valve abnormalities. Their paper does not discuss the clinical or hemodynamic effect of the

TABLE 21.1 Intraartrial Repair of Transposition of the Great Arteries 1964 – 1984

Procedure	Simple TGA	TGA, VSD
Mustard	407	155
Senning	121	42
Total	523	197

Abbreviations: TGA = transposition of the great arteries; VSD = ventricular septal defect.

morphological changes described where the abnormality is specifically associated with ventricular septal defect.

The 10 patients in our series with great artery transposition with significant tricuspid regurgitation fell into three groups: *(a)* those with iatrogenic damage; *(b)* those with congenital tricuspid insufficiency; and *(c)* those with late insufficiency associated with diminished tricuspid function.

IATROGENIC DAMAGE

Iatrogenic damage was present in two patients. One patient was a neonate who was transferred to our unit at the age of 3 days with detachment of the septal leaflet of the tricuspid valve after balloon atrial septostomy the previous day. Attempted repair of the damaged valve during an arterial "switch" operation the next day (4 days of age) was unsuccessful.

The second, a 13-year-old boy who had previously undergone a Blalock-Taussig operation, underwent a Rastelli repair for transposition of great arteries, ventricular septal defect, and pulmonary stenosis. The tricuspid valve straddled the ventricular septal defect, and to achieve competence after closure of the ventricular septal defect the tricuspid valve was replaced. It had, however, not been regurgitant pre-operatively. The repair was completed with a valved conduit from right ventricle to pulmonary artery. The child did not survive the operation.

CONGENITAL TRICUSPID INSUFFICIENCY

Six patients were noted to have severe tricuspid regurgitation at the time of their original investigation in infancy. This led to tricuspid valve replacement at the time of Mustard operation in two; in the other four patients tricuspid valve replacement was undertaken at age 3 years, 6 years, 7 years, and 9 years, respectively, after the Mustard operation; one of these children had a ventricular septal defect that was closed at the time of the Mustard operation.

Three of these children survived tricuspid valve replacement; one for 4 years, and the other two children are alive and well 8 years later. The course, however, has not been uncomplicated: both children have had a succession of valve replacements; the initial Hancock valve being replaced by an Ioenescu-Shiley valve and finally by a Björk-Shiley valve.

A different approach was used for the fourth patient, in whom the degree of tricuspid regurgitation was the most severe. The pulmonary artery was banded in accordance with the then-current policy to prepare for an arterial "switch" procedure; but the infant died with severe biventricular failure.

LATE INSUFFICIENCY ASSOCIATED WITH DIMINISHED RIGHT VENTRICULAR FUNCTION

The final patient developed tricuspid regurgitation as the right ventricle failed, and he, too, did not survive tricuspid valve regurgitation. He had been referred back to our unit 15 months after undergoing Mustard operation with evidence of severe superior and inferior vena caval pathway obstruction in addition to right ventricular failure.

CONCLUSIONS

The conclusion of our study is that tricuspid valve function is maintained after the Senning and Mustard procedures. There are a very small number of infants with congenital tricuspid insufficiency of such a magnitude that replacement is necessary, but our data, both for incidence and risks involved in valve replacement in childhood, are in accord with the published experience.[3] These data indicate that valve replacement does carry a significant risk and that the risk is higher when the tricuspid valve is the systemic rather than the pulmonary atrioventricular valve. These data should be compared with an incidence of six left atrioventricular valve replacements in 84 patients with atrioventricular and ventriculoarterial discordance (two deaths, and one survivor, 5 years post-operatively) in a total of 19 tricuspid replacements for all lesions. A corollary to the study remains the question of the most appropriate valve to use in childhood.

Still unanswered is the very long-term effect of the Mustard-and-Senning modified circulation in transposition. One may still face deterioration of right ventricular function in the third and fourth decades after operation, with associated tricuspid regurgitation. This entity is analogous to mitral regurgitation occuring as left ventricular function fails in the end stage of ischoemic or other myopathic disease. This is not a failure of the valve itself, so much as failure of the subvalve mechanism as part of the general myocardial failure. Our experience does not suggest that this is an early phenonmenon in transposition of the great arteries.

REFERENCES

1. Huhta JC, Edwards WD, Danielson GK, Feldt RH. Abnormalities of the tricuspid valve in complete transposition of the great arteries with ventricular septal defect. J Thorac Cardiovasc Surg 1982;83:569.
2. Macartney FJ, Taylor JFN, Graham GR, de Leval M, Stark J. The fate of survivors of cardiac surgery in infancy. Circulation 1980;62:80.
3. Berry BE, Ritter DG, Wallace RB, McGoon DC, Danielson GK. Cardiac valve replacement in children. J Thorac Cardiovasc Surg 1974;68:705.

Section IV

THE TRICUSPID VALVE

CHAPTER 22

Congenital Malformations of the Morphologically Tricuspid Valve

Robert H. Anderson, MD, FRC Path,
James R. Zuberbuhler, MD, FACC, and
Siew Yen Ho, PhD

SUMMARY

In this chapter we will consider the morphology of Ebstein's malformation and tricuspid atresia. Other lesions such as isolated dysplasia, clefts, and parachute malformation can affect the tricuspid valve, but these rarely produce hemodynamic problems and will not be considered in detail; neither will straddling and/or overriding, although the latter lesion is of major clinical importance. Ebstein's malformation can deform the tricuspid valve irrespective of the segmental arrangement of the heart. Thus, in hearts with usual atrial arrangement, it is the right-sided valve that is involved when the atrioventricular connection is concordant but the left-sided valve when it is discordant. The septal and mural leaflets are most deformed. They are not delaminated from the myocardium, thus producing downward displacement of the effective orifice of the valve. The valve closes at the junction of the inlet with the rest of the ventricle, the inlet becoming incorporated into the right atrium hemodynamically and morphologically when its wall is thinned, although the atrioventricular junction stays at its anticipated site. The major feature concerning repair of the valve is the distal attachment of the anterosuperior leaflet, which may be focal or linear.

In the most common variant of tricuspid atresia, the entire tricuspid valve apparatus and atrioventricular junction is absent. The muscular flow of the right atrium is separated by the adipose tissue of the atrioventricular groove from the ventricular mass. Rarely, the lesion can be produced by an imperforate valve membrane in any segmental setting. The variant with absent connection can also exist with the left atrium connected to a dominant right or a solitary indeterminae ventricle, but almost always the left ventricle is dominant. The major variants of surgical significance are the ventriculoarterial connection and the presence or absence of subarterial outflow tract obstruction, which most frequently exists at the ventricular septal defect.

INTRODUCTION

The spectrum of lesions afflicting the morphologically tricuspid valve is lim-limited in comparison with those that deform the mitral valve (see Chapter 20). In this chapter we will consider in depth the anatomy of Ebstein's malformation and that of tricuspid atresia; this will set the scene for the clinical contributions that follow. Brief mention should be made, however, of other lesions that affect the valve. Dysplasia almost always occurs as an integral part of Ebstein's malformation,[1] but it can occur in isolation (Fig. 22.1). Clefts and other lesions that deform the leaflets can occur, but rarely produce the hemodynamic disturbances that they do when found in the

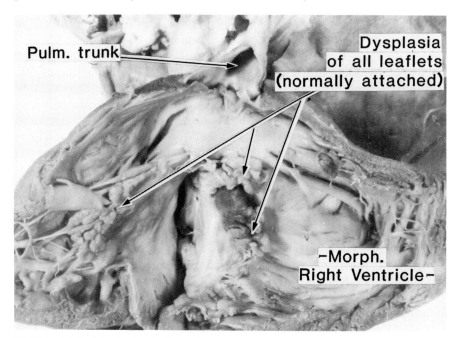

FIGURE 22.1 Dysplasia of the leaflets of a normally positioned morphologically tricuspid valve.

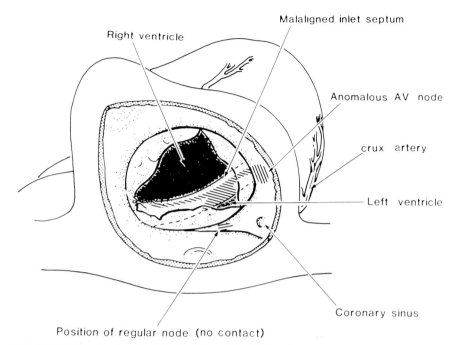

Malaligned inlet septum

Right ventricle

Anomalous AV node

crux artery

Left ventricle

Coronary sinus

Position of regular node (no contact)

FIGURE 22.2 A drawing showing the disposition of the atrioventricular conduction axis as it might be visualized by the surgeon operating through the morphologically right atrium in a patient with straddling bicuspid valve.

setting of the mitral valve. Similarly, a "parachute" malformation can be found with all the tendinous chords inserting to a solitary papillary muscle,[2,3] but this does not usually give problems during life. The most significant lesion (other than Ebstein's malformation or atresia) is straddling of the valve tension apparatus and/or overriding of the atrioventricular junction.[4] These lesions, existing either in combination or in isolation, present a major surgical problem[5,6] in no small part due to the grossly abnormal disposition of the atrioventricular conduction axis (Fig. 22.2). Because of these surgical implications, it is important to diagnose straddling and/or overriding of the tricuspid valve. This can be accomplished angiocardiographically,[7] but echocardiographic diagnosis is probably easier and more reliable.[8,9]

THE NORMAL MORPHOLOGICALLY TRICUSPID VALVE

As with all the other cardiac valves, in order to appreciate the morphology of the deformed tricuspid valve it is necessary first to examine the normal anatomy. In most normal hearts it is possible to distinguish the anticipated three leaflets. These are located in septal, antero-superior and inferior (or

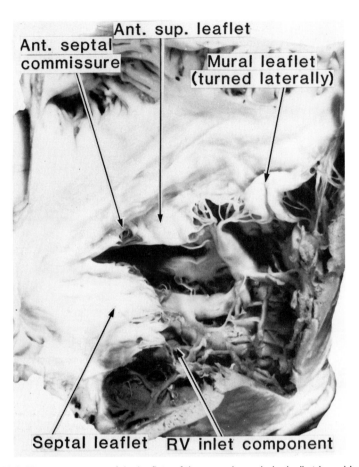

FIGURE 22.3 The arrangement of the leaflets of the normal morphologically tricuspid valve as seen with the right atrioventricular junction opened through the inferior commissure.

mural) position (Fig. 22.3). The leaflet segments are divided by commissures atop the medial, anterior, and inferior papillary muscles. Often the anterior muscle (the most prominent of the three) inserts directly to the midpoint of the anterosuperior leaflet. The inferior muscle is frequently duplicated, producing prominent scallops in the mural leaflets. The medial papillary muscle ("muscle of Lancisi," conal papillary muscle) is the most constant and most easily recognized. It is a relatively small structure, sometimes represented only by a fibrous chord, but it is often being multiple. The muscle (or muscle complex) arises from the posteroinferior limb of the prominent septomarginal trabeculation. It supports the anteroseptal commissure beneath the supraventricular crest (ventriculoinfundibular fold of the right ventricle). It is "round the corner" from the area of the membranous septum. The septal leaflet itself is often deeply cleft in the area of the membranous septum. It is here that its junctional attachment divides the fibrous septum into atrioventricular and interventricular components. The junctional attachment of the septal leaflet posteroinferior to the membranous septum forms the inferior margin of the triangle of Koch. The atrial component of the atrioventricular conduction axis is exclusively contained within this vital landmark area. The distal extent of the septal leaflet is tethered by multiple short tendinous chords to the inlet component of the muscular ventricular septum. It is these septal attachments that are the most reliable morphological markers of the tricuspid valve. They persist in virtually all malformed hearts. Other features, such as offsetting of the proximal attachment of the valve leaflets, are lacking in several significant lesions (such as a perimembranous inlet ventricular septal defect). The anterosuperior leaflet in the normal valve hangs like a curtain from the underside of the ventriculoinfundibular fold. The blood is propelled from the inlet to the outlet component of the right ventricle beneath its leading edge (Fig. 22.4).

EBSTEIN'S MALFORMATION

Ebstein's malformation can deform the morphologically tricuspid valve irrespective of its position within the heart. Although the basic morphology of the lesion is comparable in all circumstances, subtle differences exist when the malformation is found in the setting of a concordant atrioventricular connection on the one hand and a discordant connection on the other.

With Concordant Atrioventricular Connection

The essence of Ebstein's malformation is a downward (distal) displacement of the annular attachment of the valve leaflets. Almost always the leaflets are additionally deformed and dysplastic.[1,10] Indeed, it is possible that the initial case described by Wilhelm Ebstein had valve dysplasia as the prominent lesion.[11] Dysplasia can, however, exist without any downward displacement; it would not then be considered as Ebstein's malformation (Fig. 22.1). It is the displacement, then, that is the hallmark of the malformation.

By virtue of the normal anatomy, this displacement affects mostly the septal and mural leaflets. It is most prominent at the commissure between these leaflets. There is certainly a spectrum of displacement from normality to abnormality.[12] Minimal displacement may be a chance autopsy finding (Fig. 22.5). Very rarely the attachment of the anterosuperior leaflet can be displaced along the ventriculoinfundibular fold.[13] The septal leaflet can vir-

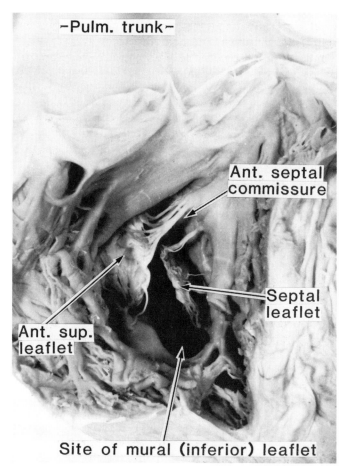

FIGURE 22.4 The infundibular aspect of the normal morphologically tricuspid valve.

tually disappear in the severest cases. The surface of the inlet component of the ventricular septum is then smooth, and the dysplastic valve tissue is found only as multiple cauliflower excresences towards the inlet-trabecular junction (Fig. 22.6). In view of this morphology, it is perhaps more accurate to describe the deformity in terms of failure of delamination of the leaflet tissue rather than "downward displacement." Be that as it may, the end result is to produce a valve mechanism (usually stenotic and often incompetent) at the inlet-trabecular rather than the atrioventricular junction. The fibrous insulation between atrial and ventricular muscle masses persists at the atrioventricular junction, although accessory atrioventricular muscular connections producing Wolff-Parkinson-White syndrome are frequent. Because the valve mechanism is depressed into the ventricular mass, the inlet component of the right ventricle hemodynamically becomes "atrialized." The inlet myocardium becomes severely thinned in severe cases. This arrangement is distinguished as anatomical atrialization (Fig. 22.7).

The most significant variant in valve morphology concerns the nature of distal attachment of the anterosuperior leaflet.[14] As described, in the normal heart this leaflet hangs down from the ventriculoinfundibular fold. Its annular attachment is hardly ever deformed in Ebstein's malformation. The variability affects its leading edge. In some cases this edge has focal commissural attachments as in the normal heart (Fig. 22.8). The blood is then able to pass from inlet to outlet in the usual fashion. In other cases the

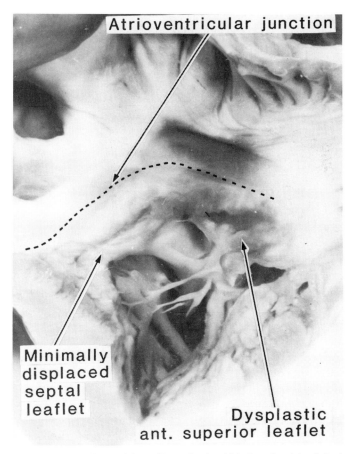

FIGURE 22.5 An example of Ebstein's malformation in which there is minimal displacement of the annular attachment of the valve leaflets. The heart is viewed from the inlet aspect (compare with Fig. 22.3).

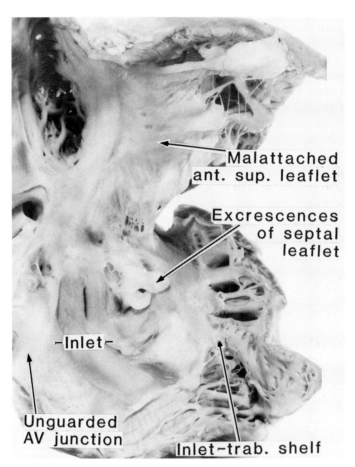

FIGURE 22.6 The inlet aspect of Ebstein's malformation with more severe displacement of the annular attachment of the leaflets, but with focal distal attachment of the anterosuperior leaflet. The heart is viewed from the inlet aspect (compare with Figs. 22.3 and 22.5).

valve leaflet has a linear attachment to a prominent muscular shelf at the inlet-apical trabecular junction (Fig. 22.9). The valve then sits as a square saillike partition between the atrialized inlet and the remainder of the right ventricle. The blood is then able to pass from inlet to outlet components only through the commissural areas of the valve. It is but a short step from such linear attachment of the antero-superior leaflet to an imperforate valve. The latter arrangement then produces an unusual form of tricuspid atresia (see below and Fig. 22.10).

Closely related to imperforate Ebstein's malformation (and also producing functional tricuspid atresia) are those cases with a muscular partition between the inlet and the remainder of the right ventricle (Fig. 22.11). In these cases, however, the atrioventricular junction is unguarded and there is no evidence of tricuspid valve tissue. It is probably more accurate to describe them as muscular tricuspid atresia in the setting of a concordant atrioventricular connection. Earlier we included them in our account of Ebstein's malformation.[15] All things considered, it seems to us that the arrangement of the distal attachment of the anterosuperior leaflet is the most significant feature determining the feasibility of valve reconstruction at surgery.

We have discussed the thinning of the ventricular inlet component, which is described as anatomical atrialization. The outlet and apical trabecu-

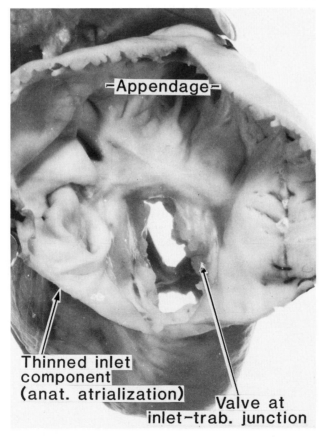

FIGURE 22.7 The major thinning of the inlet segment of the morphologically right ventricle ("anatomical atrialization") that makes up a fundamental part of the spectrum of severe Ebstein's malformation.

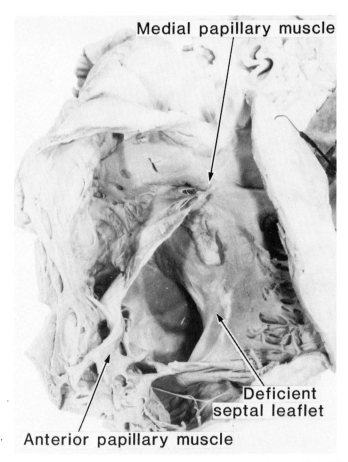

Medial papillary muscle

Deficient septal leaflet

Anterior papillary muscle

FIGURE 22.8 The infundibular aspect of the heart illustrated in Figure 22.6 with Ebstein's malformation and a focal distal attachment of the tension apparatus of the anterosuperior leaflet.

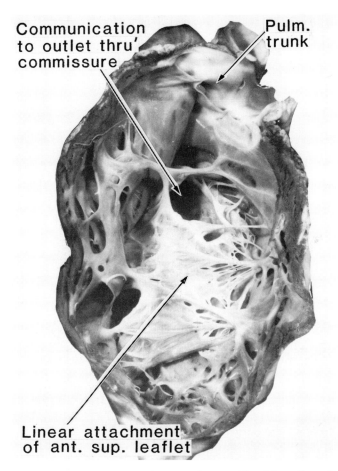

FIGURE 22.9 The infundibular aspect of a case of severe Ebstein's malformation with linear attachment of the distal extent of the anterosuperior leaflet to the junction of the inlet and apical trabecular components of the morphologically right ventricle.

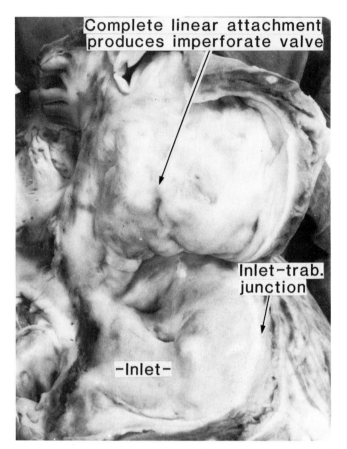

FIGURE 22.10 Ebstein's malformation with an imperforate valve as seen from the inlet aspect.

lar myocardial musculature may also be thinned and dilated, as may the right atrium. The most severe dilation and thinning is found when Ebstein's malformation presents during the neonatal period, coexisting with critical pulmonary stenosis or pulmonary atresia. These cases have "wall-to-wall" ventricles (Fig. 22.12) and a terrible prognosis. It is difficult to see what surgical options can be offered in these cases other than transplantation. In terms of categorization, they should not be grouped with Uhl's anomaly. The parietal ventricular myocardium in the latter lesion is absent, rather than thinned, and the tricuspid valve is normally attached.

Associated lesions are highly significant in the setting of Ebstein's malformation. An interatrial communication is almost always present. Most usually this is a defect within the oval fossa, but the lesion can be found in the setting of an atrioventricular septal defect.[13,16] A ventricular septal defect can also be found, usually communicating with the distal component of the morphologically right ventricle. Any lesion that is anatomically feasible should be anticipated as a possibility.

With Discordant Atrioventricular Connection

Lesions of the morphologically tricuspid valve are the third component of the triad of associated lesions anticipated with congenitally corrected trans-

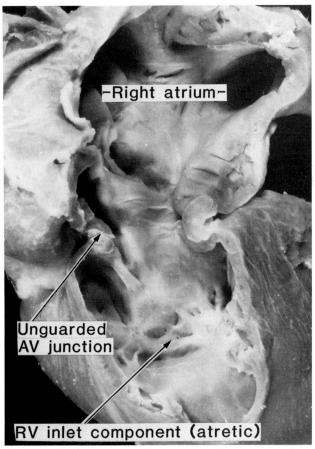

FIGURE 22.11 The blind-ending inlet component of the morphologically right ventricle in a heart with congenital absence of the leaflets of the tricuspid valve, giving an unguarded right atrioventricular junction. The hemodynamic consequence is tricuspid atresia.

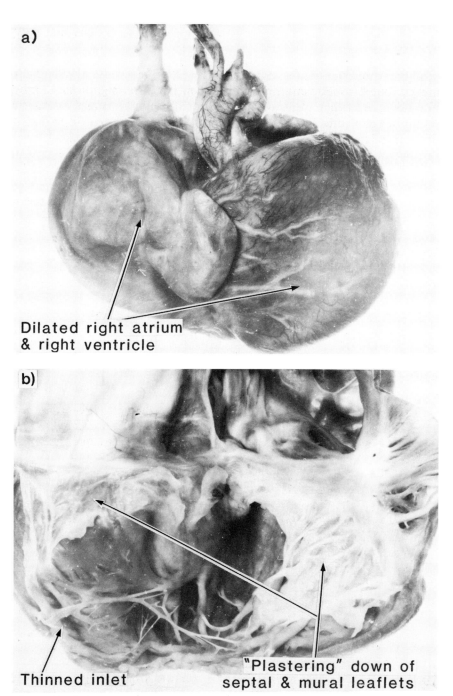

a)

Dilated right atrium
& right ventricle

b)

Thinned inlet

"Plastering" down of
septal & mural leaflets

FIGURE 22.12 The anatomy generally seen when Ebstein's malformation presents in the neonatal period. The *upper panel* shows the gross dilation of the right atrium and the inlet component of the right ventricle while the *lower panel* shows the dysplastic and plastered down leaflets as viewed from the inlet aspect.

position.[17] Ebstein's malformation is the most frequent cause of valve deformation; but straddling and/or overriding are found in a significant number of cases. The basic anatomy of Ebstein's malformation is as found in the setting of a concordant atrioventricular connection. The valve displacement (lack of delamination) affects the septal and mural leaflets and is most marked at the inferoseptal commissure.[18] Hemodynamic atrialization always exists as a consequence of the distal displacement. Anatomic atrialization is much rarer than in hearts with a concordant atrioventricular connection. A spectrum of thinning of the inlet myocardium is found (Fig. 22.13). Only a small proportion show major dilation. A focal attachment of the anterosuperior leaflet is the rule, although cases with linear attachment exist. Examples of an imperforate valve should be anticipated. The major distinction of Ebstein's malformation in the setting of a discordant atrioventricular connection is the small size of the morphologically right ventricle.[18,19] This makes replacement of the tricuspid valve a daunting procedure and, if performed, dictates the need for low profile prosthesis.

TRICUSPID ATRESIA

Atresia means occlusion of a natural channel of the body. It is nonspecific when used in the setting of the tricuspid valve. The occlusion of flow from the right atrium can be produced by an imperforate valve membrane, by an imperforate muscular partition within the ventricular mass, or by complete absence of the atrioventricular connection. The term "tricuspid" is itself also relatively nonspecific. This is because the morphologically tricuspid valve can guard the left atrioventricular junction in the setting of discordant atrioventricular connection. Similarly, a case can be made on embryological grounds for an absent left atrioventricular connection to represent "tricuspid" atresia when the right atrium is connected to a dominant left ventricle and the rudimentary right ventricle is left-sided. Taken together, therefore, the term "tricuspid atresia" is remarkably imprecise. Its major value lies in its clinical usage. Here it traditionally describes the constellation of features resulting when there is no direct communication between the systemic venous atrium and the ventricular mass. All the systemic venous return then has to traverse the atrial septum so as to reach the ventricles. It is in this sense that the term will be used in this chapter.

Attempts were made previously to give some specificity to the anatomic variants by using an alphanumeric system.[20] This accounted for the ventriculoarterial connection (A through C) and the magnitude of pulmonary flow (I through III). In general terms, this simple system stands the test of time well, despite the inherent deficiencies of alphanumeric systems which, by

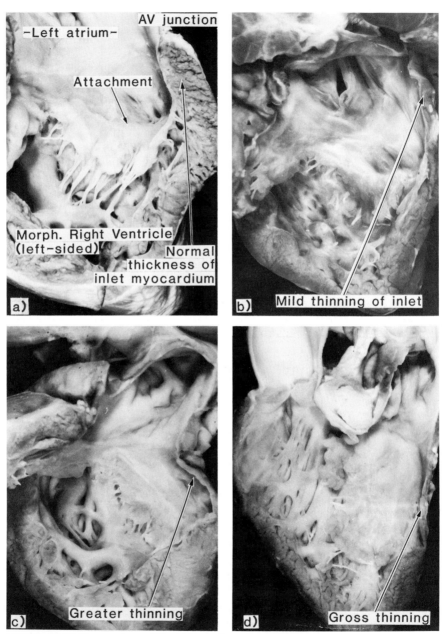

FIGURE 22.13 The spectrum of Ebstein's malformation as it affects the left-sided morphologically tricuspid valve in congenitally corrected transposition. The sequence of **(a)** through **(d)** shows increasing degrees of thinning ("atrialization") of the inlet component of the morphologically right ventricle.

their very nature, must be cryptic. It is attempts to expand this approach[21,22] to account for further variability which have led to confusion. The variability is too great to lend itself to procrustean classification. In this chapter, therefore, we will describe a sequential anatomical approach to the varied morphology of tricuspid atresia. The most significant variable is unequivocally the nature of the atrioventricular junction. We will describe first the possibilities before considering the detailed morphology of the commonest variant, the so-called "classical tricuspid atresia."

Variability at the Atrioventricular Junction

Atresia at the right atrioventricular junction can be produced either by an imperforate valve membrane or by absence of the atrioventricular connection. The rare muscular position within the right ventricle (Fig. 22.11) also produces functional tricuspid atresia. Although the term tends to conjure up the concept of an imperforate valve, by far the greater majority of cases are the consequences of absence of the right atrioventricular connection. The anatomical distinction between the different forms is striking. The atrioventricular junction in presence of an imperforate membrane is formed, but unpassable. In other words, there is a potential communication between the floor of the right atrium and the ventricular mass that is blocked by the valve membrane (Fig. 22.14). Removal of the membranes restores the continuity of the circulation. There is then the potential for much more variability according to the precise atrioventricular connection present. Imperforate membranes are rare in the overall setting of tricuspid atresia.[23] When found, they may be seen either in the context of imperforate Ebstein's malformation with a concordant atrioventricular connection (Fig. 22.10) or else double inlet left ventricle (Fig. 22.15) Imperforate membranes must also be anticipated, however, in the setting of discordant or ambiguous atrioventricular connection or with double inlet right or solitary and indeterminate ventricle. If found with a discordant atrioventricular connection, then it is the morphologically mitral valve that would be imperforate so as to block flow from the systemic venous atrium. This would then be anticipated to coexist with pulmonary atresia and hypoplasia of the right-sided morphologically left ventricle.

By far the commonest cause of tricuspid atresia as here defined is absence of the right atrioventricular connection. This exists when the floor of the atrium is exclusively muscular and there is no vestige of the atrioventricular junction (Fig. 22.16). Sectioning in "four-chamber" plane confirms the absence of the connection, showing how the fibro-fatty tissue of the atrioventricular groove (sulcus tissue) extends into the central fibrous body (Fig. 22.17). A dimple, if present, is also muscular and overlies the atrioventricular component of the membranous septum. It points into the outflow tract of

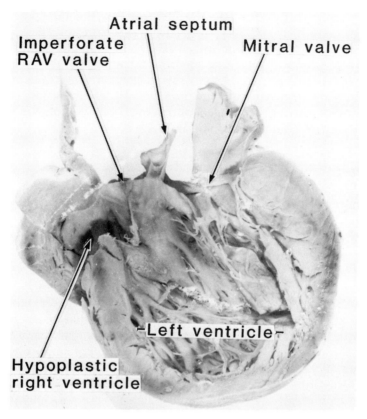

FIGURE 22.14 The very rare lesion of an imperforate right atrioventricular valve, which is normally attached to the atrioventricular junction. The heart is shown in simulated four-chamber section. The arrangement produces "tricuspid atresia."

the left ventricle and not to the rudimentary right ventricle.[24,25] If a fibrous membrane does exist in the floor of the atrium, then there is no longer absence of the atrioventricular connection (Fig. 22.15). It is necessary to traverse the extracardiac space in hearts with absent atrioventricular connection so as to pass from the right atrium into the ventricular pass.

As with imperforate membranes, variability can occur in hearts with absent right atrioventricular connection according to the morphology of the ventricles. The left atrium in classical tricuspid atresia connects to a dominant morphologically left ventricle, almost always in presence of a rudimentary right ventricle. Cases then exist with the left atrium connected to a dominant right ventricle. These usually have a right-sided rudimentary left ventricle along with straddling of the left atrioventricular valve. Because of the left-hand morphological pattern of the ventricular mass, they have much in common with congenitally corrected transposition. Embryologically they would be considered to have been "mitral" atresia. Anatomically and hemodynamically, however, their right atrial features are indistinguishable from classical tricuspid atresia (Fig. 22.18). Rare cases also exist in which the right atrioventricular connection is absent and the left atrium is connected to a solitary and indeterminate ventricle. Of necessity, these cases must have either double or single outlet ventriculoarterial connection.

CLASSICAL TRICUSPID ATRESIA

The essential anatomy of the most frequent morphological variant of tricuspid atresia is absence of the right atrioventricular connection. The left atrium is connected to a dominant left ventricle (Fig. 22.16) in presence of an anterosuperiorly located rudimentary right ventricle (Fig. 22.19). The sys-

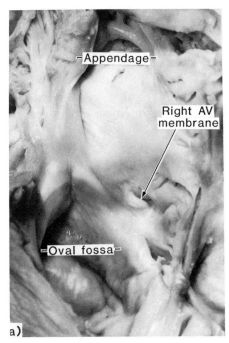
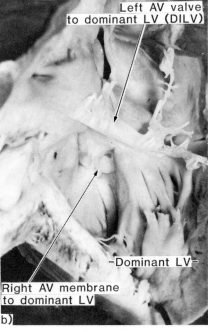

FIGURE 22.15 "Tricuspid atresia" produced by an imperforate and hypoplastic valve membrane in the setting of double inlet left ventricle. The left hand panel **(a)** shows the small right atrioventricular junction while the right hand panel **(b)** shows the imperforate membrane herniated into the dominant left ventricle.

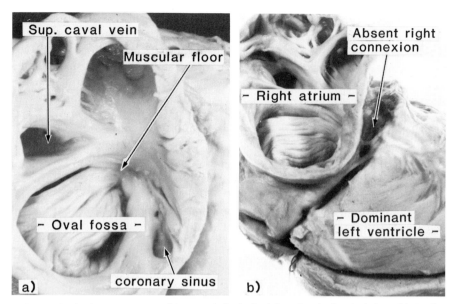

FIGURE 22.16 The appearance of the morphologically right atrium in classical tricuspid atresia. The left hand panel **(a)** shows the muscular floor of the atrium while the right hand panel **(b)** shows how the atrioventricular groove separates the atrial chamber completely from the ventricular mass.

temic and pulmonary venous connections are almost with exception normal (the most common anomaly is connection of a persistent left superior caval vein to the enlarged coronary sinus). The only egress for the systemic venous return is across the atrial septum into the left atrium. Most frequently this occurs through the oval foramen, which may be probe patent (Fig. 22.20a). Alternatively, its floor may be deficient, resulting in a atrial septal defect within the oval fossa (Fig. 22.20b). Rarely there may be a deficiency of the inferior limbus of the oval fossa producing an "ostium primum" defect.[21,25] It could be argued that such a lesion would produce a common atrioventricular junction connected exclusively to the left ventricle. The left valve, however, has the morphology of a left rather than a common valve, with the "cleft" pointing into the right atrium. The morphology is, therefore, that of absent right atrioventricular connection with an "ostium primum" defect rather than a common atrioventricular junction. We have never seen a sinus venosus defect, but there is no reason why one should not coexist with tricuspid atresia. The right atrial myocardium is usually hypertrophied, considerably more so than in the setting of double inlet left ventricle.[23,26]

Sometimes the floor of the oval fossa is herniated into the left atrium (Fig. 22.21) and then tends to create excessive right atrial hypertrophy. The

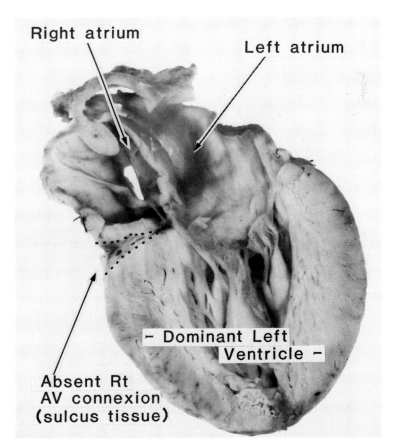

Right atrium

Left atrium

Dominant Left
Ventricle -

Absent Rt
AV connexion
(sulcus tissue)

FIGURE 22.17 A simulated "four chamber" section (showing only three chambers) which illustrates how the commonest example of tricuspid atresia is due to complete absence of the right atrioventricular connection.

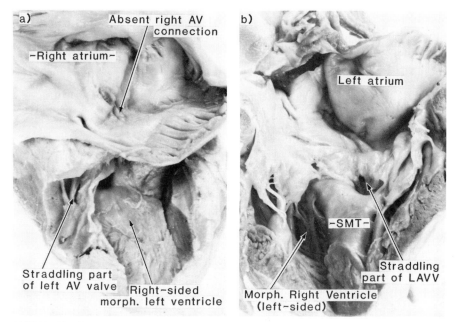

FIGURE 22.18 Absence of the right atrioventricular connection **(a)** with the left atrium connected primarily to a left-sided dominant right ventricle **(b)**. Note that the left valve straddles through a small ventricular septal defect into the right-sided rudimentary left ventricle as illustrated in **(a)**. Abbreviation: SMT = septomarginal trabeculation.

valve of the inferior caval vein (Eustachian valve) is frequently well formed and forms a curtain between the venous sinus and the appendage of the right atrium. If present, it should be preserved during a Fontan procedure. The "dimple" is a muscular depression anterior to the coronary sinus, which overlies the atrioventricular component of the membranous septum. It "points" to the left ventricular outflow tract. The commissure of the Eustachian and Thebesian valves (tendon of Todaro) inserts at the dimple, making it a good landmark for the site of the atrioventricular node.

The most significant associated lesion affecting the atrial chambers is juxtaposition of the atrial appendages. The right appendage lies in the transverse sinus so that its tip protrudes beyond the arterial pedicle to lie alongside the left appendage (Fig. 22.22). This arrangement distorts the internal anatomy of the right atrium so that the orifice of the juxtaposed appendages lies in the anticipated site of the oval fossa. The oval fossa itself tends to be a posteriorly displaced slitlike structure. The absence of the appendage in its usual position means that surgical access to the right atrium is limited, particularly since the sinus node lies in the terminal groove much closer to

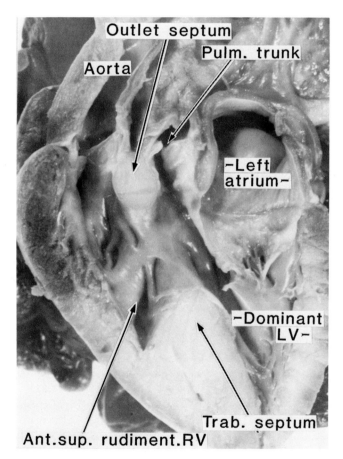

FIGURE 22.19 A long-axis cut of the ventricular mass in classical tricuspid atresia showing how the atrial chambers are connected exclusively to the dominant left ventricle in presence of an antero-superior rudimentary right ventricle.

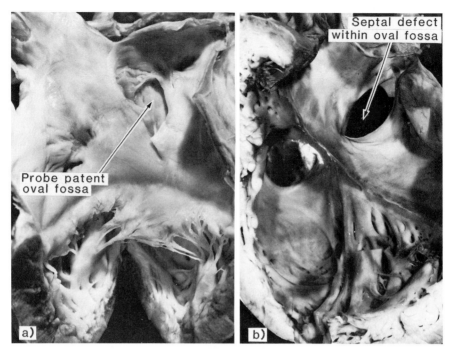

FIGURE 22.20 The left atrial view of the septum in classical tricuspid atresia showing **(a)** a probe-patent oval foramen and **(b)** a defect within the oval fossa.

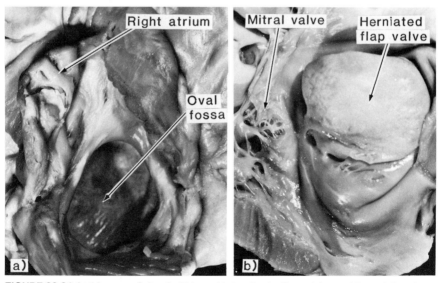

FIGURE 22.21 In this case of classical tricuspid atresia; the floor of the oval fossa is herniated into the left atrium. The heart is viewed **(a)** from the right and **(b)** from the left atrial aspects.

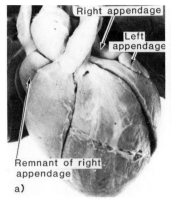
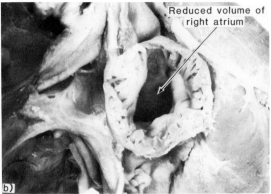

FIGURE 22.22 Juxtaposition of the atrial appendages to the left of the arterial pedicle. The anterior view of the heart is shown in **(a)** with a small part of the right appendage still protruding in its expected position. Opening this part **(b)** reveals its small volume.

the atrioventricular groove than usual.[27] The juxtaposed position of the appendage within the traverse sinus, however, places it directly adjacent to the pulmonary trunk. This facilitates direct atriopulmonary connection as a variant of the Fontan procedure.

The location of the sinus node and the course of its arterial blood supply are equally significant for the surgeon when the appendage is normally positioned. The node then lies laterally in the terminal groove immediately below the crest of the appendage. It is the course of the artery to the node that places it at risk if a direct atriopulmonary connection is performed through the atrial roof. The artery usually originates from the proximal portions of either the right or the circumflex coronary arteries. It then runs through the interatrial groove toward the cavoatrial junction, often burrowing itself deeply within the atrial walls (Fig. 22.23). It is, therefore, potentially at risk if deep incisions are made across the interatrial furrow. Care should also be taken to preserve the lateral right arteries during surgery for tricuspid atresia, particularly if one supplies the sinus node.[28]

The left atrium is almost always morphologically normal. It is connected by a morphologically mitral valve to the dominant left ventricle. The mitral valve is also almost always normal. Rarely it may be cleft, may exhibit a parachute malformation, or may straddle and/or override the ventricular septum. The basic arrangement of the ventricular mass is that of a dominant left ventricle with an anterosuperior rudimentary right ventricle. Almost always the right ventricle is right-sided. It may be directly anterior on occasion or even to the left.[25] The ventricular septum has only apical trabecular and outlet components (Fig. 22.19). It extends to the acute margin of the

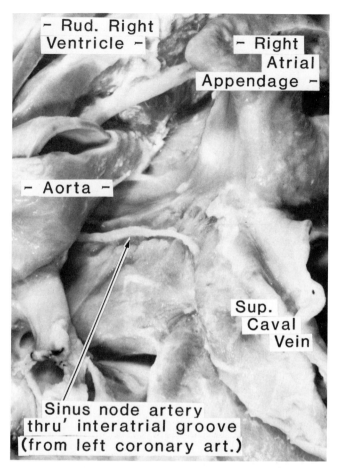

FIGURE 22.23 Dissection showing the course of the artery to the sinus node through the interatrial groove.

ventricular mass. Its position is marked externally by the anterior interventricular and marginal coronary arteries (Fig. 22.24). The ventricular septal defect has exclusively muscular margins, and usually it is situated between the crest of the apical trabecular septum and the lower edge of the outlet septum. The atrioventricular conduction axis descends posteroinferiorly to the defect, being carried on the left ventricular aspect of the septum (Fig. 22.25). Rarely there may be a muscular defect within the apical septum which can coexist with the usual defect or be the only interventricular communication. The conduction axis runs in the roof of such apical defects.[23]

The precise morphology of the ventricular septal defect and the rudimentary right ventricle is related to the ventriculoarterial connection.

Usually the connection is concordant. Then the apical trabecular component of the right ventricle is right-sided. The septal defect is centrally located, and the extensive infundibulum runs up to the left-sided pulmonary valve (Fig. 22.26). The size of the defect varies markedly and is directly proportional to the size of the rudimentary ventricle, which has a well-developed apical trabecular component. More usually the defect is restrictive (Fig. 22.27a). The right ventricle is then smaller. Rarely, however, the defect can be atretic (Fig. 22.27b), and then the ventricle is tiny. In the cases discussed thus far, the great arteries have all been presumed to be normally related. In other words, they take a spiraling course and the pulmonary trunk is anterior

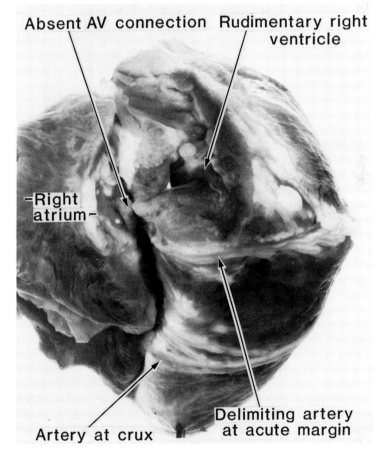

FIGURE 22.24 A case of classical tricuspid atresia photographed from infero-posteriorly to show the delimiting coronary arteries marking the site of the rudimentary right ventricle.

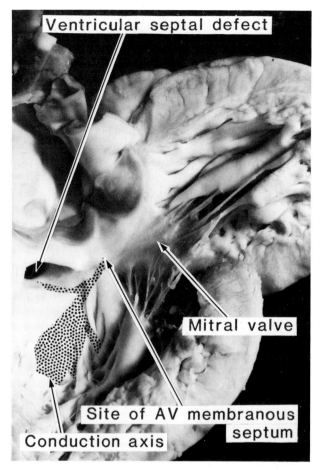

FIGURE 22.25 A view of the dominant left ventricle in a case of classical tricuspid atresia opened anteriorly to show the relationship of the atrioventricular conduction axis *(stippled)* to the ventricular septal defect.

and left-sided. The great arteries are unusually related in a small proportion of cases with a concordant atrioventricular connection. In these cases the aorta arises from the dominant left ventricle in anterior and left-sided position, usually with its valve supported by a complete muscular infundibulum. The rudimentary right ventricle is right-sided and supports a right-sided pulmonary trunk, which is usually stenotic or atretic. This arrangement (termed anatomically corrected malposition) is often associated with juxtaposed atrial appendages.[29]

The ventriculoarterial connection is discordant in about a one-fifth of cases. The pulmonary trunk arises from the dominant left ventricle, usually with pulmonary-mitral valvar fibrous continuity. The aorta has a complete muscular infundibulum and usually arises in right-sided position from the anterior rudimentary right ventricle; it may sometimes be left-sided. The rudimentary right ventricle tends to have a different morphology in this setting. The apical trabecular component is relatively longer than the outlet component, although in absolute terms it is usually smaller than in cases with a concordant ventriculoarterial connection. The ventricular septal defect is immediately beneath the aortic valve (Fig. 22.28). Should it be necessary to enlarge the defect, it is the segment of apical septum closest to the anterior descending interventricular artery which can safely be resected.

Other ventriculoarterial connections may be encountered. A double outlet can be found either from the dominant left or the rudimentary right ventricle. A bilateral infundibulum is often found with a double-outlet right

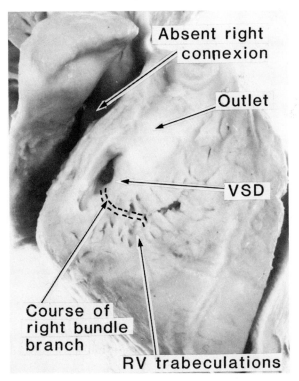

FIGURE 22.26 A view of the rudimentary right ventricle as typically seen in classical tricuspid atresia with a concordant ventriculoarterial connection. The course of the right bundle branch *(dotted line)* has been superimposed on the photograph.

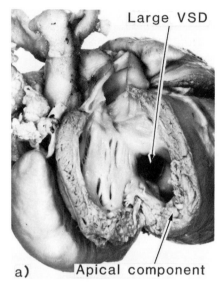

Large VSD

Apical component

a)

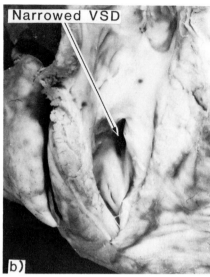

Narrowed VSD

b)

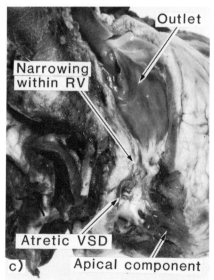

Outlet

Narrowing within RV

Atretic VSD

Apical component

c)

FIGURE 22.27 The varying morphology of the rudimentary right ventricle in classical tricuspid atresia with concordant ventriculo-arterial connection with **(a)** a large, **(b)** a narrowed, and **(c)** an atretic ventricular septal defect. The apical trabecular component of the ventricle is well formed in each, as is the extensive outlet component.

ventricle, while a bilaterally deficient infundibulum is frequently seen with a double-outlet left ventricle. A single-outlet ventricle is by no means infrequent. When the heart is available for study, then pulmonary atresia is almost always found to be in the setting of a concordant connection. In a clinical setting, however, it is often not possible to be sure of the connection of the atretic pulmonary trunk. The arrangement may then be categorized as

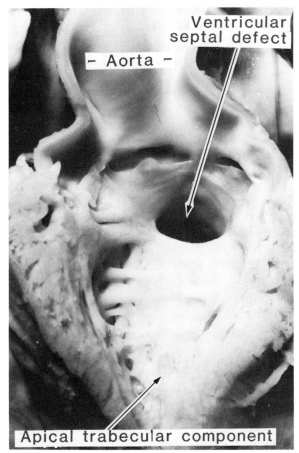

FIGURE 22.28 The morphology of the rudimentary right ventricle in classical tricuspid atresia with discordant ventriculoarterial connection differs because of the much shorter outlet component (compare with Fig. 22.27).

single outlet. A common arterial trunk can exist, but it is rare, as is a solitary pulmonary trunk with aortic atresia.

The most significant associated lesions are those that obstruct the ventricular outflow tract. This is usually due to stenosis of the ventricular septal defect. This results in subpulmonary stenosis with a concordant ventriculoarterial connection. Often there is an additional stenotic area at the junction of apical trabecular and outlet components of the rudimentary right ventricle. A restrictive ventricular septal defect in the setting of a discordant ventriculoarterial connection produces subaortic stenosis. This is frequently associated with coarctation or interruption of the aortic arch. Subpulmonary stenosis with a discordant ventriculoarterial connection is usually due either to posterior deviation of the outlet septum[30] fibrous tissue tags[31] or anomalous attachment of the tension apparatus of the mitral valve.

TRICUSPID ATRESIA AND THE UNIVENTRICULAR HEART

It would be inappropriate to conclude this chapter without clarifying the confusion that has arisen around our concepts concerning tricuspid atresia and the "univentricular heart."[32] When we developed these concepts, we took double-inlet left ventricle as our paradigm of a "univentricular heart." We did this fully cognizant of the fact that double-inlet left ventricle possessed a rudimentary right ventricle. Conventional wisdom at the time dictated that this lesion was considered a "single ventricle" despite the presence of an "outlet chamber" within the ventricular mass. The point we made was that the rudimentary right ventricle in tricuspid atresia was morphologically identical to the "outlet chamber" in single ventricle. To appreciate the similarity in ventricular morphology it was necessary to compare examples of each lesion with the same ventriculoarterial connection, that is tricuspid atresia and double inlet left ventricle both with a concordant or discordant ventriculoarterial connection respectively.[33] It was not our intention to imply that tricuspid atresia possessed a solitary ventricular chamber. Neither does a double-inlet left ventricle, but most at that time were happy to describe it as a "single ventricle" (and possibly still are).

It soon became clear to us that our concept was not widely understood and appreciated; neither was it logical. The basis of our concept was that all hearts could be divided into two groups. On the one hand, there are all those hearts with each atrium connected to its own ventricle (concordant, discordant, and ambiguous atrioventricular connections). On the other hand are those hearts with the atrial chambers connected to only one ventricle (double-inlet and absence of one atrioventricular connection). There was no need for us to describe the latter group in terms of "univentricular hearts." What they had in common was a univentricular atrioventricular connection.[34] Thus, classical tricuspid atresia is comparable with double-inlet left ventricle insofar as both lesions possess a dominant left ventricle with a rudimentary right ventricle. Neither is an example of a univentricular heart or a single ventricle. Not all hearts with tricuspid atresia are of this type: Some may indeed be true examples of double inlet left ventricle with an imperforate right atrioventricular valve; others may have right atrioventricular valve atresia in the setting of concordant, discordant or ambiguous atrioventricular connections. It is simply not possible to describe accurately all this varied morphological information under the simple banner of tricuspid atresia.

Sequential segmental description is needed for full and adequate description. Nonetheless, tricuspid atresia remains an exceedingly useful term in a clinical situation for description of all those hearts lacking any direct communication between the systemic venous atrium and the ventricular mass.

ACKNOWLEDGEMENTS
We are grateful to all our colleagues with whom we have collaborated in the study of lesions of the tricuspid valve. We are particularly indebted to Professor Anton E. Becker, University of Amsterdam, the Netherlands, who permitted us to reproduce Figures 22.15, 22.20, 22.21, 22.25, and 22.28 from his unpublished work.

REFERENCES

1. Becker AE, Becker MJ, Edwards JE. Pathologic spectrum of dysplasia of the tricuspid valve. Arch Pathol 1971;91:167–178.
2. Milo S, Stark J, Macartney FJ, et al. Parachute deformity of the tricuspid valve (case report). Thorax 1979;34:543–546.
3. Maitre Azcarate MJ. Parachute deformity of the tricuspid valve (lett). Thorax 1980;35:240.
4. Milo S, Ho SY, Macartney FJ, et al. Straddling and overriding atrioventricular valves morphology and classification. Am J Cardiol 1979;44:1122–1134.
5. Tabry IF, McGoon DC, Danielson GK, et al. Surgical management of straddling valve. J Thor Card Surg 1979;77:191–201.
6. Pacifico AD, Soto B, Bargeron LM Jr. Surgical treatment of straddling tricuspid valves. Circulation 1979;60:655–664.
7. Soto B, Ceballos R, Nath PH, et al. Overriding atrioventricular valves. An angiographic–anatomical correlate. Int J Cardiol 1985;9:327–340.
8. Smallhorn JF, Sutherland G, Anderson RH, et al. Cross-sectional echocardiographic assessment of conditions with atrioventricular valve leaflets attached to the atrial septum at the same level. Br Heart J 1982;48:331–341.
9. Rice MJ, Seward JB, Edwards WD, et al. Straddling atrioventricular valve: two-dimensional echocardiographic diagnosis, classification and surgical implications. Am J Cardiol 1985;55:505–513.
10. Pechstein J. Beitrag zur Ebsteinschen Anomalie der Valvula tricuspidalis. Arch Kreisforsch 1957;26:282–337.
11. Schiebler GL, Gravenstein JS, Van Mierop LHS. Ebstein's anomaly of the tricuspid valve. Translation of original description with comments. Am J Cardiol 1968;22:867–873.
12. Gussenhoven EJ, Stewart PA, Becker AE, et al. "Offsetting" of septal tricuspid leaflet in normal hearts and in hearts with Ebstein's anomaly. Anatomic and echocardiographic correlation. Am J Cardiol 1984;54:172–176.
13. Zuberbuhler JR, Becker AE, Anderson RH, et al. Ebstein's malformation and the embryological development of the tricuspid valve. With a note on the nature of "clefts" in the atrioventricular valves. Pediatr Cardiol 1984;5:289–296.
14. Taussig HB. Congenital Malformations of the Heart, 2nd ed, Vol 2. The Commonwealth Fund, Harvard University Press, Cambridge, Mass, 1960, pp 466–489.
15. Zuberbuhler JR, Allwork SP, Anderson RH. The spectrum of Ebstein's anomaly of the tricuspid valve. J Thorac Cardiovasc Surg 1979;77:202–211.

16. Caruso G, Losekoot TG, Becker AE. Ebstein's anomaly in persistent common atrioventricular canal. Br Heart J 1978;40:1275–1279.
17. Van Praagh R. What is congenitally corrected transposition. N Engl J Med 1970;282:1097–1098.
18. Anderson KR, Zuberbuhler JR, Anderson RH, et al. Ebstein's anomaly: a review of the pathologic anatomy. Mayo Clin Proc 1979;54:174–180.
19. Sharma S, Zuberbuhler JR, Anderson RH. Abnormalities of the morphologically tricuspid valve in atrioventricular discordance—an autopsy study. Ind Heart J 1984;36:396–400.
20. Edwards JE, Burchell HB. Congenital tricuspid atresia: a classification. Med Clin North Am 1949;33:1117–1119.
21. Tandon R, Edwards JE. Tricuspid atresia. A re-evaluation and classification. J Thorac Cardiovasc Surg 1974;67:530–542.
22. Rao PS. A unified classification for tricuspid atresia. Am Heart J 1980;99:799–804.
23. Scalia D, Russo P, Anderson RH, et al. The surgical anatomy of hearts with no direct communication between the right atrium and the ventricular mass—so-called tricuspid atresia. J Thorac Cardiovasc Surg 1984;87:743–755.
24. Rosenquist GC, Levy RJ, Rowe RD. Right atrial–left ventricular relationships in tricuspid atresia; position of the presumed site of the atretic valve as determined by transillumination. Am Heart J 1970;80:493–497.
25. Anderson RH, Wilkinson JL, Gerlis LM, et al. Atresia of the right atrioventricular orifice. Br Heart J 1977;39:414–428.
26. Quero Jimenez M. Discussion. In, Anderson RH, Shinebourne EA (eds): Paediatric Cardiology. Churchill Livingstone, Edinburgh. 1977, p 402.
27. Ho SY, Monro JL, Anderson RH. The disposition of the sinus node in left-sided juxtaposition of the atrial appendage. Br Heart J 1979;41:129–132.
28. Busquet J, Fontan F, Anderson RH, et al. The surgical significance of the atrial branches of the coronary arteries. Int J Cardiol 1984;6:223–234.
29. Freedom RM, Harrington DP. Anatomically corrected malposition of the great arteries. Report of 2 cases, one with congenital asplenia; frequent association with juxtaposition of atrial appendages. Br Heart J 1974;36:207–215.
30. Ottenkamp J, Wenink ACG, Rohmer J, et al. Tricuspid atresia with overriding imperforate tricuspid membrane: an anatomic variant. Int J Cardiol 1984;6:599–610.
31. Gerlis LM, Anderson RH, Scott O. Interventricular and subarterial obstruction in tricuspid atresia due to a tissue tag. Am J Cardiol 1984;54:236–237.
32. Rao PS. Terminology: tricuspid atresia or univentricular heart. In, PS Rao (ed):Tricuspid Atresia. Futura Publishing Company, Mount Kisco, New York, 1982, p 3–6.
33. Deanfield JE, Tommasini G, Anderson RH, et al. Tricuspid atresia: an analysis of the coronary artery distribution and ventricular morphology. Br Heart J 1982;48:485–492.
34. Anderson RH, Becker AE, Tynan M, et al. The univentricular atrioventricular connection: getting to the root of a thorny problem. Am J Cardiol 1984;54:822–828.

CHAPTER **23**

Ebstein's Malformation

Albert D. Pacifico, MD

There are a number of aspects of the surgical treatment of Ebstein's malformation that are quite controversial. I am afraid that I cannot resolve all of those controversies.

It is interesting to look for a moment at some of the historical aspects of the surgical treatment of Ebstein's malformation. A systemic to pulmonary artery shunt, interestingly enough, was initially done and it was unsuccessful for a patient with Ebstein's malformation and cyanosis in 1950. Soon after that, however, there were several reports of the use of a Glenn shunt for similar patients with cyanosis and these were successful. In 1954 at the Mayo Clinic, John Kirklin closed the atrial septal defect of a patient with Ebstein's malformation. Lillihei et al in 1958[1] and Hardy et al in 1964[2] first described tricuspid valve repair, and Barnard in 1963[3] described the replacement of the tricuspid valve with the coronary sinus inferior or downstream to the placement of the valve in order to avoid the conduction tissue.

The natural history of untreated patients with Ebstein's malformation is demonstrated in a report by Giuliani et al[4] from the Mayo Clinic in 1979. This was an experience with 67 patients over a period of 12 years. When first identified, 39% of these patients were in the New York Heart Association class 1 or 2, and 61% in the New York Heart Association class 3 or 4. Over the follow-up period, death occurred in 21%. The factors related to premature death were the presence of New York Heart Association class 3 or 4 at the time of presentation, a large heart evidenced by cardiothoracic ratio of greater than 0.65, and systemic arterial desaturation below 90%. A small percentage of these patients were infants when they were diagnosed, and 50% of these patients died before age 2 years.

Similar data is reported from the Greenlane Hospital in Aukland, New Zealand.[5] This is an experience with 35 (surgically untreated) patients with

Ebstein's malformation with an 18-year follow-up. Nineteen patients presented beyond the first week of life — with a late survival of about 60% at 18 years; this is quite similar to the data from the Mayo Clinic. In contrast, 16 patients presented in the first week of life. The majority died soon after presentation and then there was a rather stable late survival of about 45% out to 12 years. Again, the incremental risk factors for premature death in patients with surgically untreated Ebstein's malformation are the degree of cyanosis, the magnitude of cardiomegaly, and the degree of congestive heart failure. New York Heart Association class 3 or 4 is a grave prognostic sign.

The surgical options for these patients include *(a)* closure of the atrial septal defect alone; *(b)* replacement or repair of the incompetent tricuspid valve; *(c)* atrial–pulmonary artery connection — a modified Fontan; and *(d)* surgery for Wolff-Parkinson-White, which can be accomplished in a small group of patients.

INDICATIONS FOR OPERATION

We believe that valve replacement or repair and ASD closure should be done when important tricuspid incompetence is present and there is moderate or severe cyanosis and symptoms of congestive heart failure. These patients should be operated before they reach New York Heart Class 4 when the risk is very high. Atrial septal defect (ASD) closure alone is beneficial when the tricuspid valve is either competent or mildly incompetent and when there is significant atrial shunting either right to left or left to right. Division of the Kent bundle for Wolff-Parkinson-White syndrome is appropriate in selected patients.

In replacing the valve, we prefer to place the suture line proximal to the location of the coronary sinus posteriorly to avoid conduction tissue. What to do with the atrialized ventricle is quite controversial. Some surgeons believe that it should be always plicated at the time of repair or replacement, and some believe that plication is never necessary. A middle of the road approach is to advise plication at the time of valve repair or replacement when this portion is very thin, aneurysmal, and has paradoxical motion. This is present in about 10% – 15% of patients with Ebstein's malformation. We observe the atrialized portion of the right ventricle externally for the paradoxical motion. If the patient is large enough, we examine the tricuspid valve digitally through the right atrial appendage. It is of interest that when there is very severe tricuspid incompetence, the regurgitant jet is not really palpable, but instead it is kind of a turbulence that one feels. The operation of course is done with cardiopulmonary bypass, excising the tricuspid valve and leaving a generous remmant of it near the conduction tissue and the prosthesis is sutured proximal to the coronary sinus, and in most patients, because the atrial septum is thin, a patch is used to close the interatrial communication.

For the purpose of this report, our experience at University of Alabama between 1967 and 1980 is combined with those from Greenlane Hospital in Aukland, New Zealand between 1958 and 1981. There are only 29 cases over these years from two relatively experienced surgical groups indicating the rather uncommon nature of surgery for Ebstein's malformation. There were 16 patients in New York Heart Association class 3 who received valve replacement and ASD closure with one death, a mortality of 6%. This occurred in a patient who had an associated partial AV septal defect. There were four patients in New York Heart Association class 4 with three surgical deaths, a mortality of 75%, significant at the 0.01 level. Nine patients had ASD closure alone with no mortality. The group is too small to analyze for its late results in a meaningful way, but a review of the literature indicates that most patients who have the tricuspid valve replacement and ASD closure are in New York Class Association class 1 or 2 late postoperatively. There is a late mortality of between 10%–15%. Supraventricular tachycardia persists in about 15% of patients, and there seems to be no clear difference among those who have undergone plication of the atrialized portion of the right ventricle at the time of valve replacement versus those in whom this portion is left alone. When the atrial septal defect is closed as the sole procedure, the late results are good when the indication is appropriate.

Now I think that you can find in the literature a number of papers that indicate that tricuspid valve replacement for patients with other types of valvular disease not as a part of Ebstein's malformation is not particularly good because of an increased set of problems with prosthetic valves in the tricuspid position. So I thought I would show a bit of our data from 1967 thru 1981 in this category of patients. There were 103 hospital survivors of tricuspid valve replacement, either alone or combined with mitral or mitral and aortic valve replacement or other procedures. None of these patients had Ebstein's malformation. There were five reoperations among the 103 patients over the follow-up period – a reoperation rate of 5%.

The indications for reoperation were *(a)* one case of prosthetic valve endocarditis of a Starr-Edwards ball valve 9.3 years after implantation; *(b)* two cases of valve thrombolic encapsulation, one with a Björk-Shiley valve and one with a Braunwald-Cutter valve 6 and 8 years, respectively, after operation; and *(c)* two cases of heterograft degeneration requiring replacement of the tricuspid valve heterograft prosthesis.

The reoperation-free rate was 88% over 15 years. So overall we believe that prostheses placed in the tricuspid position have problems that are similar to prostheses placed in the mitral position and without an increased incidence. Currently, our approach is to try to repair the tricuspid valve in Ebstein's malformation when its anatomy seems suited to such a repair, and, in the absence of doing that, to replace the tricuspid valve with a mechanical device because it will provide a good late result.

REFERENCES

1. Lillihei CW, Kalbe BR, Carlson RC. Evaluation of corrective surgery for Ebstein's anomaly. Circulation 1967;35–36:111.
2. Hardy KL, Mary IA, Webster CA, Kimball KA. Ebstein's anomaly. A functional concept and successful definitive repair. J Thorac Cardiovasc Surg 1964;48:927.
3. Barnard CN, Schire Y. Surgical correction of Ebstein's malformation with a prosthetic tricuspid valve. Surgery 1963;54:302.
4. Giuliani ER, Fuster V, Brandenburg RD, Mair DD. Ebstein's anomaly. The clinical features and natural history of Ebstein's anomaly of the tricuspid valve. Mayo Clin Proc 1979;54:163.
5. Kirkin JW, Barratt Boyes BG. Cardiac Surgery. Wiley and Sons, New York, 1986, p 899.

CHAPTER 24

The Use of Valves in the Fontan Circulation

Catherine Bull, MD, MRCP

SUMMARY

Contrary to the early conception of the right atrium as the pump for the pulmonary circulation, the atrium in fact pumps poorly. Valves incorporated in an atriopulmonary connection close very briefly or not at all. They are at best dispensible and at worst deleterious because they can introduce obstruction between the right atrium and the pulmonary artery. Valves in atrioventricular connections can however be useful in cases were the rudimentary ventricular chamber grows to contribute substantially to pulmonary blood flow.

INTRODUCTION

The question of the usefulness of valves in the Fontan operation relates to the concept of the right atrium as the pump for the pulmonary circulation. The theoretical implications of assuming that the function of the right atrial pump is necessary and sufficient to allow for right ventricular bypass led to caval and right atrial outlet valves being incorporated in early Fontan operations. Since then, changing surgical fashions have helped differentiate what is dispensable from what is mandatory in this rather special circulation.

The Fontan circulation differs from the normal in which there are two major pumps, the left and right ventricles (Fig. 24.1a). The left ventricle takes in blood at low pressure and ejects it at higher pressure (aortic pressure), which is sufficient to perfuse the systemic vascular resistance and

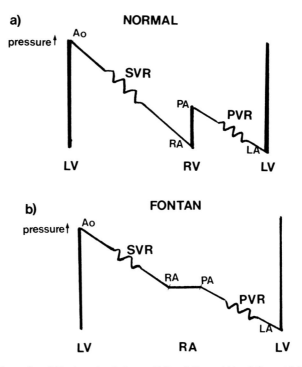

FIGURE 24.1 Normal and Fontan circulations. Abbreviations: LV = left ventricle; RV = right ventricle; LA = left atrium; RA = right atrium; Ao = aorta; PA = pulmonary artery; SVR = systemic vascular resistance; PVR = pulmonary vascular resistance.

return blood to the right atrium. The right ventricle takes in blood at low pressure and ejects it at a higher pressure (pulmonary artery pressure), which is sufficient to perfuse the pulmonary vascular resistance and return blood to the left side of the heart. In normal circulation, both atrial pressures are low, the left slightly exceeding the right due to a greater thickness of its corresponding ventricle.

In the Fontan circulation (Fig. 24.1b) there are also two pumps, the left ventricle and the right atrium. The left ventricle ejects blood at aortic pressure sufficient to perfuse the systemic vascular resistance and return blood to the right atrium. The right atrial and pulmonary artery pressures are comparable, and the pulmonary artery pressure is sufficient to perfuse the pulmonary vascular bed and return blood to the left atrium. The right atrial pressure is thus higher than the left, and it is the sequelae of this high right atrial pressure that characterizes the postoperative physiology after the Fontan operation.

The absolute height of the right atrial pressure depends on the resistance to right atrial outflow and, because the whole cardiac output must pass through each element in the circulatory pathway, the resistances summate (Fig. 24.2). Blood must cross any resistance in the atriopulmonary connection, pass through the lungs from pulmonary artery to left atrium (the pulmonary vascular resistance), and, because most of left ventricular filling occurs before atrial systole, blood must cross any obstruction at the mitral valve and overcome resistance to left ventricular filling. If any of these resistances is inordinately high — if left ventricle is stiff, if the mitral valve is stenotic, if the pulmonary vascular resistance is excessive or if there is any gradient in the atriopulmonary connection — the right atrial pressure will be driven up. The right atrial pressure cannot be held chronically much above 20 mm Hg because venous capillaries begin to leak. Thus, if the resistance to right atrial outflow should correspond to a higher right atrial pressure, instead the flow through the circuit (cardiac output) falls giving the picture of a swollen patient in fixed low cardiac output.

Remembering that the resistance in the atriopulmonary connection is one determinant of the right atrial pressure, we return to the place of valves in the Fontan circuit. Incorporation of valves is seen as a method of increasing the efficiency of the right atrium as a pump. At Great Ormond Street, our first Fontan operation was done in 1975, and we have never used caval valves. Until 1982, however, we regularly incorporated outlet valves (almost exclusively homografts) in atriopulmonary connections. We have studied the movement of these valves and the flow patterns in the conduits of 16 such patients.[1] In assessing the usefulness of a valve, valve closure is the important issue: If the valve does not close, a tube would be more appropriate. Figure 24.3a shows an M-mode echocardiogram of a normal aortic valve. During left ventricular systole, the aortic valve is open, its leaflets flattened against the aortic wall. In left ventricular diastole the valve functions by closing for a large proportion of the cardiac cycle. Figure 24.3b shows the form of M-

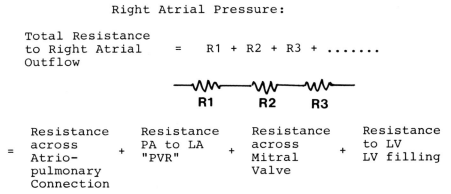

FIGURE 24.2 Determinants of right atrial pressure.

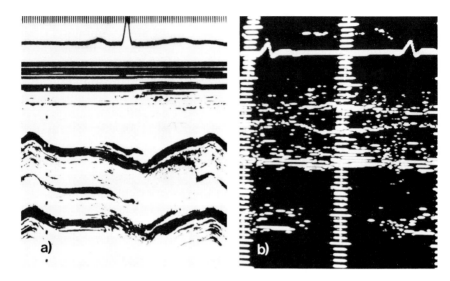

FIGURE 24.3 (a) Normal aortic valve, M-mode echo. (b) Valve in atriopulmonary conduit.

mode studies of the conduit valves. In 14 of the 16 patients our series, the conduit valves floated more or less open throughout the cardiac cycle with Doppler documentation of continuous forward flow, irrespective of atrial systole. In other words the valves did not work. In the other two children, the valves closed only very briefly — for less than one-tenth of the cardiac cycle.

Even if caval valves had been incorporated it seems unlikely that these would have closed. The right atrium is an inadequate pump. Its stroke volume is less than the stroke volume of the pump on the other side of the heart (the left ventricle) so that blood must reach the pulmonary artery with timing other than atrial systole. When the atrium is relaxed, blood flows forward from cavae to pulmonary artery without the benefit of atrial kick and leaving no time for valve closure.

We know the atrium is dispensable; cavopulmonary connections have been performed in patients with anomalous systemic venous return diverting all the caval blood directly into the pulmonary artery (Fig. 24.4). Here, unequivocally, the left ventricle perfuses the systemic and pulmonary vascular resistances in series.

If the atriopulmonary conduit valve is not useful, can it be deleterious? Obstruction can occur at valve or conduit level and increase the resistance to right atrial outflow. Posieuille's law (Fig. 24.5) governs flow in tubes and points a proportionality between the gradient between two points and flow, viscosity, and length of tube, but it relates the gradient inversely to the fourth

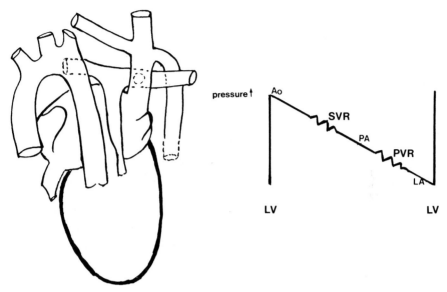

FIGURE 24.4 Left ventricular-dependent systemic and pulmonary circulations.

power of the diameter of the tube. Thus, as the tube becomes narrower, the gradient increases steeply. This law is the basis of most valve area formulas and can be used to derive a theoretical relationship between the diameter of an atriopulmonary connection and the gradient across it (Fig. 24.6).

Illustrated are the theoretical gradients with increasing flow for two atriopulmonary connections: one, the size of the tricuspid valve; one, the size of the pulmonary valve appropriate for a 0.85 m² child. Though unimportant at rest, gradients increase sharply with exercise, and we can understand that a small atriopulmonary connection would impair the success of a Fontan procedure especially if other elements of resistance to right atrial outflow were high or if the tube became more stenotic by formation of an intimal peel.

$$\text{grad} = \frac{128\,m\,Q\,l}{\pi\,d^{4}}$$

FIGURE 24.5 Posieuilles Law.

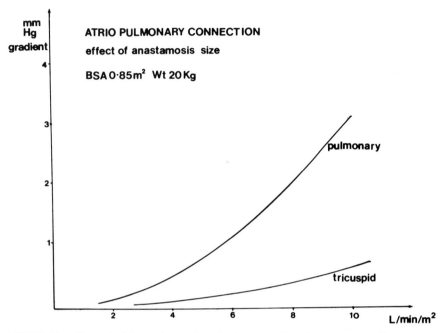

FIGURE 24.6 Theoretical dependence of gradient across atriopulmonary connection on anastomosis size.

Apart from the tube, a conduit valve itself may become obstructive, and in our series of 66 Fontan procedures (53 survivors), three reoperations have been required for valve-related problems. It is now our view that valves in the atriopulmonary connection are dispensable and can be deleterious. In the last 11 Fontan procedures, we have performed direct atriopulmonary connections, anastomosing the roof of the right atrium to the pulmonary artery with or without deviation of the atrial septum into the left atrium to further enlarge the dimension of the anastomosis. In the two such patients we have restudied, this maneuver has been associated with a gradient-free connection.

The atrioventricular connection is conceptually slightly different: in this circuit (tricuspid valve interposition for tricuspid atresia with normally related great arteries) there is a small true right ventricle. The stroke volume of this small ventricle is never as great as the stroke volume of the left ventricle, so that soon after operation atrial systole must push blood through the conduit, open the pulmonary valve, and produce forward flow into the pulmonary artery. Pressure peaks corresponding to ventricular systole and to atrial systole are present in the pulmonary artery pressure trace after this

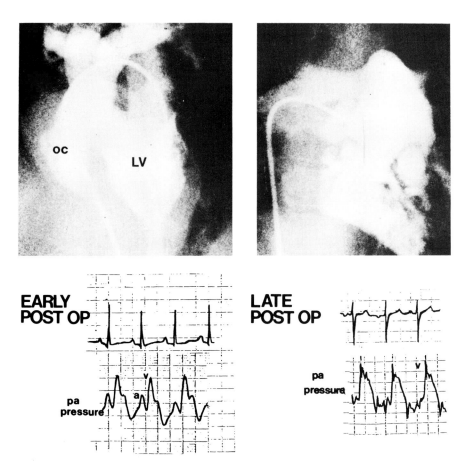

FIGURE 24.7 Atrioventricular connection. The small right ventricle may grow, and clinical deterioration occurs if the valve deteriorates.

procedure (Fig. 24.7). Some of these ventricles can grow; illustrated is a right ventricular angiogram 1 year after operation with the catheter passed through a valved conduit. The pressure trace in the pulmonary artery shows only a peak corresponding to ventricular systole, and the child had a low right atrial pressure, suggesting that his right and left ventricular stroke were equal. Unfortunately, 2 years later this child's atrioventricular conduit valve deteriorated and he developed signs of tricuspid regurgitation and atrial arrhythmias related to his tense atrium. He and one other similar patient have required replacement of their conduit valves. Thus, for an atrioventricular conduit, the connection must never be stenotic, as the right atrial kick must be able to reach the pulmonary artery; if the right ventricle is large the connection must also not be incompetent. A tube will probably not suffice in the long run.

In summary, we have found the valveless atriopulmonary connection is satisfactory, but if in tricuspid atresia with normally related great arteries, a rudimentary right ventricle seems large and is incorporated in the repair, a valve should be included in an atrioventricular connection.

REFERENCES

1. Bull C, de Leval MR, Stark J, Taylor JFN, Macartney FJ. Use of a subpulmonary ventricular chamber in the Fontan circulation. J Thorac Cardiovasc Surg 1983;85:21 – 31.

Section V

PROSTHETIC VALVES IN CHILDREN

CHAPTER 25

Mechanical Prosthetic Heart Valves

Timothy J. Gardner, MD, and
A. Michael Borkon, MD

In the 30 years since cardiac valve substitutes were first implanted, refinements in prosthesic design and manufacture, as well as improvements in implantation techniques, have allowed the safe use of these devices even in very young children. Valve replacement has been carried out successfully in children of all ages with marked deformities of their native cardiac valves and great vessels. Mechanical valve prostheses currently available can be expected to remain functional indefinitely after implantation, and the risk of mechanical valve failure of FDA-approved prostheses is believed to be low. Furthermore, intrinsic hemodynamic function is usually near normal in most patients receiving artificial heart valves, and it is anticipated that this feature will provide long-term protection of cardiac function. The major limitation of mechanical heart valve implantation in children relates to the risk of thrombus formation, which may result in lethal or disabling thromboembolic complications. Although such complications have been reported in virtually all series of patients who receive mechanical heart valve prostheses, the use of warfarin-type anticoagulation can significantly reduce this risk. Other concerns related to the use of mechanical prostheses in children include the absence of specific information regarding long-term durability, as well as the possibility that somatic growth will result in an inadequate sized prosthesis for the child in later life.

   The era of cardiac valve replacement began even before the availability of cardiopulmonary bypass techniques made open heart surgery feasible. In

1954, Hufnagel[1] implanted a ball valve mechanism in the descending thoracic aorta of a patient with aortic valve incompetence, resulting in striking clinical improvement for the patient. As the development of open heart surgery progressed, direct heart valve replacement was attempted using a wide array of devices, including substitute leaflets made of a variety of materials and ball-cage valve prostheses that bore some design resemblance to the original Hufnagel valve.[2] The first successful mechanical cardiac valve substitutes were of the ball-cage design.[3,4]

STARR-EDWARDS PROSTHESIS

Among the most successful prosthetic devices used during this early era of open heart surgery were those designed by Starr and Edwards.[4] First used in 1960 (Fig. 25.1), the Starr-Edwards valve was a ball-valve mechanism utilizing a Silastic poppet and a bare open-wire cage. Minor design variations were incorporated, depending upon whether the valve will be used for aortic or mitral valve replacement. Over the past 25 years, the Starr-Edwards prosthesis has undergone a number of design modifications in an attempt to reduce the likelihood of valve-related thromboemboli, as well as to improve its hemodynamic characteristics.[5] Interestingly, virtually all of these design changes have been abandoned in favor of the early original 1260/6120

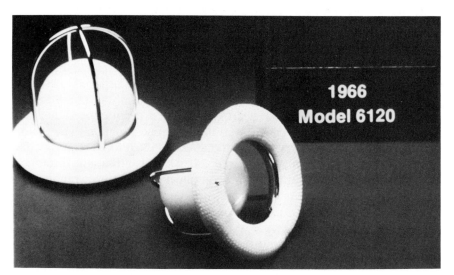

FIGURE 25.1 The Starr-Edwards model 6120 valve prosthesis for mitral valve replacement. There are four bare stellite wire struts enclosing a radiopaque silicone ball poppet. Cloth covering extends into inflow orifice.

models.[6] This prosthesis has proven to be functionally reliable and extremely durable.[7,8] Although valve failure rates and valve-related mortality are low, and sustained improvement in the patient's clinical status occurs after valve replacement, the risk of thromboembolic complications with these prostheses is significant, ranging from just under 2% per patient-year with aortic valve replacement to 5% per patient-year following mitral valve replacement.[9,10] These results are found even in patients who are anticoagulated with warfarin. Based on actuarial estimates from such follow-up data, it is obvious that the risk of thromboembolic complications with this prosthesis is substantial and that nearly 50% of adult patients having the Starr-Edwards prosthesis implanted in the mitral position would be expected to suffer a thromboembolic episode within the first 10 years after valve placement.[10]

Late follow-up information from children after valve replacement with the Starr-Edwards prosthesis was provided in a recent report by Schaff et al[11] from the Mayo Clinic. Fifty children operated on between 1963 to 1978 were reviewed with respect to long-term performance of the Starr-Edwards valve. The mean age of patients at the time of valve replacement was just over 10 years; equal numbers of children had aortic and mitral valve replacements. The mean follow-up interval was 7.9 ± 4.9 years. Actuarial survival was 90% for aortic valve recipients and 76% for children having replacement of an atrioventricular valve at 10 years. In this group of 50 patients, there were 11 deaths, four of which were valve-related. Seven of the patients had major thromboembolic events while an additional five patients had transient neurological symptoms suggesting a thromboembolism. It is unclear why the incidence of late thromboembolism was nearly twice as high (5.3% per patient-year) among children having aortic valve replacement compared with those receiving the Starr-Edwards prostheses in the systemic atrioventricular position (2% per patient-year). Most of the children with major thromboembolic events had mitral prostheses, however, and several of these children were not receiving therapeutic anticoagulation at the time of the thromboembolic event.

Although this relatively long-term series confirms that the Starr-Edwards prosthesis can be used safely in children, some theoretical disadvantages remain. Because of its high profile and caged housing, its use in the small aortic root or in a patient with a small left ventricular cavity may be difficult and possibly dangerous. In addition, the ball-cage design can be moderately obstructive due to lack of central flow and increased turbulent blood flow across the prosthesis may lead to hemolysis or neointimal proliferation around the valve. The Starr-Edwards prosthesis, however, remains attractive as a potential valve substitute because of the simplicity of its mechanical design and function coupled with nearly 20 years of clinical experience and reliability.

BJÖRK-SHILEY PROSTHESIS

The description of a tilting disc valve prosthesis by Wada in 1968 and Björk in 1969 introduced a second generation of mechanical prostheses with important new and improved design features.[12,13] The major advantages of the tilting disc prostheses are central flow and a low-profile. The Wada-Cutter valve, although hemodynamically successful, was removed from clinical use because of complications related to the occluder disc.[14] Björk's original tilting disc valve employed a Delrin disc occluder that demonstrated size variance.[15] This problem was apparently eliminated with the development and use of pyrolytic carbon for construction of the occluder disc, and this material has been incorporated in the production of the Björk-Shiley valve since 1971.

The basic design features of the Björk-Shiley standard spherical disc prosthesis involves the opening and closing movement of a pyrolytic carbon disc between two wire struts fixed to the valve housing. The disc opens to about 60 degrees, allowing blood to pass through both a major and minor valve orifice (Fig. 25.2). As a result, hemodynamic function even with small valve sizes has been good.[16] A more recent refinement incorporated into the Björk-Shiley valve has been the use of a curved or convex/concave occluder disc held within the valve housing in the same manner, but resulting in increased opening of the valve with improved central flow. Poppet escape, which was an extremely rare occurrence with the standard spherical Björk-Shiley tilting disc valve, has occurred much more often with the convex/concave model due to fracture of the struts holding the disc in place.[17]

Perhaps the major shortcoming of the valve, however, has been the fact that there is a marked discrepancy in the area between the major and minor valve orifices. With additional impingement on the minor orifice by the wire strut, turbulent flow across the Björk-Shiley valve results and there is a significant risk of thrombus formation occurring in the vicinity of the minor orifice. Sudden valve occlusion from thrombus formation has been seen and, the risk of thromboembolism with this prosthesis remains significant even when the patient is well-managed on anticoagulation therapy.[18]

The Björk-Shiley valve has been used for valve replacement in children with reasonable success. Late follow-up reports suggest that thromboembolic and thrombotic complications may be somewhat lower in children than in adults.[19] Fewer thromboembolic complications have been observed with these valves than the Starr-Edwards model.[20] Nevertheless, incidences of thrombosis of the Björk-Shiley valve vary between 1.2% and 2.7% per patient-year with aortic prostheses and 1.8% and 7% per patient year with mitral valve replacement.[21,22] Enthusiasm for the use of this prosthesis in children has not been high. Furthermore, although the convex/concave disc

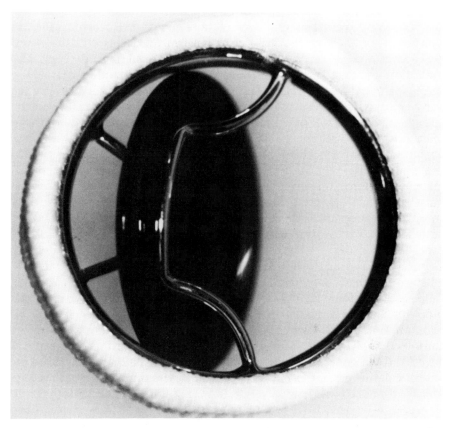

FIGURE 25.2 The Björk-Shiley spherical tilting disc prosthesis. The pyrolytic carbon occluder disc rotates and is secured by the two wire struts. Flow through the valve orifice is eccentric.

modification may reduce this thrombotic risk, the development of strut fractures and catastrophic poppet escape have further diminished interest in using this model of the Björk-Shiley valve in children.

ST. JUDE MEDICAL PROSTHESIS

A third-generation valve prosthesis, the design of which was originally introduced by Gott in the mid-1960s,[23] is the centrally hinged, bi-leaflet valve prosthesis.[24] The St. Jude Medical valve is the only currently FDA-approved prosthesis of this type, and this valve substitute has been enthusiastically adopted for use in children because of several favorable design characteristics. The valve is composed of two centrally hinged disc occluders that tilt upward at an angle of about 30 degrees when the valve is in the closed position. With complete opening, these occluders open to nearly 90 degrees and allow for excellent central flow through three channels. (Fig. 25.3) Because the two occluders are virtually perpendicular to the plane of the valve annulus when the prosthesis is in the open position, there is little of the turbulent flow seen with the Björk-Shiley or Starr-Edwards valves. Both the valve ring and the occluding leaflets are made of pyrolytic carbon. Although the durability of this prosthesis is felt to be excellent based on in vitro materials testing,[24] the St. Jude Medical prosthesis has the theoretical disadvantage of nonrotating occluder discs that interface at fixed points with the valve ring, such that the areas of friction and stress are constant. Furthermore, the regurgitant fraction, or the amount of blood that will cross the prosthesis in a retrograde fashion during valve closure, is relatively high, exceeding 5%.[25]

Reports examining the long-term follow-up of patients with the St. Jude Medical prosthesis suggest a lower risk of thromboembolic complications than is seen with the Björk-Shiley prosthesis.[26,27] Furthermore, there is one report of children with the St. Jude Medical prosthesis who have been managed without warfarin anticoagulation and in whom there has been a low thromboembolic incidence.[28] The follow-up interval for this group of just over 30 children is relatively short, but the results to date support the observation that this prosthesis may be significantly less thrombogenic than previously available prosthetic valve substitutes. In addition, the hemodynamic

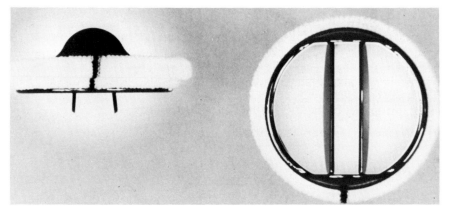

FIGURE 25.3 The St. Jude Medical prosthesis, with two stationary occluding discs of pyrolytic carbon which open fully at a 90-degree angle. This prosthesis has a very low profile and allows for central flow with little turbulence.

features of the St. Jude Medical prosthesis have been demonstrated to be quite satisfactory.[29,30]

The St. Jude Medical prosthesis has been implanted in 28 children at the Johns Hopkins Hospital since 1979, with the mean age of these children being 10 years.[31] Six of the children underwent valve replacement during the first two years of life. Fourteen of these patients had mitral valve replacement, 13 underwent aortic valve replacement, and one child underwent replacement of the pulmonary valve. There were two early deaths in this series, both occurring in infants, but neither death was believed to be related to the prosthetic valve. In both infants, good prosthetic valve function was observed up until the time of the deaths. Four late deaths have occurred and, of these, one was associated with prosthetic valve thrombosis, while two others were felt to be the result of sudden fatal cardiac dysrhythmias. The fourth death, which occurred in an 8-month-old child 2 months after mitral valve replacement for congenital mitral stenosis, was not explained and could be due to prosthetic valve dysfunction. Most of these children have been receiving warfarin for anticoagulation. Eight of the children, however, including six infants, have been therapeutically managed with aspirin alone because of difficulties encountered when attempting to use warfarin anticoagulation in these young patients. The single patient who developed valve thrombosis was in this group of children receiving only aspirin.

Although the St. Jude Medical prosthesis is thought by many to be an ideal valve substitute for use in children, it has some potentially negative features. Reports of leaflet escape which, while explained by the manufacturer to be the result of improper handling during implantation, nonetheless demonstrates the potential weakness of the hinge mechanism.[32] Leaflet entrapment has been reported with this prosthesis, but is a problem common to any tilting-disc valve substitute.[33] The valve is not radiopaque, which precludes identification of the prosthesis with a chest x-ray and eliminates the possibility of fluoroscopic examination of valve function. Also, the valve is constructed in such a way that it cannot be rotated after it is seated in place. If there is a problem with leaflet entrapment that might be obviated by simple rotation of the prosthesis, as is possible with other disc prostheses, such rotation is not possible with the St. Jude Medical valve, which instead must be removed and reimplanted in a more suitable orientation.

TILTING DISC PROSTHESES

Both the Medtronic-Hall,[34] a valve originally designed and known as the Hall-Kaster prosthesis, and the Omniscience valve[35,36] are available for implantation after being approved for clinical use by the Food and Drug

Administration. Both prostheses are tilting-disc valve substitutes; the Medtronic-Hall, as shown in Figure 25.4, utilizes a guide strut, and the Omniscience (Fig. 25.5) is a simpler design with short struts projecting from the valve ring itself. There is little clinical information available at this time to allow for a reliable comparative evaluation of these prostheses with other valve substitutes currently in use. Both of these prostheses do incorporate design and manufacturing features that have theoretical value, but the usefulness of these prostheses in children remains to be established.

SUMMARY

A variety of prosthetic valves are available for use in children, with the St. Jude Medical prosthesis favored by many surgeons today because of its

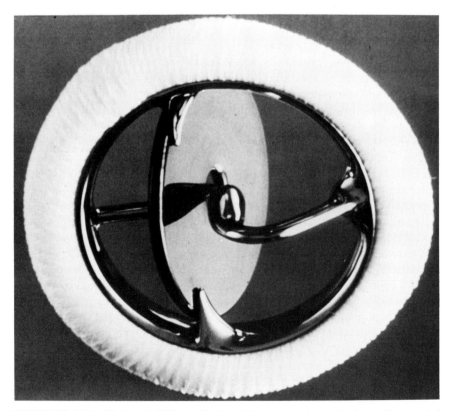

FIGURE 25.4 The Medtronic Hall prosthesis which incorporates a freely rotating pyrolytic carbon disc occluder mounted on a titanium wire strut. The full opening angle of the occluder is about 75 degrees.

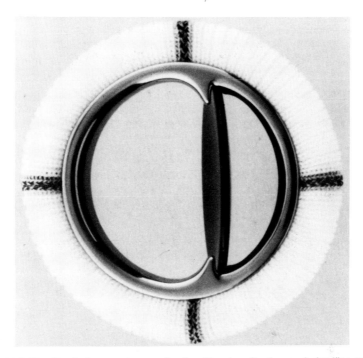

FIGURE 25.5 The Omniscience valve prosthesis with a free floating occluder disc and very small struts holding the disc in place. The opening angle of this low profile prosthesis is about 80 degrees.

excellent hemodynamic features, low profile, and apparent thromboresistance. Nonetheless, all of the currently available prostheses have been associated with thromboembolic complications despite seemingly adequate warfarin anticoagulation therapy, all have been associated with valve thrombosis, and virtually all have had a low incidence of mechanical failure. In addition, the consequences of increasing body size may result in severe patient–prosthesis mismatch with somatic growth.[37] Because of these considerations, the repair of native valves should be attempted whenever possible. If valve replacement with a mechanical prosthesis must be undertaken in a child, long-term management should include warfarin anticoagulation unless otherwise contraindicated.

REFERENCES

1. Hufnagel, CA. Aortic plastic valvular prosthesis. The Bulletin of Georgetown University Medical Center. 1951;4:128–130.

2. Merendino, KA (ed). Prosthetic Valves for Cardiac Surgery. Thomas, Springfield, 1961.
3. Starr A, Edwards ML. Clinical experience with a ball-valve prosthesis. Ann Surg 1961;154:726–740.
4. Harken DE, Soroff HS, Taylor WJ, et al. Partial and complete prostheses in aortic insufficiency. J Thorac Cardiovasc Surg 1960;40:744–762.
5. Bonchek LI, Starr A. Ball valve prostheses: current appraisal of late results. Am J Cardiol 1975;35:843–854.
6. Macmanus Q, Grunkemeier GL, Lambert LE, Starr A. Non-cloth-covered caged-ball prostheses the second decade. J Thorac Cardiovasc Surg 1978;76:788–794.
7. Tepley JF, Grunkemeier GL, Sutherland HD, et al. The ultimate prognosis after valve replacement: an assessment at twenty years. Ann Thorac Surg 1981;32:111–119.
8. Macmanus Q, Grunkemeier G, Thomas D, et al. The Starr-Edwards model 6000 valve; a fifteen-year follow-up of the first successful mitral prosthesis. Circulation 1977; 56:623–625.
9. Miller DC, Oyer PE, Mitchell RS, et al. Performance characteristics of the Starr-Edwards model 1260 aortic valve prosthesis beyond ten years. J Thorac Cardiovasc Surg 1984;88:193–207.
10. Miller DC, Oyer PE, Stinson EB, et al. Ten to fifteen year reassessment of the performance characteristics of the Starr-Edwards model 6120 mitral valve prosthesis. J Thorac Cardiovasc Surg 1983;85:1–20.
11. Schaff HV, Danielson GK, DiDonato RM, et al. Late results after Starr-Edwards valve replacement in children. J Thorac Cardiovasc Surg 1984;88:583–589.
12. Wada J, Komatsu S, Ikeda K, et al. A new hingeless valve. In, Brewer LA III (ed): Prosthetic Heart Valves. Springfield, Thomas, 1969;304–314.
13. Björk VO: A new tilting disc valve prosthesis. Scand J Thorac Cardiovasc Surg 1969;3:1–7.
14. Roe BB, Fishman NH, Hutchinson JC, Goodenough SH. Occluder disruption of Wada-Cutter valve prosthesis. Ann Thorac Surg 1975;20:256–264.
15. Björk VO. Delrin: an implant material for valve occluders. Scand J Thorac Cardiovasc Surg 1972;6:103–110.
16. Schaff HV, Borkon AM, Hughes C, et al. Clinical and hemodynamic evaluation of the 19 mm Björk-Shiley aortic valve prosthesis. Ann Thorac Surg 1981;32:50–57.
17. Complications of convexo-concave heart valves. FDA Drug Bulletin 1984;14:22.
18. Wright JO, Hiratzka LF, Brandt B, Doty DB. Thrombosis of the Björk-Shiley prosthesis: illustrative cases and review of the literature. J Thorac Cardiovasc Surg 1982;84:138–44.
19. Iyer KS, Reddy KS, Rao IM, et al. Valve replacement in children under twenty years of age. Experience with the Björk-Shiley prosthesis. J Thorac Cardiovasc Surg 1984;88:217–24.
20. Murphy DA, Levine FH, Bulkley MJ, et al. Mechanical valves: A comparative analysis of the Starr-Edwards and Björk-Shiley prosthesis. J Thorac Cardiovasc Surg 1983;86:746–52.
21. Karp RB, Cyrus RJ, Blackstone EH, et al. The Björk-Shiley valve. Intermediate-term follow-up. J Thorac Cardiovasc Surg 1981;81:602–614.
22. Björk VO, Henze A. Ten years' experience with the Björk-Shiley tilting disc valve. J Thorac Cardiovasc Surg 1979;78:331–342.
23. Gott VL, Daggett RL, Whiffen JD, et al. A hinged-leaflet valve for total replacement of the human aortic valve. J Thorac Cardiovasc Surg 1964;48:713–723.
24. Emery RW, Nicoloff DM. St. Jude Medical cardiac valve prosthesis: in vitro studies. J Thorac Cardiovasc Surg 1979;78:269–276.
25. Yoganathan AP, Chaux A, Gray RJ, et al. Bileaflet, tilting disc and porcine aortic valve substitutes: in vitro hydrodynamic characteristics. J Am Coll Cardio 1984;3:313–320.
26. Horstkotte D, Korfer R, Seipel L, et al. Late complications in patients with Björk-Shiley and St. Jude Medical heart valve replacement. Circulation 1983;68(suppl 3):175–84.

27. Baudet EM, Oca CC, Roques XF, et al. A 5½ year experience with St. Jude Medical cardiac valve prosthesis. J Thorac Cardiovasc Surg 1985;90:137–144.
28. Pass HI, Sade RM, Crawford FA, Hohn AR. Cardiac valve prostheses in children without anticoagulation. J Thorac Cardiovasc Surg 1984;87:832–835.
29. Wortham DC, Tri TB, Bowen TE. Hemodynamic evaluation of the St. Jude Medical valve prosthesis in the small aortic anulus. J Thorac Cardiovasc Surg 1981;81:615–620.
30. Nicoloff DM, Emery RW, Arom KV, et al. Clinical and hemodynamic results with the St. Jude Medical cardiac valve prosthesis. J Thorac Cardiovasc Surg 1981;82:674–683.
31. Borkon AM, Reitz BA, Donahoo JS, Gardner TJ. St. Jude Medical valve replacement in infants and children. In, Matloff JM (ed): Cardiac Valve Replacement. Martinus Nighoff, Boston, 1985, pp 129–135.
32. Hjelms E. Escape of a leaflet from a St. Jude Medical prosthesis in the mitral position. In, Matloff JM (ed): Cardiac Valve Replacement. Martinus Nighoff, Boston, 1985, pp 285–289.
33. Sharma A, Johnson DC, Cartmill TB. Entrapment of both leaflets of St. Jude Medical aortic valve prosthesis in a child. J Thorac Cardiovasc Surg 1983;86:453–4.
34. Nitter-Hauge S, Semb B, Abdelnoor M, Hall V. A 5 year experience with the Medtronic-Hall disc valve prosthesis. Circulation 1983;68(suppl II):II 169–74.
35. DeWall R, Pelletier C, Panebianco A, et al. Five-year clinical experience with the Omniscience cardiac valve. Ann Thorac Surg 1984;38:275–80.
36. Rabago G, Martinell J, Fraile J, et al. Results and complications with the Omniscience prosthesis. J Thorac Cardiovasc Surg 1984;87:136–40.
37. Friedman S, Edmunds LH, Cuaso CC. Long-term mitral valve replacement in young children. Influence of somatic growth on prosthetic valve adequacy. Circulation 1978; 57:981–986.

CHAPTER **26**

Heterograft Valves in Children

Louis M. Marmon, MD,
James W. Buchanan, DVM, M Med Sci, and
Jeffrey M. Dunn, MD

In the search for the ideal prosthetic valve for use in the pediatric population, a number of different prosthetic devices have been utilized. Although older children with large hearts can often have adult-sized prosthesis inserted, the problem of diminutive annulus and small outflow tracts in infants and young children limit the types of prosthesis that can be used. The energetic lifestyle of children would predispose to the hemorrhagic complications associated with long-term anticoagulation therapy. In addition, the earlier the valve replacement is performed, the more likely it is that the prosthesis will need to be replaced at a later date as the heart grows or as the valve performance declines. The rewarding use of bioprosthetic tissue valves, such as the preserved porcine aortic or the bovine pericardial grafts, in adults has lead to their implantation in children. These low-profile valves can be fabricated into the small sizes required for the infant heart without sacrificing performance. Yet these bioprosthetic valves are not without serious complications when implanted into children; tissue valves are subject to severe dystrophic calcification via unknown mechanisms that result in valvular failure within years after implantation.

Since the first implantation of an artificial cardiac valve in an adult, there have been a myriad of mechanical prosthesis designed and evaluated. As experience and postoperative follow-up data increased, so did the cardiac surgeons' awareness that the mechanical valve prosthesis was not a panacea. Complications related to hemodynamics and thrombogenicity resulted in the use of allogenic aortic valves in 1962.[1] However, difficulties related to durability and availability of human tissue valves lead to the fabrication of autograft and homograft tissue valves from material such as fascia lata,

334

human dura, and untreated pericardium. These early devices were found to degenerate rapidly and fail soon after implantation. Formaldehyde pretreatment of tissue preparations was found to cause collagen cross-linking and thereby increase valve durability; however, these valves continued to deteriorate rapidly after implantation. Carpentier et al[2] found that gluteraldehyde pretreatment produced greater collagen cross-linking and significantly improved tissue valve durability without sacrificing flexibility. Gluteraldehyde preservation has become the current preferred method for preparation of both porcine aortic and bovine pericardial valves.

The ideal prosthetic device would have normal hemodynamics, be nonthrombogenic and nonembolic, have a low profile, require no anticoagulation therapy, and have the durability to function normally for the patient's entire life. With adults, who could be expected to have a rather sendentary lifestyle and a fixed cardiac output, compromises in some of these ideal valve characteristics could be expected to have little effect on the outcome and long-term performance of the valve replacement. In contrast, the pediatric patient should live an active lifestyle with wide variations in cardiac output. The small annulus and heart size frequently encountered in pediatric patients require small prosthesis, and the earlier a valve implantation is performed the more likely the patient will eventually outgrow the prosthetic device and require a replacement. Although the adult valve may need to function for 10–20 years, the ideal pediatric cardiac valve prosthesis should be durable enough to last for two to three times as long.

Thus the ideal pediatric valve prosthesis would exhibit the previously mentioned characteristics, but to a much greater degree. The flow characteristics would demonstrate no obstruction at expected outputs even in small annular sizes. Because the ventricular chamber and the outflow tract is often small, a low profile is manditory. The thrombogenicity of the ideal pediatric valve must be zero because the long life expectancy of a child would increase the accumulative risk of thrombosis or embolization of even a minimally thrombogenic prosthesis. The risk of significant hemorrhage associated with chronic anticoagulation therapy is greatly increased in the active child who is prone to injuries. An additional difficulty associated with chronic anticoagulation therapy is the management of a female patient contemplating pregnancy because of the teratogenicity of Coumadin on the fetus, the risk of third-trimester bleeding, and the inconvenience of chronic heparin therapy.

CLINICAL EVALUATION

After the successful use of tissue valves in adults, these devices were implanted in children. Many of these valve-related problems appeared to have been eliminated. Tissue valves are moderately low profile, exhibit excellent central hemodynamics, can be manufactured in small sizes, and, in general, do not require anticoagulation therapy. Braunwald et al[4] demonstrated that tissue valves with sewing rings in the range of 12–20 mm could be configured, which would allow for adequate blood flow without development of a significant gradient. The currently available tissue valves exhibit central flow with minimal turbulance and a gradient range midway between the mechanical ball valve and the newer tilting-disc designs. Clinical evaluation of adults after implantation of bovine pericardial valves or porcine aortic valves have demonstrated marked improvement in New York Heart Association (NYHA) classification and improved hemodynamics.[3,5] After implantation of pericardial valves the transvalvular gradients ranged from 8 mm Hg at rest to 17.5 mm Hg during exercise.[6] Except in cases of small aortic root, hemodynamic and clinical performance of the porcine valve is comparable to the pericardial valves and to mechanical prosthesis, despite the poor orifice-to-annulus ratio of the porcine valve.[7,8]

Adult patient survival data after tissue valve implantation has demonstrated the clinical performance of these bioprosthetic valves. Actuarial survival 8 years after porcine valve implantation in both the aortic and mitral position is 80%. The projected freedom from thromboembolism at 8 years is 97% in the aortic and 82% in the mitral position. The actuarial probability of the porcine valve being free from dysfunction at 8 years in both positions is 90%, with an overall incidence of primary valve dysfunction of only 4%.[9] Likewise, follow-up evaluation of adult patients with bovine pericardial valves implanted in the aortic position demonstrate an actuarial survival at 8 years of 77.1%, with actuarial freedom of dysfunction at 91.4%, and freedom from emboli at 98.5%.[3] An 11-year follow-up of bovine xenograft valves implanted in the mitral position in adults demonstrated an overall survival of 74.8% and an actuarial freedom from valve failure of 90.4% at 11 years. The actuarial freedom from thromboembolism is 96.4%, with an incidence of emboli of 0.6% per patient year.[10] When directly compared with a tilting-disc prosthetic the porcine bioprosthetic valve is found to have a lower incidence of thromboembolism, valve thrombosis, and anticoagulant-related hemmorrhagic complication than the tilting-disc when implanted in the aortic position. The rate of valve failure is higher in the bioprosthesis, (0.79% per patient year) as compared with 0% for the tilting-disc prosthesis.[11]

As the smaller heterograft valves designed for implantation in children have shown the same central flow characteristics as the larger valves implanted in adults, the expectation was that when implanted into the pediatric population these bioprosthetic valves would demonstrate the same freedom from complications. Unfortunately, the durability of the tissue valves after implantation into children has been poor with a linearized incidence of primary tissue failure in children of 9.8% per patient year as compared to 0.2% in adults.[12] We initially reported spontaneous failure of a porcine valve implanted in an 11-year-old boy. Extensive calcification resulted in valve failure only 3 years after surgery.[13] Our review of a multiinstitutional experience with porcine valves in pediatric patients found that only 40% of mitral and aortic valves remained functional 5 years after implantation.[14] (Figs. 26.1 and 26.2) Morphologic examination of the explanted valves revealed extensive fibrosis and calcification, confirming that the valve failure was due to dysfunction and not the result of the child outgrowing the prosthesis. None of the porcine valves implanted in the tricuspid or pulmonary position failed. A comparison of patients younger than age 15 years at the time of surgery with similar patients 15 years and older clearly demonstrated that the porcine valves in the younger patients degenerated more rapidly (Fig. 26.3). Valved conduits in the pulmonary position had a durability of 73% at 5 years, while the apical–aortic conduits had a significantly decreased durability. Similar results have been reported from other institutions. Geha et al[15] have reported that of 25 children who underwent porcine valve implantations, 20% developed calcific dysfunction 10–54 months after surgery. In another series, three of nine patients, ages 2 to 15 years, who had porcine mitral valve replacements developed calcific degeneration of their valves at

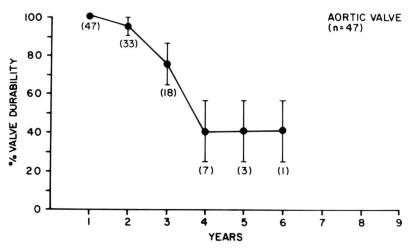

FIGURE 26.1 Aortic valve durability: Actuarial durability of porcine prosthetic aortic valves in children. (From Dunn JM: Porcine valve durability in children, Ann Thorac Surg 1981;32:357–368, with permission.)

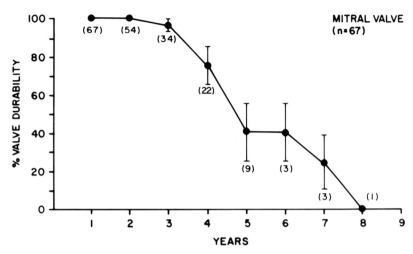

FIGURE 26.2 Mitral valve durability: Actuarial durability of porcine prosthetic mitral valve durability in children. (From Dunn, JM: Porcine valve durability in children, Ann Thorac Surg 1981;32:357–368, with permission.)

3.5, 3.6, and 4.8 years after implantation.[16] An actuarial analysis of 34 pediatric patients who underwent either a mitral or aortic valve replacement with a porcine bioprosthesis revealed that only 37% of the valves remained intact after 50 months.[17]

Thrombogenicity of the bioprosthetic valves has been minimal in the pediatric population. These valves are designed with a minimum of thrombogenic components and anticoagulation therapy can usually be eliminated or limited to the first 3 months after implantation to allow for endothelialization of the supports and sewing ring. Longer anticoagulation therapy is indicated in patients with atrial fibrilation, a massive left atrium, or a history of embolic incidents. Both the bovine pericardial valves and the porcine valves have been demonstrated to have low rates of thromboembolism. An 8-year retrospective comparative study found that the bovine pericardial valve demonstrates a lower actuarial incidence of thromboembolic complications (97% vs 81%) than do the porcine valves after mitral valve replacement in adults managed without long-term anticoagulation therapy.[18] The risk of hemorrhage due to anticoagulation therapy in children has been reported to be as high as 5.6% per patient-year, but more recent figures have been considerably lower when only selected patients underwent anticoagulation therapy.[19,20] The incidence of thromboembolism in children receiving porcine valve implants is as low as 1.3% per patient year.[21]

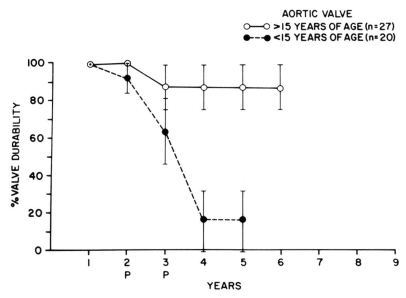

FIGURE 26.3 Aortic valve durability and age. Actuarial durability of porcine bioprosthesis. Population is divided into two groups: children under 15 years *(closed circles)* and children between 15 and 21 years *(open circles)*. Note the significantly lower durability of valves implanted in the younger age group.

MECHANISMS OF CALCIFIC DEGENERATION

The etiology of the rapid calcification of tissue valves after implantation in children has yet to be elucidated. Structural alterations in tissue valves can be seen as early as 1 month after implantation. Seventy percent of the porcine xenografts removed 30 days after implantation had significant fibrin deposits upon the valve leaflets. In valves implanted for as long as 75 months, there were other histologic alterations such as inflammatory cell infiltration and focal collagen disruption.[16] A failed porcine mitral valve removed from a 14-year-old child 12 months after implantation showed severe calcification of extending through all three layers of each cusp that was associated with the deposition of an amorphous material at areas of collagen fibril disruption.[23] Ultrastructural changes in a porcine valve explanted after 3 years include degeneration and disruption of the collagen fibrils and edematous changes in the extracellular matrix.[13] Calcium deposition has been found within the graft tissue and along the commissures in 11 of 18 porcine valves removed from children (Fig. 26.4a and 26.4b). This malignant calcific process is not

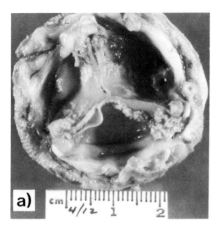
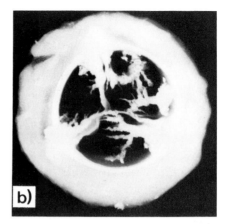

FIGURE 26.4 Explanted degenerated porcine valve: Porcine valve explanted 28 months after implantation. **(a)** Outflow surface demonstrates leaflet thickening and mineralization, especially near commissural support areas. **(b)** Roentgenogram of the same valve demonstrating calcific mineralization.

limited to porcine valves: Silver et al[25] have reported evidence of calcification within both porcine and bovine pericardial tissue valves.

Normal calcium mineralization occurs within a collagen and proteoglycan matrix in the form of the crystal hydroxyapatite. Calcium and phosphate do not spontaneously crystalize in the extracellular fluid but exist as a metastable solution.[26] Once crystalization is initiated, proliferation occurs rapidly and is normally limited to the teeth and bone.

The initial stimulus for normal calcium crystal formation is unknown, but it appears to be cell mediated. Extracellular submicroscopic particles of cellular origin are found within the calcifying matrix. These so-called matrix vesicles are apparently composed of cell or mitochondrial membranes.[27] The mitochondria activity accumulates calcium from the cytosol and may be the site of crystalization initiation. In addition, ossifying tissues are more permiable to calcium and have a higher intracellular calcium concentration.[28] The calcium within the mitochondria is transferred to cytoplasmic extensions that appear to bud off the cell membrane and be released as the matrix vesicle.[29] The vesicles contain high concentrations of several minerals besides calcium, and they are also rich in enzymes that have been associated with calcification.[30] Vesicles actively calcifying tissues contain twice the amount of calcium as do the vesicles isolated from premineralizing zones.

Dystrophic calcification, which is mineralization that occurs within damaged or abnormal tissues, may be initiated by damaged cell membranes that could sequester calcium by methods similar to normally functioning matrix vesicles. Damaged cell membranes have altered permiabilities and permit increased intracellular calcium concentrations to develop. The higher intracellular calcium stores could predispose to the formation of insoluble crystals. Indeed the formation of intracellular calcium crystals is an early sign of irreversible cellular damage.[31]

There are several other materials that are found within damaged tissues, as well as within the leaflets of bioprosthetic valves that could act as templates for the deposition of calcium. Collagen can promote calcification through stimulation of platelet aggregation, but it does not appear to be a good initiator of calcification.[32] Similarly, elastic fibers have been suggested to be a site of crystal formation, but the association is weak because of the presence of cellular debris near most specimens of calcified elastic fibers.[33] The presence of aldehydes that remain after the fixative process may lead to calcification by damaging blood cells and causing adherence to the valve leaflets, eventually resulting in calcium crystal formation.

The role of cellular debris in the mechanism of calcification of gluteraldehyde-treated materials has been investigated in our laboratory. We have implanted bovine pericardium, mounted on a rigid flange, into the atrium and ventricles of young sheep and have used this model to evaluate the calcification process. Early after implantation, the blood-contacting surface of the pericardium developed an adherent thrombus that accumulated cellular debris and eventually became more organized to form a pseudoneoinitma (PNI). Time-dependent calcification occured within the pericardium associated with elevation of alkaline phosphatase and phosphate content. Ultrastructural studies of implanted pericardium revealed that calcium deposition occurred at four distinct sites: within the pericardium in association with collagen, within the PNI, at the junction of PNI and pericardium, and along the blood-contacting surface.[34] The type of fixative buffer used to preserve the pericardium also appeared to influence the rate of calcium deposition. Phosphate buffered gluteraldehyde treated pericardium calcifies more rapidly than does pericardium treated with acetate buffered fixative[35] (Fig. 26.5).

The presence of γ-carboxyglutamic acid (GLA) proteins in association with normal calcification has lead to the investigation of the role of these compounds in ectopic crystal formation. The GLA protein component of prothrombin acts to bind calcium and phospholipid and the major noncollagen element of the calcifying matrix is a GLA protein, osteocalcin.[36,37] In ectopically calcifying tissues, such as aortic plaque, the calcium and GLA protein content correlate to their respective concentrations in normal bone.[38,39] γ-Carboxyglutamic acid is also found within calcified porcine heterografts. Whether or not GLA acts to initiate calcification or is a result of mineral deposition has not been determined. Fishbein et al[40] has implanted

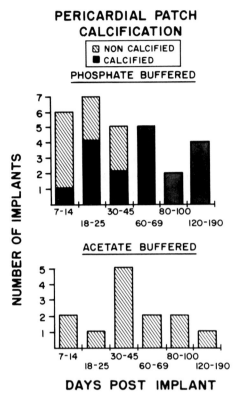

DAYS POST IMPLANT

FIGURE 26.5 Experimental pericardial patch calcification: Intracardiac bovine pericardial patch samples examined from 7 to 190 days after implantation in sheep. Demonstrates inhibition of calcification in pericardium treated with acetate buffer as opposed to standard phosphate buffer.

porcine aortic valve leaflets subcutaneously in rabbits and has found that the GLA and calcium content began to increase 2 months after implantation. The calcium and GLA ratios were similar to those found in bone and the increase in GLA was accompanied by morphologic evidence of calcium deposition along collagen fibrils.[40]

Another factor that may predispose to calcium deposition is the mechanical stress that occurs during flexion of the leaflet. Thubrikar et al[41] found that the bioprosthetic leaflet was subject to more total mechanical stress than a natural valve leaflet and that the maximum stress occurred along the areas of greatest flexion. The sites of greatest stress for both the bovine pericardium and porcine valves were also the sites of greatest calcium deposition after implantation in young animals.[42] As in other models, the calcification occurred at sites of collagen damage.

CONCLUSIONS

Despite the good hemodynamic characteristics and the remarkable freedom from thromboembolic complications associated with bioprosthetic valves, the use of heterograft valves in children is limited by the tendency of these prosthesis to fail early after implantation secondary to calcification. While the exact mechanism of calcification remains unclear, current research suggests that further modifications of these tissue valves — such as eliminating cellular debris with detergents, reducing leaflet stress or the utilization of calcium inhibitors such as diphosphatases or calcium chelating agents — could improve the durability of the heterograft valves. While not the ideal prosthetic device, with modification designed to prevent early failure, the tissue valves may become the valve of choice in the pediatric population. At present, however, we cannot advocate their use in the aortic or mitral positions.

REFERENCES

1. Duran Co, Gunning AJ. Total homologous aortic valve in the subcoronary position. Lancet 1962;2:488–489.
2. Carpentier A, Deloche A, Reland J, et al. Six year follow-up of gluteraldehyde-preserved heterografts. J Thorac Cardiovasc Surg 1974;68:771–782.
3. Ionescu MI, Tandon AP. Long term clinical and hemodynamic evaluation of the Ionescu-Shiley pericardial xenograft heart valve. Art Organs 1980;4:13–19.
4. Braunwald NS, Brais M, Castaneda A. Considerations in the development of artificial heart valve substitutes for use in infants and small children. J Thorac Cardiovasc Surg 1976;72:539–546.
5. Ionescu MI, Tandon AP, Mary DAS, Abid A. Heart valve replacement with the Ionescu-Shiley pericardial xenograft. J Thorac Cardiovasc Surg 1977;73:31–42.
6. Gabbay S, Uortolotti U, Wasserman F, et al. Long-term follow-up of the Oinescu-Shiley mitral pericardial xenograft. J Thorac Cardiovasc Surg 1984;88:758–763.
7. Cohn LH, Mudge GH, Prater F, et al. Five to eight year follow-up of patients undergoing porcine heart-valve replacement. N Engl J Med 1981;304:258–2.
8. Gray RJ, Chaux A, Matlof, et al. Bileaflet, tilting disc and porcine aortic valve substitutes: in valve hemodynamic characteristics. J Am Coll Cardiol 1984;3:321–325.
9. Magilligan DJ Jr, Lewis JW Jr, Jara FM, et al. Spontaneous degeneration of porcine bioprosthetic valves. Ann Thorac Surg 1980;30:259–266.
10. Ionescu MI, Smith DR, Hasen SS, et al. Clinical durability of the pericardial xenograft valve. Ten years' experience with mitral replacement. Ann Thorac Surg 1982;34:265–277.
11. Cohn LH, Allred EN, DiSesa VS, et al. Early and late risk of aortic valve replacement. J Thorac Cardiovasc Surg 1984;88:695–705.
12. Oyer PE, Miller DC, Stinson EG, et al. Clinical durability of the Hancock porcine bioprosthetic valve. J Thorac Cardiovasc Surg 1980;80:824–833.
13. Brown JW, Dunn JM, Spooner E, Krish MM. Late spontaneous disruption of a porcine xenograft mitral valve. J Thorac Cardiovasc Surg 1978;75:606–611.
14. Dunn JM. Porcine valve durability in children. Ann Thorac Surg 1981;32:357–368.

15. Geha AS, Laks H, Stansel HC, et al. Late failure of porcine valve heterografts in children. J Thorac Cardiovasc Surg 1979;78:351–364.
16. Kutsche LM, Oyer P, Shumway N, Baum D. An important complication of Hancock valve replacement in children. Circulation 1979;(suppl 1)60:98–103.
17. Sanders SP, Freed MD, Norwood WI, et al. Early failure of porcine valves implanted in children Abstr. Am J Cardiol 1980;45:449.
18. Gonzalez-Lavin L. Tandon AP, Chi S, et al. The risk of thromboembolism and hemorrhage following mitral valve replacement. J Thorac Cardiovasc Surg 1984;87:340–351.
19. Mathews RA, Park SC, Neches DH, et al. Valve replacement in children and adolescents. J Thorac Cardiovasc Surg 1977;73:872–876.
20. Gardner TJ, Roland J-MA, Neill CA, Conahoo JS. Valve replacement in children: a fifteen year perspective. J Thorac Cardiovasc Surg (in press).
21. Miller DC, Stinson EB, Billingham ME, et al. The durability of porcine xenograft valves and conduits in children (in press).
22. Spray TL, Roberts WC. Structural changes in porcine xenografts used as substitute cardiac valves. Am J Cardiol 1977;40:319–330.
23. Rose AG, Forman R, Bowen RM. Calcification of gluteraldehyde fixed porcine xenograft. Thorax 1978;33:111–114.
24. Rocchini AP, Weesner KM, Heidelberger K, et al. Porcine xenograft failure in children: An immunologic response. Circulation 1981;(suppl 2)64:162–171.
25. Silver MM, Pollock J, Silver MD, et al. Calcification in porcine xenografts in children. Am J Cardiol 1980;45:685–689.
26. Felix R, Hermann W, Fleisch H. Stimulation of precipitation of calcium phosphate by matrix vesicles. Biochem J 1978;170:681.
27. Wuthier RE. A review of the primary mechanism of endochondrial calcification with special emphasis on the role of cells, mitochondria and matrix vesicles. Clin Orthopedics 1982;169:219–242.
28. Lee NH, Shapiro IM. Ca-transport by chondrcyte mitochondria of the epiphyseal growth plate. J Membrane Biol 1978;41:349–360.
29. Cecil RNA, Anderson HC. Freeze-fracture studies of matrix vesicle calcification in epiphyseal growth plate. Metab Bone Dis 1978;1:89–95.
30. Wutheir RE. Electrolytes of isolated epiphyseal chondrocytes, matrix vesicles and extracellular fluid. Calif Tiss Res 1977;23:125–133.
31. Anderson HC. Normal and abnormal mineralization in mammals, Trans Am Soc Art Intern Organs 1981;27:702–708.
32. Bachra BN, Sobel AE, Stanford JW. Calcification XXIV. Mineralization of collagen and other fibers. Arch Biochem 1959;84:79–95.
33. Kim KM. Matrix vesicle calcification of rat aorta in millipore chambers. Metab Bone Dis 1978;1:213–217.
34. Frasca P, Buchanan JW, Soriano RZ, Dunn JM, Marmon LM, Melbin J, Buchanan SJ, Chang SH, Golub EE, Shapiro IM. Mineralization of short term pericardial cardiac patch grafts. Scanning Electron Microsc 1984;2:973–977.
35. Buchanan JW, Dunn JM, Marmon LM, et al. Implanted aneurysm: a new animal model for the study of cardiovascular biomaterials (Unpublished data, in preparation).
36. Lian JB, Skinner M, Glimcher MJ, Gallop P. The presence of gamma-carboxyglutamic acid in the proteins associated with ectopic calcification. Biochem Biophys Res Com 1976;73:349–355.
37. Lian JB, Levy RJ, Berhard W, Szycher M. LVAD mineralization and gamma-carboxyglutamic acid containing proteins in normal and pathologically mineralized tissues. Trans Am Soc Art Intern Organs 1981;27:683–689.

38. Levy RJ, Lian JB, Gallop P. Atherocalcin, a gammacarboxyglutamic acid containing protein from atherosclerotic plaque, Biochem Biophys Res Com 1979;91:41–49.
39. Levy RJ, Zenker JA, Lian JB. Vitamin-K dependent calcium binding proteins in aortic valve calcification. J Clin Invest 1980;65:563–566.
40. Fishbein MC, Levy RJ, Ferrans VJ, et al. Calcification of cardiac valve bioprosthesis. J Thorac Cardiovasc Surg 1982;83:602–609.
41. Thurbrikar M, Piepgrass WC, Deck DJ. Nolan SP. Stresses of natural versus prosthetic aortic valve leaflets in vivo. Ann Thorac Surg 1980;30:230–239.
42. Thurbrikar MJ, Deck JD, Aouad J, Nolan SP. Role of mechanical stress in calcification of aortic biosynthetic valves. J Thorac Cardiovasc Surg 1983;86:115–125.

CHAPTER **27**

Homograft Prosthetic Heart Valves

Walter H. Merrill, MD,
Marc R. de Leval, MD,
Catherine Bull, MD, MRCP,
F. J. Macartney, MA, MB, BCh, FRCP, FACC,
James F. N. Taylor, MD, FRCP, FACC,
and Jaroslav Stark, MD, FRCS

Between July 1971 and December 1982, 249 children received extracardiac valved conduits in the treatment of complex congenital heart defects. Survivors of the operations were reviewed between January and April 1985, follow-up ranging between 2–13.5 years.

The diagnoses and operative procedures are listed on Table 27.1. The most common were operations for truncus arteriosus, transposition the great arteries, or double-outlet right ventricle associated with ventricular septal defect and left ventricular outflow tract obstruction.

The conduits were placed either between the right ventricle and the pulmonary artery, between the morphologically left, but subpulmonary ventricle and the pulmonary artery, or between the right atrium and the right ventricle or pulmonary artery (Table 27.2).

The types of conduit used are listed in Table 27.3. We have used homografts preserved in antibiotics rather than irradiated homografts.[1] The surgeons at the Mayo Clinic used homografts sterilized by irradiation and then deep frozen. Subsequently, they reported a high incidence of obstructions in their patients.[2] Early in our experience we placed the homograft inside a short segment of knitted Dacron tube (Fig. 27.1). This was extended on both sides with woven Dacron (Fig. 27.2) and then preclotted; this technique has also been used by others.[3] Later we tried using aortic homografts without Dacron extension. Anastomosis with the ventricle can be achieved by using

346

TABLE 27.1 Extracardiac Conduits 1971–1982

Diagnosis/Operation	Number of Patients
Truncus arteriosus	70
Transposition of the great arteries and/or double outlet right ventricle with ventricular septal defect and left ventricular outflow tract obstruction	64
Fontan operation	37
Pulmonary atresia and ventricular septal defect	29
Corrected transposition of the great arteries	22
Left ventricle to pulmonary artery conduit	11
Other	16
Total	249

the anterior cusp of the mitral valve, which is "harvested" with the homograft, as recommended by Ross and Sommerville[4]; alternatively, a small pericardial patch can be used. However, this technique is not always feasible. In some conditions, such as congenitally corrected transposition of the great arteries, the conduit must be quite long because high ventriculotomy should be avoided for risk of complete atrioventricular block (Fig. 27.3). In such patients we have extended the homograft with a tube of woven Dacron (Figs. 27.4 and 27.5).

TABLE 27.2 Extracardiac Conduits 1971–1982

	Number of Patients	Totals
Truncus arteriosus	70	
Transposition of the great arteries and/or double outlet right ventricle with ventricular septal defect and left ventricular outflow tract obstruction	64	
Pulmonary atresia and ventricular septal defect	29	
Absent pulmonary valve syndrome	4	
Fallot's tetralogy	3	
Other	9	
Total		179
Transposition of the great arteries and left ventricular outflow tract obstruction	11	
Corrected transposition of the great arteries and left ventricular outflow tract obstruction	22	
Total		33
Fontan procedure	37	37
Total of all patients		249

TABLE 27.3 Extracardiac Conduits 1971–1982

Type of Conduit	Number
Aortic homograft	108
Hancock porcine	94
Ross' pericardial	24
Carpentier-Edwards	13
Ionescu-Shiley	4
Valveless	6
Total	249

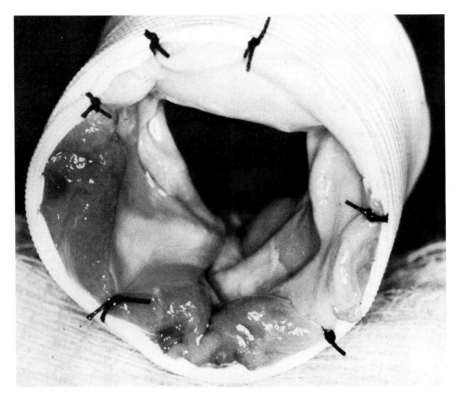

FIGURE 27.1 Aortic homograft is prepared. Coronary ostia are oversewn and excess muscle trimmed off. It is then sutured into a short segment of knitted Dacron tube.

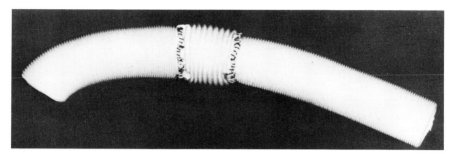

FIGURE 27.2 The segment containing the homograft is extended on both sides with a woven Dacron tube. The whole conduit is then preclotted.

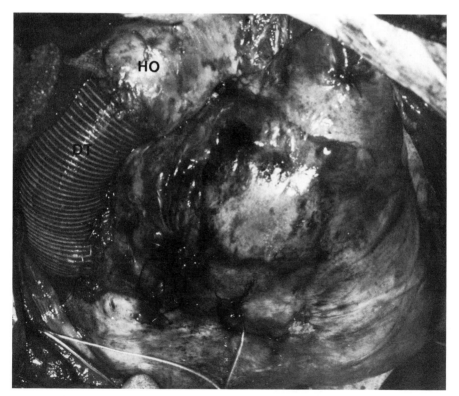

FIGURE 27.3 Homograft *(HO)* is sutured to the pulmonary artery. Dacron tube *(DT)* extending the homograft is attached near the apex of the left ventricle (in congenitally corrected transposition).

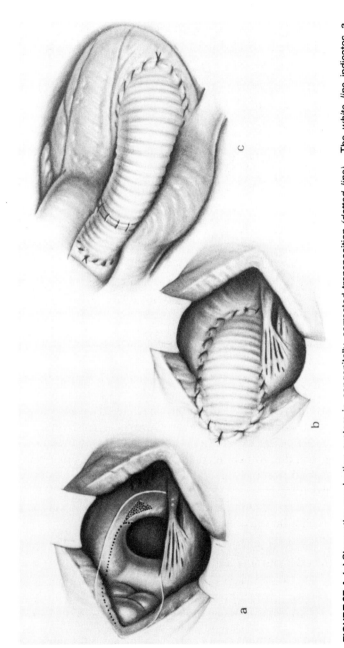

FIGURE 27.4 **(a)** Shows the conduction system in congenitally corrected transposition *(dotted line)*. The *white line* indicates a possible placement of a suture to avoid conduction mechanisms. **(b)** Illustrates completed intracardiac patch closing the ventricular septal defect. The patch incorporates the pulmonary valve. To complete the repair, the pulmonary artery has to be occluded and the conduit placed from the lower part of the left ventricle to the pulmonary artery **(c)**.

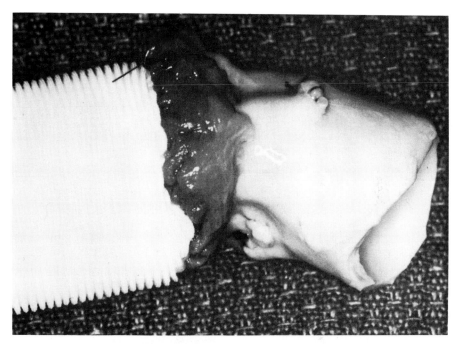

FIGURE 27.5 If a longer conduit is required, aortic homograft is extended with a segment of Dacron tube. The tube is either presealed with fibrinogen (Tisseel) or preclotted.

When conduits containing heterograft valves (such as porcine valves or pericardial valves) became commercially available, we started to use them. Their easier availability (compared with homografts) and a wide selection of sizes were the obvious advantages. However, Dunn et al[5] and others[6,7] soon noted the rather short "life span" of heterografts when used in children. In addition, obstructions due to peel formation in the Dacron tube were also reported.[8] A thickened porcine valve and peel inside a Dacron conduit is illustrated in Figure 27.6.

So in the light of these results and our own experience, we have modified our policies. These can be summarized as follows:

1. Aortic or pulmonary homograft preserved in a nutrient solution and antibiotic sterilized is our first choice for an extracardiac valved conduit.

2. Whenever possible, the homograft is used without a Dacron extension.

3. Should a longer conduit be required, the homograft is extended with a double velour, knitted Dacron graft, which is presealed with Tisseel.[9,10]

The long-term performance of a valved conduit does not only depend on the conduit and valve; to achieve the best results, careful techniques

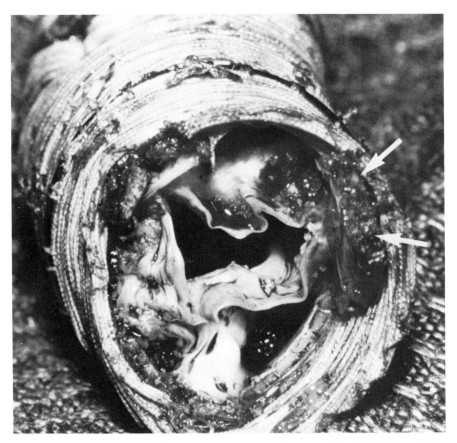

FIGURE 27.6 Porcine heterograft removed 5 years after insertion. Note the thickened valve and a thick peel inside the Dacron tube *(arrows)*.

should be used during all stages of conduit insertion. Anastomosis with the pulmonary artery should be performed with fine monofilament suture material to avoid bleeding (Fig. 27.7). If extensive reconstruction of the pulmonary arteries is needed, such as in complex pulmonary atresia or banded truncus arteriosus, we prefer to reconstruct the pulmonary artery with pericardium before attaching the conduit (Fig. 27.8). To avoid bleeding from such complex anastomoses, careful suture techniques should be used and anastomosis can be treated with Tisseel. The anastomosis between the conduit and the right ventricle must be very wide and gradient free (Fig. 27.9). The conduit should not be placed directly under the sternum so as to avoid external compression. If these criteria are observed, excellent and long-lasting results can be achieved. An example of a good anatomic repair of a truncus arteriosus, banded at age 10 months and repaired with homograft conduit at age 6 years, is shown on angiocardiogram (Fig. 27.10) obtained 5 years after operation.

All 249 patients operated on between 1971 and 1982 were followed up and their status reviewed between January to April, 1985. Of those discharged from the Hospital after the conduit repair, actuarial survival at 5

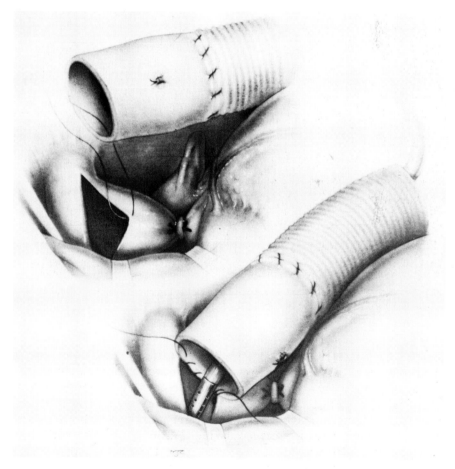

FIGURE 27.7 The homograft is sutured to the pulmonary artery with a fine monofilament suture material. When the posterior anastomosis is completed a sump may be placed through the conduit into the pulmonary artery to facilitate suturing.

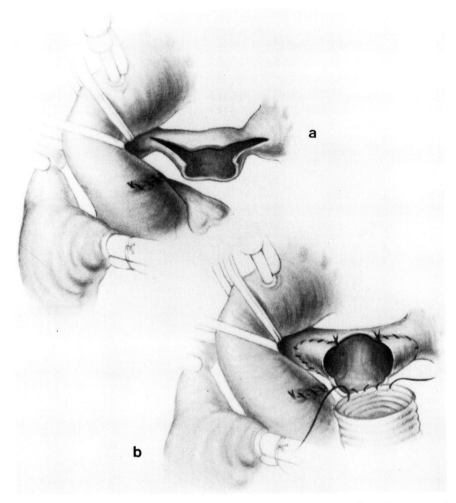

FIGURE 27.8 Pulmonary artery is reconstructed **(a)** after previous banding with a piece of pericardium *(arrows)*. The conduit is then sutured to the reconstructed pulmonary artery **(b)**.

years was 90% for patients with pulmonary atresia and ventricular septal defect; 80% for those with transposition of the great arteries and/or double-outlet right ventricle with ventricular septal defect and left ventricular outflow tract obstruction; and 78% for those who required repair of truncus arteriosus. Survival at 10 years was 78%, 50%, and 68% respectively. The lower late survival rate in patients with transposition of the great arteries/double-outlet right ventricle was mainly due to arrhythmias and, in those with truncus arteriosus, progression of pulmonary vascular obstructive disease.

When the conduit survival was analyzed, the following information was obtained: The probability to survive 5 years with the original conduit was 85% in patients with the pulmonary atresia, 70% in those with transposition of the great arteries and/or double-outlet right ventricle with ventricular septal and left ventricular outflow tract obstruction, and 62% those with truncus arteriosus. The 10-year survival data with the original conduit were 25%, 48%, and 22% respectively. Our interpretation of the differences between these three diagnostic groups was based on the following factors: More

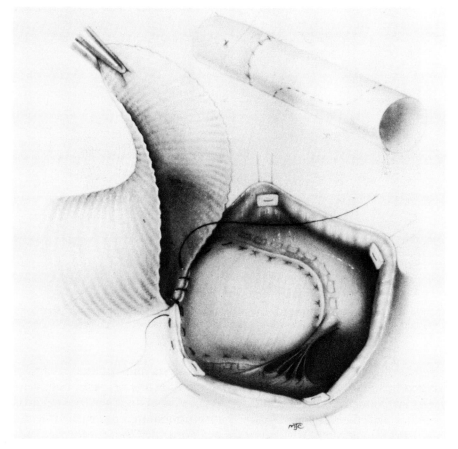

FIGURE 27.9 Anastomosis between the ventricle and the conduit must be very wide. *Insert* shows how the Dacron extension is cut.

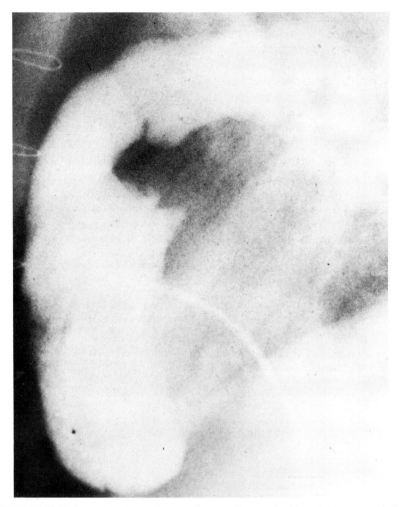

FIGURE 27.10 Right ventricular angiogram 5 years after repair of banded truncus arteriosus shows unobstructed conduit with well-functioning homograft valve.

heterografts were used in patients with pulmonary atresia and truncus arteriosus compared to those with transposition and/or double-outlet right ventricles; earlier deterioration of the heterografts, compared with homografts, would explain the difference. However, the situation is complicated by the fact that some aortic homografts were extended with a tube of woven Dacron, thus the deterioration could also have been due to the obstruction of the tube rather than simple degeneration of the valve. Further detailed analysis of this problem is required and is currently being undertaken. In the group with truncus arteriosus, the original conduits (valve and the tube) were usually small because most operations were performed in infants. Therefore, patients may outgrow the conduits before they actually obstruct. This point is also being investigated.

When all conduits were analyzed in two groups; homografts and other, the figures for survival with the original conduits are 72% at 5 years and 50% at 10 years for homografts, and 78% at 5 years and 30% at 10 years for heterografts.

We conclude that external cardiac conduits allow surgical repair of many complex congenital heart defects. Although the risks of such operations are decreasing, significant long-term problems remain. With regard to the type of conduit, our data support the findings of others[11-14] that conduits made of homograft aortic valve and preserved in antibiotic solution survived longer than any other valved conduits currently available. We believe that continued follow-up of these patients and research into better and more durable conduits is still required.

REFERENCES

1. Breckenridge IM, Stark J, Bonham-Carter RE, Oeelert H, Graham GR, Waterston DJ. Mustard's operation for transposition of the great arteries. Review of 200 cases. Lancet 1972;1:1140-2.
2. Merin G, McGoon DC. Reoperation after insertio of aortic homograft as a right ventricular outflow tract. Ann Thorac Surg 1973;16:122.
3. Kouchoukos NT, Barcia A, Bageron LM, Kirklin JW. Surgical treatment of congenital pulmonary atresia with ventricular septal defect. J Thorac Cardiovasc Surg 1971;61:70-84.
4. Ross DN, Somerville J. Correction of pulmonary atresia with a homograft aortic valve. Lancet 1966;2:1146.
5. Dunn J. Porcine valve durability in children. Ann Thorac Surg 1981;32:357-368.
6. Geha AS, Laks H, Stansel HC Jr, Cornhill JF, Kilman JW, Buckley MJ, Roberts WC. Late failure of porcine valve heterografts in children. J Thorac Cardiovasc Surg 1979;78:351-364.
7. Miller DC, Stinson EB, Oyer PE, Billingham ME, Pitlick PT, Reitz BA, Jamieson SW, Bamgartner WA, Shumway NE. The durability of porcine xenograft valves and conduits in children. Circulation 1982;66:(suppl I):172-85.
8. Agarwal KC, Edwards WD, Feldt RH, Danielson GK, Puga FJ, McGoon DC. Clinicopathological correlates of obstructed right-sided porcine valved extracardiac conduits. J Thorac Cardiovasc Surg 1981;81:591-601.
9. Haverich A, Borst HG. Fibrin glue for treatment of bleeding in cardiac surgery. In, Bircks W, Ostermeyer J, Schulte HD (eds): Cardiovascular Surgery. Springer-Verlag, New York, 1980, p 621.
10. Stark J, de Leval M. Experience with fibrin seal (Tisseel) in operations for congenital heart defects. Ann Thorac Surg 1984;38:411-3.

11. Fontan F, Choussat A, Deville C, Doutremepuich C, Coupillaud J, Vosa C. Aortic valve homografts in the surgical treatment of complex cardiac malformation. J Thorac Cardiovasc Surg 1984;87:649–57.

12. Barratt-Boyes B. Discussion to: Fontan F, Choussat A, Deville C, Doutremepuich C, Coupillaud J, Vosa C. Aortic valve homografts in the surgical treatment of complex cardiac malformations. J Thorac Cardiovasc Surg 1984;87:649–57.

13. Moore CH, Martelli V, Ross DN. Reconstruction of right ventricular outflow tract with a valved conduits in 75 cases of congenital heart disease. J Thorac Cardiovasc Surg 1976;71:11.

14. Ahmed M, Yacoub M. Late results of aortic homograft reconstruction of right ventricular outflow tract in infants and children. Thorachir Vasc Chir 1975;23:445–459.

CHAPTER 28

Anticoagulation for Children Requiring Heart Valve Replacement

Timothy J. Gardner, MD

For children undergoing prosthetic heart valve replacement, long-term anticoagulation with warfarin is widely accepted as the best means of avoiding thromboembolic complications related to the valve prosthesis. Although some groups of young patients with prosthetic heart valves have been managed with warfarin, the safety of this approach has not been conclusively demonstrated by careful late follow-up. Warfarin and similar anticoagulant compounds are effective primarily by interfering with vitamin K activity, which results in prolongation of the prothrombin time. Problems associated with the use of this type of drug include variable degrees of therapeutic activity with resultant instability of the prothrombin time prolongation and occasional hemorrhagic complications due to excessive extension of the prothrombin time. In addition, warfarin-type compounds appear to have a teratogenic action with administration early during pregnancy in some patients. Pregnancy in women receiving chronic warfarin therapy may be complicated further by hemorrhagic complications, including intrauterine bleeding and premature placental separation. Because of these problems associated with warfarin therapy during pregnancy, the use of tissue valve substitutes for older adolescent women approaching child-bearing age should be considered, in spite of the known limited durability of tissue valve substitutes.

Chronic anticoagulation therapy to avoid late thromboembolic complications in the child or adolescent undergoing valve replacement may limit the extent of rehabilitation achieved with the heart surgery. Warfarin, the most commonly prescribed oral anticoagulant agent in the United States,

359

requires daily ingestion and regular surveillance of prothrombin time to maintain a stable state of anticoagulation. Regulation of warfarin dosages can be extremely difficult in young children, making these patients susceptible to wide swings in the prothrombin time prolongation. Furthermore, the fully anticoagulated child may be at a significantly increased risk of serious hemorrhagic complications when he or she is exposed to the normal physical activities of childhood and adolescence. As a result, rather stringent activity limitations often are imposed on the young patient with a prosthetic valve, such that the quality of the child's life may be adversely affected.

The possibility that a child with an artificial heart valve might be freed of the burden of anticoagulation therapy was raised when tissue valve substitutes, both porcine and bovine heterograft valves, were first implanted in children in the mid- and late 1970s.[1] By 1981, however, there was ample clinical evidence of premature tissue valve calcification and degeneration in children, with the result that most people became convinced that tissue valve substitutes are not suitable for routine use in children.[2]

Although there is general agreement that patients with prosthestic heart valves should receive anticoagulation therapy with warfarin to reduce the risk of prosthesis-related thromboembolic complications, a few groups managing children after valve replacement are omitting warfarin therapy. In a 1982 report from the University of California, San Francisco, it was suggested that aspirin, an antiplatelet agent, might replace conventional anticoagulation with warfarin in children having valve replacement. Weinstein, et al[3] reported on 18 children who after valve replacement received either aspirin or aspirin and dipyridamole. Twelve of these patients had mechanical valve prostheses (Björk-Shiley) implanted and were followed-up clinically for a total of 168 patient-months.

Although none of these patients developed any evidence of definite thromboembolic complications during the follow-up interval, there was one late death 9 months after surgery whose cause of death was unknown; a second patient required replacement of the prosthetic valve because of the development of apparent "tissue overgrowth."[3] It is at least possible that the tissue proliferation around the valve orifice may have developed secondary to a thrombotic focus on the prosthesis. Given that these two patients, cannot be definitely shown to free of thromboembolic complications, and given that six of the remaining patients were followed-up for no more than 6 months when this report was prepared, conclusions about the safety of the non-warfarin approach used in these 12 patients would appear to be unwarranted.

There has been a more recent report by Pass et al[4] from the Medical University of South Carolina describing a group of children with St. Jude Medical prostheses who are not receiving warfarin anticoagulation therapy.

The 34 children in this group ranged in age from 9 months to 21 years, and had valve prostheses placed in either the aortic, mitral or pulmonary positions. Of those who survived the operation, one patient died suddenly at home 5 weeks after valve insertion. The cause of this death is not described in the report, but it was assumed by the authors not to be valve-related. The 30 remaining patients were followed-up from 1 to 50 months (a total of 646 patient-months) without warfarin anticoagulation therapy. There was no evidence of any thromboembolic occurrence during this time period.

With publication of this report, additional updated follow-up information was provided by the authors, describing 33 patients who had been observed for a total of 923 patient-months. In this larger group of patients, there was one incidence of valve thrombosis in the pulmonary position, which occurred in a 4-year-old girl 18 months after surgery. The other complication was that of an apparent major embolic event, resulting in an acute myocardial infarction in a 17-year-old male 6 months after aortic valve replacement. Out of the original group, then, there were three major complications: one death, the cause of which is not known, and two definite thrombotic occurrences.[4]

In our own experience is with 26 patients in whom the St. Jude Medical prosthesis was implanted and who were discharged from the hospital over the past 5 years. Eighteen of these patients were received warfarin therapy immediately after surgery and are still being maintained on the anticoagulant. One of them suffered a significant hemorrhagic complication that resulted in a peripheral neuropathy.

The remaining eight patients were discharged from the hospital receiving either aspirin or aspirin and dipyridamole. Six of these eight patients were less than 5 years of age at the time of valve replacement and were found to be very difficult to anticoagulate in a stable fashion using daily oral warfarin dosing. One of these eight patients developed prosthetic valve thrombosis 2 months after surgery and died. This individual had complicated congenital heart disease, had undergone a Fontan procedure and replacement of a left-sided systemic atrioventricular valve with a St. Jude Medical prosthesis. This child, who was 4 years old, developed gastroenteritis while at home several weeks after surgery, became dehydrated, and, presumably under these circumstances, developed valve thrombosis.

The current approach taken at this hospital with children who have mechanical prostheses implanted, including the apparently relatively thromboresistant St. Jude Medical prosthesis, is to maintain the patients on aspirin and dipyridamole therapy only when the use of warfarin poses a significant risk or when warfarin therapy is difficult to regulate. The recommended aspirin dosage is 6–10 mg/kg daily, with a maximum of 675 mg per day; the recommended dipyridamole dosage is 2–3 mg/kg daily.

It should be emphasized that in four recent clinical series describing prosthestic valve replacements in children, the reported rate of major thrombotic or thromboembolic complications ranged between 1.1% and 2.9% per patient-year. The incidence of thromboembolic complications in Pass's patient group not receiving warfarin and excluding the child who died suddenly at home, was 2.6% per patient-year.[4] Schaff et al,[5] reporting on the experience from the Mayo Clinic with children receiving Starr-Edwards prostheses, noted a thromboembolic incidence of 2.9% per patient-year, with most of the patients receiving warfarin therapy. Similar incidences of thromboembolism were described by Henze et al[6] and Iyer et al[7] in groups of children in whom the Björk-Shiley valve was implanted and warfarin-type anticoagulants used.

The primary mechanism of action of warfarin and other anticoagulants is to interfere with vitamin K-mediated formation of clotting factors, including prothrombin as well as factors VII, IX, and X; warfarin may also block the release of prothrombin from the liver. Although warfarin therapy is a reliable means of minimizing the risk of thromboembolism in patients with prosthetic heart valves, maintenance of the patient who requires long-term warfarin anticoagulation therapy and regulation of the patient's prothrombin time can be problematic because warfarin works primarily by blocking vitamin K-mediated activity in the liver. A marked change in dietary vitamin K will likely affect the prothrombin time in the patient receiving warfarin. The absorption of vitamin K, as well as warfarin, is influenced by bile salts and, therefore, changes in the dietary fat content can also significantly affect the absorption of vitamin K. In addition, if the patient has a very rapid gastrointestinal tract transient time, vitamin K absorption may be inhibited, thereby affecting the stability of the prothrombin time prolongation. Another factor that may affect warfarin activity is the patient's intrinsic hepatic function. An individual with chronic hepatic congestion is generally more sensitive to lower doses of warfarin than is the patient with normal liver function. Furthermore, because lower intestinal tract bacteria result in vitamin K production, the use of oral antibiotics that alter the gut flora may affect warfarin activity. Finally, there are a variety of drugs, including some antihypertensive medications and oral contraceptives, that cause alterations in warfarin activity and prothrombin time.

In addition to the fact that excessive warfarin use may result in internal bleeding or other hemorrhagic complications, another major concern with chronic warfarin therapy is its teratogenic potential. A specific warfarin-type of embryopathy has been described, characterized by facial deformity and, in particular, nasal hypoplasia, as well as the development of stippled and calcified long-bone epiphyses. The occasional affected child may also have short limbs, and cases of optic nerve atrophy have also been described.

Although not present in every child affected with warfarin embryopathy, central nervous system abnormalities, including the development of significant mental retardation, have been described.[8,9] It appears that the maximum teratogenic action of warfarin occurs between 6 and 9 weeks of pregnancy. This time period of major warfarin teratogenesis is especially problematic for people receiving chronic warfarin therapy. During this early stage of the pregnancy, conception might not yet be diagnosed, and the patient may still be receiving warfarin without realizing that she is pregnant.

In a review of the effects of anticoagulation therapy during pregnancy recently reported by Hall et al[10] in the *American Journal of Medicine*, 418 pregnancies occurring in patients taking warfarin-type medications resulted in abortion and stillbirth rates of about 15%; an additional 15% of the pregnancies resulted in delivery of abnormal infants. Of 135 pregnancies in which subcutaneous heparin was used for anticoagulation, there was a significant incidence of stillbirths and prematurity, presumably related to abnormal intrauterine bleeding and early placental separation. The premature babies in this group had a significant perinatal mortality, but compared to patients managed with warfarin throughout the pregnancy, there was an apparent lack of any teratogenic effects with heparin.

In a report by Larrea et al[11] in 1983, 47 pregnancies in 38 women who were taking warfarin during the pregnancy were reviewed. There was a 23% incidence of spontaneous abortion, 17% of the births were premature, and two of the newborns (4.3%) were affected with typical warfarin-type embryopathy. In addition, three of the mothers developed valve thrombosis during the course of the pregnancy, one of whom suffered a major peripheral embolus. It has been suggested by some that pregnant women are relatively hypercoagulable and are even more prone to thrombosis of a valve substitute and to thromboembolic complications during pregnancy.

Recently, there was the publication of an extensive review of the experience of a large group of women with artificial heart valves who became pregnant. This report from the National Cardiology Institute in Mexico encompassed the period 1966–1984. In the first group of 68 women, dipyridamole was substituted for warfarin as soon as the pregnancy was diagnosed. In the second group of 128 patients, warfarin was maintained until the last two weeks of gestation, at which point the mothers were treated with subcutaneous heparin therapy. The third group of patients received subcutaneous heparin from the time of the diagnosis of pregnancy until the end of the thirteenth week of gestation, in an attempt to avoid the maximum teratogenic effects of warfarin, after which warfarin therapy was resumed until the final two weeks of the pregnancy. The last group of patients in the review had tissue valves in place and were thought not to require anticoagulant therapy.

Examination of maternal mortality and morbidity in this group of more than 200 patients revealed that in the first group, the patients who received dipyridamole only during pregnancy, there were three maternal deaths, a 25% incidence of major cerebral embolism, and an additional 4.5% occurrence of major systemic embolization during the course of the pregnancy; all deaths were due to valve thrombosis. In the second group, for patients receiving warfarin throughout the pregnancy, maternal health was much better maintained with no deaths and only a 2.3% incidence of cerebral embolization; there was, however, an increased incidence of significant peripartum bleeding. In the third group, those who received subcutaneous heparin initially, followed by warfarin and then resumption of subcutaneous heparin near partuition, the incidence of cerebral embolism was higher. The only death among patients with a tissue valve and no anticoagulation was unrelated to the valve substitute itself.[12]

Fetal and infant mortality were examined in these same pregnancies and the number of abortions and stillbirths was 10% and 7%, respectively, in the group receiving dipyridamole, while 35% of patients receiving warfarin aborted or experienced stillbirths. In addition, there were three neonatal deaths in the warfarin group. Although no valve thromboses occurred in the 128 patients receiving warfarin therapy throughout the pregnancy, there were three major thromboembolic events in spite of apparently adequate anticoagulation; there were also three children born with congenital anomalies consistent with warfarin embryopathy.

Clearly, these data and those reported by Hall et al[10] emphasize that the use of warfarin during pregnancy is likely to result in a significant number of spontaneous abortions, stillbirths, and newborns with congenital anomalies. Without warfarin therapy, however, the mother is placed at a significant risk of valve thrombosis, making pregnancy an extremely hazardous time for the young woman with an artificial heart valve.

With all of the above information available, several considerations should influence the use of conventional warfarin anticoagulation therapy in children with mechanical heart valves. Valve thrombosis and significant thromboembolism have been reported in virtually all series of valve replacements in children, with the incidence of serious thromboembolic complications apparently higher in patients who were not receiving warfarin. In addition, the manufacturers of valve prosthesis in the U.S. have specifically advised that therapeutic warfarin be used in order to avoid thromboembolic complications. In view of this information, one may feel constrained to manage these young patients with warfarin therapy because of medical – legal considerations. On the other hand, it has been our experience and that of others that the attempted use of warfarin to achieve a stable level of anticoagulation in young children less than 5 years of age can be extremely difficult. Furthermore, many children and their parents are poorly compliant with the anticoagulation regimens, with the result that the level of anticoagulation achieved is either uncertain or inadequate. In some other instances, the risk of hemorrhage may exceed the risk of thrombus formation, and under these circumstances, warfarin anticoagulation therapy should be omitted. Finally, the whole issue of how best to manage the pregnant woman with an artificial valve prosthesis remains unanswered.

For all of these considerations, the issue of what type of valve substitute to use for older children, especially for young women, is unresolved. Warfarin is associated with significant hemorrhagic complications in active children and is associated with a significant incidence of teratogenesis in women who take the drug early during pregnancy. It might be reasonable to conclude, therefore, that tissue valve substitutes, in spite of known limited durability, may be preferable for adolescent girls who are likely to become pregnant and for adolescent boys who are physically very active, in order to relieve them of the need to take warfarin during this high risk period.

REFERENCES

1. Sade RM, Ballinger JR, Hohn AR, et al. Cardiac valve replacement in children. Comparison of tissue with mechanical prostheses. J Thorac Cardiovasc Surg 1979;76:123–127.
2. Dunn JM. Porcine valve durability in children. Ann Thorac Surg 1981;32:357–368.
3. Weinstein GS, Mavroudis C, Ebert PA. Preliminary experience with aspirin for anticoagulation in children with prosthetic cardiac valves. Ann Thorac Surg 1982;33:549–553.
4. Pass HI, Sade RM, Crawford FA, Hohn AR. Cardiac valve prostheses in children without anticoagulation. J Thorac Cardiovasc Surg 1984;87:832–835.
5. Schaff HV, Danielson GK, DiDonato RM, et al. Late results after Starr-Edwards valve replacement in children. J Thorac Cardiovasc Surg 1984;88:583–589.
6. Henze A, Lindblom, Björk VO: Mechanical heart valves in children. Scand J Thorac Cardiovasc Surg 1984;18:155–159.
7. Iyer KS, Reddy KS, Rao IM, et al. Valve replacement in children under twenty years of age. Experience with the Björk-Shiley prosthesis. J Thorac Cardiovasc Surg 1984;88:217–224.
8. Becker MH, Eniesser NB, Finegold M, et al. Chondrodysplasia punctata: is maternal warfarin a problem? Am J Dis Child 1975;129:356–359.
9. Sherman S, Hall BD: Warfarin and fetal abnormalities. Lancet 1976;1:692.
10. Hall JG, Paul RM, Wilson KM. Maternal and fetal sequelae of anticoagulation during pregnancy. Am J Med 1980;68:122–140.
11. Larrea JL, Nunez L, Reque JA, et al. Pregnancy and mechanical valve prostheses: a high risk situation for the mother and fetus. Ann Thorac Surg 1983;36:459–463.
12. Salazar E, Zajorias A, Gutierrez N, Iturke I. The problem of cardiac valve prostheses, anticoagulants and pregnancy. Circulation 1984;70(suppl I):I169–I177.

Index

367